Praise for *Listening to Prozac*

"Intelligent and informative."   *—The New York Times*

"One of the most important and provocative books on psychology I've seen in years . . . asks us to question all our assumptions about what the self is, what therapy has been and can be, and about the role of drugs in affecting behavior and personality."
      —Owen Lipstein, Psychology Today

"Dr. Kramer seems to be writing about the therapeutic credos of our time. The result is entertaining, provocative, irritating, and often originally insightful."   *—The New York Times Book Review*

"Kramer is a wonderful writer, and his readers will learn much about the new research on temperament and personality, biological theories of mood disorders, and the behind-the-scenes stories of how psychiatric drugs were discovered or invented."
      —Los Angeles Times Book Review

"[Kramer] has taken on in a lucid and informed manner, issues that many clinicians and academics have been unwilling to tackle. . . . His book will be truly heuristic . . . it will generate agreement or disagreement but, most importantly, it will generate thought and discussion. This is what one hopes for, but too rarely gets, in the public discussion of science and medicine."
      —The Washington Post

"Peter Kramer deals brilliantly with the complex issue of personality and questions whether a commonly used antidepressant can alter the very essence of a person's character."
      —Abraham Verghese, *Nature*

"Kramer presents a lucid and convincing demonstration that American psychiatry is not brain dead. . . . It demonstrates that conceptual brilliance and innovative thinking are alive and well in our field today."   *—American Journal of Psychiatry*

PENGUIN BOOKS

LISTENING TO PROZAC

Peter D. Kramer received his M.D. from Harvard. A clinical professor of psychiatry at Brown University, he has a private practice in Providence, Rhode Island. The author of *Moments of Engagement: Intimate Psychotherapy in a Technological Age* (Penguin), and *Should You Leave?*, his writings have appeared in *The New York Times*, *The Washington Post*, and other national publications. He also lectures internationally on topics related to psychiatry and the modern sense of self.

LISTENING TO PROZAC

PETER D. KRAMER

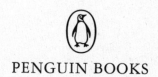

PENGUIN BOOKS

PENGUIN BOOKS
Published by the Penguin Group
Penguin Putnam Inc., 375 Hudson Street,
New York, New York 10014, U.S.A.
Penguin Books Ltd, 27 Wrights Lane, London W8 5TZ, England
Penguin Books Australia Ltd, Ringwood, Victoria, Australia
Penguin Books Canada Ltd, 10 Alcorn Avenue,
Toronto, Ontario, Canada M4V 3B2
Penguin Books (N.Z.) Ltd, 182–190 Wairau Road,
Auckland 10, New Zealand

Penguin Books Ltd, Registered Offices:
Harmondsworth, Middlesex, England

First published in the United States of America by Viking Penguin,
a division of Penguin Books USA Inc. 1993
Published in Penguin Books 1994
This edition with a new afterword by Peter D. Kramer
published in Penguin Books 1997

5 7 9 10 8 6

PUBLISHER'S NOTE:
The ideas, procedures, and suggestions contained in this book are not intended as
a substitute for medical treatment by a physician. The reader should regularly
consult a physician in matters relating to health.

Grateful acknowledgment is made for permission to reprint excerpts
from the following copyrighted works:
"Anxiety Reconceptualized" by Donald F. Klein, M.D., appearing in *Anxiety: New Research and
Changing Concepts*, edited by Donald F. Klein and Judith G. Rabkin, Raven Press, 1981.
By permission of the publisher and the author.
"Self-Portrait in Tyvek™ Windbreaker" by James Merrill. Reprinted by permission;
© 1992 James Merrill. Originally in *The New Yorker*. All rights reserved.
"On the So-Called Good Hysteric," reprinted from *The Capacity for Emotional Growth* by
Elizabeth R. Zetzel. By permission of International Universities Press, © 1970.

THE LIBRARY OF CONGRESS HAS CATALOGUED THE HARDCOVER EDITION AS FOLLOWS:
Kramer, Peter D.
Listening to Prozac: a psychiatrist explores antidepressant drugs and
the remaking of the self/Peter Kramer.
p. cm.
Includes index.
ISBN 0-670-84183-8 (hc.)
ISBN 0 14 02.6671 2 (pbk.)
1. Fluoxetine—Moral and ethical aspects.   2. Fluoxetine—Social aspects.
3. Fluoxetine—Psychotropic effects.   4. Personality change.   I. Title.
RC483.5.F55K7   1993
616.85′27061—dc20   92–50733

Printed in the United States of America
Set in Garamond No. 3
Designed by Brian Mulligan

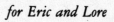

for Eric and Lore

CONTENTS

Introduction

Toward the end of 1988, less than a year after the antidepressant drug Prozac was introduced, I had occasion to treat an architect who was suffering from a prolonged bout of melancholy. Sam was a charming, quirky fellow, inclined to sarcasm, who prided himself on his independent style in sexual matters. He was of Austrian descent, cultivated a continental, nonconformist manner, and would not have been ashamed to be called a roué. A central conflict in his marriage was his interest in pornographic videos. He insisted his wife watch hard-core sex films with him despite her distaste, which he attributed to inhibition and narrow-mindedness.

As he neared forty, Sam fell into a brooding depression set off by a reversal in his business and the death of his parents. He consulted me, and we began to talk. Though he had fought with his parents, Sam had dreamed of reconciliation, of making their farm his crowning design project. But time overtook these plans. First his father, then his mother died, and the farm was sold. As we talked, Sam began to believe he understood his depression in terms of the events that preceded it, but his feelings of paralysis and deep sadness persisted. I prescribed an antidepressant; Sam responded only partially, able to function at work but left with a constant feeling of vulnerability.

In our meetings, Sam recalled having been a somewhat obsessional child, given to worrying about death and to spending hours rearranging his many collections, which ranged from stamps and coins to bottle caps, coasters, and whatever else came his way. This quality faded as he entered adulthood and focused on his career. When Sam's depression failed to respond to traditional treatments, I thought further about the hints in his history of something vaguely resembling obsessive-compulsive disorder. Prozac, then a new antidepressant with which few doctors had experience, was thought to have the potential to ameliorate compulsiveness. I shared my speculations with Sam, and he agreed to try Prozac.

The change, when it came, was remarkable: Sam not only recovered from his depression, he declared himself "better than well." He felt unencumbered, more vitally alive, less pessimistic. Now he could complete projects in one draft, whereas before he had sketched and sketched again. His memory was more reliable, his concentration keener. Every aspect of his work went more smoothly. He appeared more poised, more thoughtful, less distracted. He was able to speak at professional gatherings without notes.

I will explore later these aspects of Prozac, its ability to make certain people "better than well" and its effect on mental agility. Here I want to focus on a solitary detail that troubled Sam: though he enjoyed sex as much as ever, he no longer had any interest in pornography. In order to save face in the marriage, he continued to rent the videos that had once titillated him, but he found it a chore to watch them.

Altogether, Sam became less bristling, had fewer rough edges. He experienced this change as a loss. The style he had nurtured and defended for years now seemed not a part of him but an illness. What he had touted as independence of spirit was a biological tic. In particular, Sam was convinced that his interest in pornography had been mere physiological obsessionality. This conviction was based on a visceral sensation: on medication he felt less driven, freed of an addiction. Although he was grateful for the relief Prozac gave him from his mental anguish, this one aspect of his recovery was disconcerting, because the medication redefined what was essential and what contingent about his own personality—and the drug agreed with his wife when she was being critical.

Sam was under the influence of medication in more ways than one: he had allowed Prozac not only to cure the episode of depression but also to tell him how he was constituted. I might have been less struck by this response to Prozac had I not observed a parallel tendency in myself. Though I had never taken psychotherapeutic medication, I, too, seemed to be under its influence.

Shortly after Sam reported his loss of interest in pornography, I made two ordinary mistakes that caused me to wonder about the source of my own beliefs about people.

The first occurred in my care of a college student with a collection of problems not uncommon in young men who consult psychiatrists: He was angry at and mistrustful of authority, and at the same time he was uncertain of his identity, without goals or direction—at once asking for and resenting guidance. He was also depressed in a way that interfered with his ability to study or interact with classmates. As the situation deteriorated despite psychotherapy, I suggested he begin taking an antidepressant.

The young man accepted my prescription, and at the next session he appeared with a new collection of symptoms. Now his voice was tremulous, and when I questioned him he said his heart was racing and he was feeling markedly anxious. It is not unusual for a person beginning to take an antidepressant to experience an amphetaminelike effect on the third or fourth day—the feeling of having drunk too much coffee. Often this sensation disappears spontaneously. Sometimes it is necessary to lower the medication dose or to add a second, sedating medication at bedtime or to select a different antidepressant.

I considered these alternatives and began to discuss them with the young man when he interrupted to correct my misapprehension: He had not taken the antidepressant. He was anxious because he feared my response when I learned he had "disobeyed" me.

As my patient spoke, I was struck by the sudden change in my experience of his anxiety. One moment, the anxiety was a collection of meaningless physical symptoms, of interest only because they had to be suppressed, by other biological means, in order for the treatment to continue. At the next, the anxiety was rich in overtones. Hearing that the anxiety was not a medication side effect, I had an instantaneous sense of how I appeared to the student—demanding, judgmental, punitive, powerful in the face of his weakness—and how it must feel for him to go through life surrounded by similar figures. Here was emotion a psychoanalyst might call Oedipal, anxiety over retribution by the exigent father. The two anxieties were utterly different: the one a simple outpouring of brain chemicals, calling for a scientific response, however diplomatically communicated; the other worthy of empathic exploration of the most delicate sort.

Anxiety is at the heart of the psychological understanding of man. The "dynamic" in psychodynamic psychotherapy is anxiety; anxiety is the motor force behind psychoanalysis, a discipline replete with such phrases as "signal anxiety," "anxiety neurosis," and, of course, "castration anxiety." Beyond the profession, in the work of existential philosophers like Kierkegaard and Heidegger, the individual's struggle with anxiety is the preferred route to self-discovery. As a psychiatrist, I have spent most of my professional energy attending to psychological issues—to the significance of anxiety. Now, like Sam, I appeared changed in my perspective: I had caught myself assuming that a patient's anxiety was meaningless.

The weekend after my encounter with the depressed and anxious student, I was invited to the home of old friends I see only now and then. The husband in this couple is a fine finish carpenter; the wife, a funky graphic artist. The afternoon I was with them, I noticed about their children what one so often notices about children—

namely, how much they resemble their parents. The son was a boy mechanic, the type whose favorite toy is an old vacuum cleaner he can take apart and reassemble. The girl had her mother's ethereal manner and her fascination with ornamentation, shape, and color. I thought to myself, "Don't the genes breed true!"

I was about to say something of the sort when I remembered that these children were adopted and, beyond being human, had no genetic relationship to these parents. Evidently I had developed the habit of mistaking the psychological for the biological not just in the office but everywhere. And here, in my friends' home, the issue was not a symptom but the whole of who the children were: their style, their talents, their preferences. Since when had I—I, who make my living through the presumption that people are shaped by love and loss, and above all by their early family life—begun to assume that personality traits are genetically determined?

These three incidents occurring in conjunction—Sam's response to Prozac and my own to the college student and my friends' children —made me keenly aware of the effect of medication on my own and my patients' view of the self. This effect was not occurring in a vacuum. Our culture is caught in a frenzy of biological materialism. Newspaper columns, sit-coms, comic strips, talk shows—our public banter is replete with corollaries of the thesis that biology is destiny. When we laugh, if we do, at the claims that the genes for noticing dirty dishes, asking directions, and making commitments in relationships are absent on the Y chromosome, or that the gene for channel-surfing with the TV buzz box is present only there, it is because these beliefs are not distant from ones we actually hold.

I remember the days when you could be hounded off a college campus for suggesting that IQ is partly heritable. Recently I noticed in a *Newsweek* "Ideas" column an explanatory parenthesis—a bit of by-the-way information for those not *au courant*—containing the estimate that genes account for "half the difference in individuals' IQs and thirty percent of personality differences." What was only recently taboo is now the background assumption that sets the stage for discussion of human behavior.

My sense when I began my inquiries—and this is still my sense today—is that the new biological materialism is a cultural phenomenon that goes beyond the scientific evidence. There have always been observations favoring nature over nurture. What changes, in response to the spirit of the times, is the choice of evidence to which we attend.

It is instructive to follow the course of scientific opinion regarding the heritability of such disorders as manic-depressive illness and alcoholism. At least three times in recent years, the genes for these ailments have been discovered. In each instance, the studies proved impossible to replicate, and re-examination of the original data showed it to have been both flawed and incorrectly analyzed. My impression is that the result of each of these *failures* to demonstrate that a disorder is genetic has been a paradoxical *increase* in the conviction, both of scientists and of the informed public, that the disorder is and will soon be shown to be heritable in a simple, direct fashion.

Why have our beliefs changed faster than the evidence? The answer is probably in the province of sociology. Carl Degler, a Stanford professor who has charted the fall and rise of social Darwinism over the past century, has concluded that cultural needs influence the evidence scientists attend to. During the American civil-rights struggle, for example, the proposition that biology is destiny became unthinkable. Today, in a society filled with the material fruits of the new biology—PET and CAT and MRI scanners, genetically engineered plants and animals, recombinant-DNA probes, and so forth—the proposition may seem incontrovertible.

No doubt, in seeing my friends' children through genetic lenses I was influenced by this change in culturally permissible thought. But as a psychiatrist I was under a more particular influence—the influence of drugs.

I was used to seeing patients' personalities change slowly, through painfully acquired insight and hard practice in the world. But recently I had seen personalities altered almost instantly, by medication. This impressive, close-up view of the power of biology over an unexpectedly broad spectrum of human behavior—over a range of traits even hardened pharmacologists had thought impervious to simple physiological influence—had done a good deal to move my assumptions about how people are constituted in the direction of the contemporary zeitgeist.

Prozac—the new antidepressant—was the main agent of change. There has always been the occasional patient who seems remarkably restored by one medicine or another, but with Prozac I had seen patient after patient become, like Sam, "better than well." Prozac seemed to give social confidence to the habitually timid, to make the sensitive brash, to lend the introvert the social skills of a salesman. Prozac was transformative for patients in the way an inspirational minister or high-pressure group therapy can be—it made them want to talk about their experience. And what my patients generally said was that they had learned something about themselves from Prozac. Like Sam, they believed Prozac revealed what in them was biologically determined and what merely (experience being "mere" compared to cellular physiology) experiential.

I called this phenomenon "listening to Prozac." As I thought about it, I began to understand how far my own listening to Prozac extended. Spending time with patients who responded to Prozac had transformed my views about what makes people the way they are. I had come to see inborn, biologically determined temperament where before I had seen slowly acquired, history-laden character. I formed new beliefs about how self-esteem is maintained, how "sensitivity" functions in interpersonal relationships, and how social skills are employed. Seeing how poorly patients fared when they were cautious and inhibited, and how the same people flourished once medication had made them assertive and flexible, I developed a strong impression of how our culture favors one interpersonal style over another. I do not mean that I had thought these issues through, only that the experience of repeatedly seeing a medication catapult people into new ways of behaving had exercised a great influence on my habitual way of seeing the world.

I write a monthly column in a trade paper for psychiatrists, and in it I began musing aloud about Prozac. First I wrote about Sam and his sense that medication simultaneously transformed him and taught him how he was put together. Then I wrote about patients who became "better than well," patients who acquired extra energy and became socially attractive. My mnemonic for this effect was "cosmetic psychopharmacology."

That two-word phrase, as it happened, did for me what Prozac had done for certain of my patients: it made me instantly popular. By the time my second essay about Prozac appeared, in March 1990, the drug was hot. It had appeared on the cover of *New York* magazine and was about to hit the national media. I was the psychiatrist who had written about Prozac—I had said out loud what thousands of doctors had observed—and as a result, I was due my fifteen minutes in the limelight. I was quoted in a cover story in *Newsweek,* interviewed on talk radio, asked for opinions by any number of magazine and newspaper reporters, and finally referenced in the definitive contemporary article for physicians on the use of antidepressants, in *The New England Journal of Medicine.*

After that flurry of activity, I continued to track Prozac's fame. How extraordinary it was to see a green-and-off-white capsule on the cover of *Newsweek,* where we expect the falsely sincere phiz of a head of state, the curves of a starlet. Here was a phenomenon that required explaining. For forty years, pharmaceutical houses had been making antidepressants, a new one every three or four years on average, and where were they, Tofranil and Nardil and Wellbutrin? They were not in the rotogravure, not talked about at cocktail parties or in movie lines.

Prozac enjoyed the career of the true celebrity—renown, followed by rumors, then notoriety, scandal, and lawsuits, and finally a quiet rehabilitation. Prozac was Gary Hart, Jim Bakker, Donald Trump.

Prozac was on "Nightline" when you went to sleep and on the "Today" show when you woke up. How could a medicine preoccupy us, stimulate us so? The news stories, the sober ones that tried to describe what the drug does, told little. Prozac, they said, has fewer side effects than other antidepressants. But why did we care about side effects? Since when had we taken to reading day after day about the fine points of a medication for mental illness? No, the news was not side effects. The news was takeoff. Prozac enjoyed the fastest acceptance of any psychotherapeutic medicine ever—650,000 prescriptions per month by the time the *Newsweek* cover appeared, just over two years after Prozac was introduced.

And then the backlash began, in the great American tradition of tarnishing the idol's luster. The occasional column or feature story asked why we had jumped on the bandwagon. People were taking the drug for weight loss and for binge eating, for premenstrual tensions and postpartum blues. These were women mostly, and the question arose, was Prozac another Miltown or Librium, the "mother's little helper" from which we expect too much and about which we know too little?

Just before *Newsweek* made Prozac a star, an ominous report had appeared in a scholarly journal. Six depressed patients experienced urgent suicidal thoughts while on Prozac. Yes, some had considered suicide before. But when they took Prozac, their self-destructive drive was more persistent and more intense. Lawyers began to venture the Prozac defense in murder trials. Celebrities associating as they do, Prozac was implicated in the suicide of a celebrity, the rock star Del Shannon. Lawsuits sprouted like toadstools after rain.

Geraldo reappeared on the scene, with Donahue, Larry King, "Eye on America," "Prime Time Live," and *Time* magazine, eager to see bad where *Newsweek* had seen good, and finally *Newsweek* again, not contrite, just reporting the trends, with a cover story on violence, in which "Backlash Against Prozac" marched side by side with "Violence Goes Mainstream" (*The Silence of the Lambs, American Psycho*), and, yes, "Apocalypse in Iraq."

On the talk shows, there was word of Prozac Survivor Support Groups, as if the pill were an abuser—a molesting parent, perhaps. The Scientologists came whooping in, seeing in Prozac conspiracy, coercion, evil incarnate. Fear reigned: Macy's barred a man from a Santa Claus job because he was taking Prozac.

Time began the backlash to the backlash, with a cover exposé of the Scientologists, who were shown to be fomenting much of the anti-Prozac hysteria. Then "60 Minutes" weighed in with a balancing piece: Lesley Stahl confronted women who claimed not to have been suicidal before taking Prozac—leaders of the anti-Prozac movement—with a medical report and doctor's letter saying they had.

By now, new drugs had entered the market—Prozac wannabes. They were not Prozac, but perhaps Prozac was no longer what it had been. The craze was over. And we were free to wonder, what had the fuss been about?

My own sense was that the media, for all the attention they paid Prozac, had missed the main story. The transformative powers of the medicine—how it went beyond treating illness to changing personality, how it entered into our struggle to understand the self—were nowhere mentioned. Scientists who studied Prozac had for the most part worked to satisfy the Food and Drug Administration. They tested the medicine on seriously depressed people and reported their results: a reasonable main effect, diminished side effects. Then they spoke to the media about what had been strictly proved. These researchers were hardly likely to address questions of personality, self, transformation.

Meanwhile, clinician after clinician had written or stopped me at meetings to say he or she had seen Prozac change patients' outlook and self-image in quite fundamental ways. If researchers could not speak to the implications of this phenomenon—what it means that a medication can, even occasionally, transform personality—I thought I might be able to. I was also curious about what I call the dyer's-hand question—how I and others who see psychotherapeutic medication in action had been tainted by what we work in.

By now, not yet five years after it was introduced, eight million people have taken Prozac, over half in the United States. My concern has been with a subset of these millions: fairly healthy people who show dramatic good responses to Prozac, people who are not so much cured of illness as transformed.

I have focused on this phenomenon because I find it intriguing and because I believe it has power to influence the way we understand human nature. As a result, I have all but ignored certain issues. Side effects, for example, though they should play an important role in anyone's decision to take or forgo Prozac, have been of secondary interest to me; even if Prozac were shown to cause one or another serious physical illness, that reality would have little to say about this other question: how is it that taking a capsule for depression can so alter a person's sense of self? The controversy over Prozac and suicide or violence, stimulating though it is, I treat in an appendix. Nor do I address many of Prozac's positive results in treating major mental illnesses from psychotic depression to eating disorders to schizophrenia.

I have limited myself to exploring the impact of mood-altering drugs on the modern sense of self, a large topic and an absorbing one. My quest has led me deep into territories whose results inform my clinical work but whose culture and customs are foreign: cellular physiology, pharmacology, history of medicine, animal ethology, medical ethics, descriptive psychiatry. The research literature turns out to be compelling; theories from diverse fields overlap and mesh in tantalizing ways. But, finally, it has been my own patients' responses to medication that have shaped my conjectures. Those stories of people experiencing inner change will, I hope, take the reader with me to a frontier of contemporary thought, a point at which such concepts as mood, personality, and self become at once unstable and fascinating.

Makeover

My first experience with Prozac involved a woman I worked with only around issues of medication. A psychologist with whom I collaborate had called to say she was treating a patient who had accomplished remarkable things in adult life despite an especially grim childhood; now, in her early thirties, the patient had become clinically depressed. Would I see her in consultation? My colleague summarized the woman's history, and I learned more when Tess arrived at my office.

Tess was the eldest of ten children born to a passive mother and an alcoholic father in the poorest public-housing project in our city. She was abused in childhood in the concrete physical and sexual senses which everyone understands as abuse. When Tess was twelve, her father died, and her mother entered a clinical depression from which she had never recovered. Tess—one of those inexplicably resilient children who flourish without any apparent source of sustenance— took over the family. She managed to remain in school herself and in time to steer all nine siblings into stable jobs and marriages.

Her own marriage was less successful. At seventeen, she married an older man, in part to provide a base outside the projects for her younger brothers and sisters, whom she immediately took in. She never went to the movies alone with her husband; the children came along. The weight of the family was always on her shoulders. The husband was alcoholic, and abusive when drunk. Tess struggled to help him stop drinking, but to no avail. The marriage soon became loveless. It collapsed once the children—Tess's siblings—were grown and one of its central purposes had disappeared.

Meanwhile, Tess had made a business career out of her skills at driving, inspiring, and nurturing others. She achieved a reputation as an administrator capable of turning around struggling companies by addressing issues of organization and employee morale, and she rose to a high level in a large corporation. She still cared for her mother, and she kept one foot in the projects, sitting on the school committee, working with the health clinics, investing personal effort in the lives of individuals who mostly would disappoint her.

It is hard to overstate how remarkable I found the story of Tess's success. I had an image of her beginnings. The concrete apartment in which she cared for her younger brothers and sisters was recently destroyed with great fanfare on local television. Years earlier, my work as head of a hospital clinic had led me to visit that building. From the start, it must have been a vertical prison, a place where to survive at all could be counted as high ambition. To succeed as Tess had—and without a stable family to guide or support her—was almost beyond imagining.

That her personal life was unhappy should not have been surprising. Tess stumbled from one prolonged affair with an abusive married man to another. As these degrading relationships ended, she would suffer severe demoralization. The current episode had lasted months, and, despite a psychotherapy in which Tess willingly faced the difficult aspects of her life, she was now becoming progressively less energetic and more unhappy. It was this condition I hoped to treat, in order to spare Tess the chronic and unremitting depression that had taken hold in her mother when she was Tess's age.

———

Though I had learned some of this story before my consultation with Tess, the woman, when I met her, surprised me. She was utterly charming.

I have so far recounted Tess's history as if it were extraordinary, and it is. At the same time, people like Tess are familiar figures in a psychiatrist's practice. Often it will be the most competent child in a chaotic family who will come for help—the field even has a name for people in Tess's role, "parental children," and a good deal is written about them. Nor is it uncommon for psychiatric patients to report having had a depressed mother and an absent father.

What I found unusual on meeting Tess was that the scars were so well hidden. Patients who have struggled, even successfully, through neglect and abuse can have an angry edge or a tone of aggressive sweetness. They may be seductive or provocative, rigid or overly compliant. A veneer of independence may belie a swamp of neediness. Not so with Tess.

She was a pleasure to be with, even depressed. I ran down the list of signs and symptoms, and she had them all: tears and sadness, absence of hope, inability to experience pleasure, feelings of worthlessness, loss of sleep and appetite, guilty ruminations, poor memory and concentration. Were it not for her many obligations, she would have preferred to end her life. And yet I felt comfortable in her presence. Though she looked infinitely weary, something about Tess reassured me. She maintained a hard-to-place hint of vitality—a glimmer of energy in the eyes, a sense of humor that was measured and not self-deprecating, a gracious mix of expectation of care and concern for the comfort of her listener.

It is said that depressed mothers' children, since they have to spend their formative years gauging mood states, develop a special sensitivity to small cues for emotion. In adult life, some maintain a compulsive need to please and are thought to have a knack for behaving just as friends (or therapists) prefer, at whatever cost to themselves. Perhaps it was this hypertrophied awareness of others that I saw in Tess. But I did not think so, not entirely. I thought what I was seeing was a remarkable and engaging survivor, suffering from a particular scourge, depression.

I had expected to ask how Tess had managed to do so well. But I found myself wondering how she had done so poorly.

Tess had indeed done poorly in her personal life. She considered herself unattractive to men and perhaps not even as interesting to women as she would have liked. For the past four years, her principal social contact had been with a married man—Jim—who came and went as he pleased and finally rejected Tess in favor of his wife. Tess had stuck with Jim in part, she told me, because no other men approached her. She believed she lacked whatever spark excited men; worse, she gave off signals that kept men at a distance.

Had I been working with Tess in psychotherapy, we might have begun to explore hypotheses regarding the source of her social failure: masochism grounded in low self-worth, the compulsion of those abused early in life to seek out further abuse. Instead, I was relegated to the surface, to what psychiatrists call the phenomena. I stored away for further consideration the contrast between Tess's charm and her social unhappiness. For the moment, my function was to treat my patient's depression with medication.

I began with imipramine, the oldest of the available antidepressants and still the standard by which others are judged. Imipramine takes about a month to work, and at the end of a month Tess said she was substantially more comfortable. She was sleeping and eating normally—in fact, she was gaining weight, probably as a side effect of the drug. "I am better," she told me. "I am myself again."

She did look less weary. And as we continued to meet, generally for fifteen minutes every month or two, all her overt symptoms remitted. Her memory and concentration improved. She regained the vital force and the willpower to go on with life. In short, Tess no longer met a doctor's criteria for depression. She even spread the good word to one of her brothers, also depressed, and the brother began taking imipramine.

But I was not satisfied.

It was the mother's illness that drove me forward. Tess had struggled too long for me to allow her, through any laxness of my own, to slide into the chronic depression that had engulfed her mother.

Depression is a relapsing and recurring illness. The key to treatment is thoroughness. If a patient can put together a substantial period of doing perfectly well—five months, some experts say; six or even twelve, say others—the odds are good for sustained remission. But to limp along just somewhat improved, "better but not well," is dangerous. The partly recovered patient will likely relapse as soon as you stop the therapy, as soon as you taper the drug. And the longer someone remains depressed, the more likely it is that depression will continue or return.

Tess said she was well, and she was free of the signs and symptoms of depression. But doctors are trained to doubt the report of the too-stoical patient, the patient so willing to bear pain she may unwittingly conceal illness. And, beyond signs and symptoms, the recognized abnormalities associated with a given syndrome, doctors occasionally consider what the neurologists call "soft signs," normal findings that, in the right context, make the clinical nose twitch.

I thought Tess might have a soft sign or two of depression.

She had begun to experience trouble at work—not major trouble, but something to pay attention to. The conglomerate she worked for had asked Tess to take over a company beset with labor problems. Tess always had some difficulty in situations that required meeting firmness with firmness, but she reported being more upset by negotiations with this union than by any in the past. She felt the union leaders were unreasonable, and she had begun to take their attacks on her personally. She understood conflict was inevitable; past mistakes had left labor-management relations too strained for either side to trust the other, and the coaxing and cajoling that characterized Tess's management style would need some time to work their magic. But, despite her understanding, Tess was rattled.

As a psychotherapist, I might have wondered whether Tess's difficulties had a symbolic meaning. Perhaps the hectoring union chief and his foot-dragging members resembled parents—the aggressive father, the passive mother—too much for Tess to be effective with them. In simpler terms, a new job, and this sort especially, constitutes a stressor. These viewpoints may be correct. But what level of stress was it appropriate for Tess to experience? To be rattled even by tough negotiations was unlike her.

And I found Tess vulnerable on another front. Toward the end of one of our fifteen-minute reviews of Tess's sleep, appetite, and energy level, I asked about Jim, and she burst into uncontrollable sobs. Thereafter, our meetings took on a predictable form. Tess would report that she was substantially better. Then I would ask her about Jim, and her eyes would brim over with tears, her shoulders shake. People do cry about failed romances, but sobbing seemed out of character for Tess.

These are weak reeds on which to support a therapy. Here was a highly competent, fully functional woman who no longer considered herself depressed and who had none of the standard overt indicators of depression. Had I found her less remarkable, considered her less capable as a businesswoman, been less surprised by her fragility in the face of romantic disappointment, I might have declared Tess cured. My conclusion that we should try for a better medication response may seem to be based on highly subjective data—and I think this perception is correct. Pharmacotherapy, when looked at closely, will appear to be as arbitrary—as much an art, not least in the derogatory sense of being impressionistic where ideally it should be objective—as psychotherapy. Like any other serious assessment of human emotional life, pharmacotherapy properly rests on fallible attempts at intimate understanding of another person.

When I laid out my reasoning, Tess agreed to press ahead. I tried raising the dose of imipramine, but Tess began to experience side effects—dry mouth, daytime tiredness, further weight gain—so we switched to similar medications in hopes of finding one that would allow her to tolerate a higher dose. Tess changed little.

And then Prozac was released by the Food and Drug Administration. I prescribed it for Tess, for entirely conventional reasons—to terminate her depression more thoroughly, to return her to her "premorbid self." My goal was not to transform Tess but to restore her.

But medications do not always behave as we expect them to.

Two weeks after starting Prozac, Tess appeared at the office to say she was no longer feeling weary. In retrospect, she said, she had been depleted of energy for as long as she could remember, had almost not known what it was to feel rested and hopeful. She had been depressed, it now seemed to her, her whole life. She was astonished at the sensation of being free of depression.

She looked different, at once more relaxed and energetic—more available—than I had seen her, as if the person hinted at in her eyes had taken over. She laughed more frequently, and the quality of her laughter was different, no longer measured but lively, even teasing.

With this new demeanor came a new social life, one that did not unfold slowly, as a result of a struggle to integrate disparate parts of the self, but seemed, rather, to appear instantly and full-blown.

"Three dates a weekend," Tess told me. "I must be wearing a sign on my forehead!"

Within weeks of starting Prozac, Tess settled into a satisfying dating routine with men. She had missed out on dating in her teens and twenties. Now she reveled in the attention she received. She seemed even to enjoy the trial-and-error process of learning contemporary courtship rituals, gauging norms for sexual involvement, weighing the import of men's professed infatuation with her.

I had never seen a patient's social life reshaped so rapidly and dramatically. Low self-worth, competitiveness, jealousy, poor inter-personal skills, shyness, fear of intimacy—the usual causes of social awkwardness—are so deeply ingrained and so difficult to influence that ordinarily change comes gradually if at all. But Tess blossomed all at once.

"People on the sidewalk ask me for directions!" she said. They never had before.

The circle of Tess's women friends changed. Some friends left, she said, because they had been able to relate to her only through her depression. Besides, she now had less tolerance for them. "Have you ever been to a party where other people are drunk or high and you are stone-sober? Their behavior annoys you, you can't understand it. It seems juvenile and self-centered. That's how I feel around some of my old friends. It is as if they are under the influence of a harmful chemical and I am all right—as if I had been in a drugged state all those years and now I am clearheaded."

The change went further: "I can no longer understand how they tolerate the men they are with." She could scarcely acknowledge that she had once thrown herself into the same sorts of self-destructive relationships. "I never think about Jim," she said. And in the con-sulting room his name no longer had the power to elicit tears.

This last change struck me as most remarkable of all. When a patient displays any sign of masochism, and I think it is fair to call Tess's relationship with Jim masochistic, psychiatrists anticipate a protracted psychotherapy. It is rarely easy to help a socially self-destructive patient abandon humiliating relationships and take on new ones that accord with a healthy sense of self-worth. But once Tess felt better, once the weariness lifted and optimism became pos-sible, the masochism just withered away, and she seemed to have every social skill she needed.

Tess's work, too, became more satisfying. She responded without defensiveness in the face of adamant union leaders, felt stable enough inside herself to evaluate their complaints critically. She said the medication had lent her surety of judgment; she no longer tortured herself over whether she was being too demanding or too lenient. I found this remark noteworthy, because I had so recently entertained the possibility that unconscious inner conflicts were hampering Tess in her dealings with the labor union. Whether the conflicts were real or illusory, the problem disappeared when the medication took effect. "It makes me confident," Tess said, a claim I since have heard from dozens of patients, none of whom had been given a hint that this medication, or any medication, could do any such thing.

Tess's management style changed. She was less conciliatory, firmer, unafraid of confrontation. As the troubled company settled down, Tess was given a substantial pay raise, a sign that others noticed her new effectiveness.

Tess's relations to those she watched over also changed. She was no longer drawn to tragedy, nor did she feel heightened responsibility for the injured. Most tellingly, she moved to another nearby town, the farthest she had ever lived from her mother.

Whether these last changes are to be applauded depends on one's social values. Tess's guilty vigilance over a mother about whom she had strong ambivalent feelings can be seen as a virtue, one that medication helped to erode. Tess experienced her "loss of seriousness," as she put it, as a relief. She had been too devoted in the past, at too great a cost to her own enjoyment of life.

In time, Tess's mother was given an antidepressant, and she showed a modest response—she slept better, lost weight, had more energy, displayed a better sense of humor. Tess threw her a birthday party, a celebration of the mother's survival and the children's successes. In addition to the main present, each child brought a nostalgic gift. Tess's was a little red wagon, in memory of a time when the little ones were still in diapers, and the family lived in a coldwater flat, and Tess had organized the middle children to wheel the dirty linens past abandoned tenements to the laundromat many times a week. Were I Tess's psychotherapist, I might have asked whether the gift did not reveal an element of aggression, but on the surface at least the present was offered and received lovingly. In acknowledging with her mother how difficult the past had been, Tess opened a door that had been closed for years. Tess used her change in mood as a springboard for psychological change, converting pain into perspective and forgiveness.

There is no unhappy ending to this story. It is like one of those Elizabethan dramas—Marlowe's *Tamburlaine*—so foreign to modern audiences because the Wheel of Fortune takes only half a turn: the patient recovers and pays no price for the recovery. Tess did go off medication, after about nine months, and she continued to do well. She was, she reported, not quite so sharp of thought, so energetic, so free of care as she had been on the medication, but neither was she driven by guilt and obligation. She was altogether cooler, better controlled, less sensible of the weight of the world than she had been.

After about eight months off medication, Tess told me she was slipping. "I'm not myself," she said. New union negotiations were under way, and she felt she could use the sense of stability, the invulnerability to attack, that Prozac gave her. Here was a dilemma for me. Ought I to provide medication to someone who was not depressed? I could give myself reason enough—construe it that Tess was sliding into relapse, which perhaps she was. In truth, I assumed I would be medicating Tess's chronic condition, call it what you will: heightened awareness of the needs of others, sensitivity to conflict, residual damage to self-esteem—all odd indications for medication. I discussed the dilemma with her, but then I did not hesitate to write the prescription. Who was I to withhold from her the bounties of science? Tess responded again as she had hoped she would, with renewed confidence, self-assurance, and social comfort.

I believe Tess's story contains an unchronicled reason for Prozac's enormous popularity: its ability to alter personality. Here was a patient whose usual method of functioning changed dramatically. She became socially capable, no longer a wallflower but a social butterfly. Where once she had focused on obligations to others, now she was vivacious and fun-loving. Before, she had pined after men; now she dated them, enjoyed them, weighed their faults and virtues. Newly confident, Tess had no need to romanticize or indulge men's shortcomings.

Not all patients on Prozac respond this way. Some are unaffected by the medicine; some merely recover from depression, as they might on any antidepressant. But a few, a substantial minority, are transformed. Like Garrison Keillor's marvelous Powdermilk biscuits, Prozac gives these patients the courage to do what needs to be done.

What I saw in Tess—a quick alteration in ordinarily intractable problems of personality and social functioning—other psychiatrists saw in their patients as well. Moreover, Prozac had few immediate side effects. Patients on Prozac do not feel drugged up or medicated. Here is one place where the favorable side-effect profile of Prozac makes a difference: if a doctor thinks there is even a modest chance of quickly liberating a chronically stymied patient, and if the risk to the patient is slight, then the doctor will take the gamble repeatedly.

And of course Prozac had phenomenal word of mouth, as "good responders" like Tess told their friends about it. I saw this effect in the second patient I put on Prozac. She was a habitually withdrawn, reticent woman whose cautious behavior had handicapped her at work and in courtship. After a long interval between sessions, I ran into her at a local bookstore. I tend to hang back when I see a patient in a public place, out of uncertainty as to how the patient may want to be greeted, and I believe that, while her chronic depression persisted, this woman would have chosen to avoid me. Now she strode forward and gave me a bold "Hello." I responded, and she said, "I've changed my name, you know."

I did not know. Had she switched from depression to mania and then married impulsively? I wondered whether I should have met with her more frequently. She had, I saw, the bright and open manner that had brought Tess so much social success.

11

"Yes," she continued, "I call myself Ms. Prozac."

There is no Ms. Asendin, no Ms. Pamelor. Those medicines are quite wonderful—they free patients from the bondage of depression. But they have not inspired the sort of enthusiasm and loyalty patients have shown for Prozac.

No doubt doctors should be unreservedly pleased when their patients get better quickly. But I confess I was unsettled by Ms. Prozac's enthusiasm, and by Tess's as well. I was suspicious of Prozac, as if I had just taken on a cotherapist whose charismatic style left me wondering whether her magic was wholly trustworthy.

The more rational component to my discomfort had to do with Tess. It makes a psychiatrist uneasy to watch a medicated patient change her circle of friends, her demeanor at work, her relationship to her family. All psychiatrists have seen depressed patients turn manic and make decisions they later regret. But Tess never showed signs of mania. She did not manifest rapid speech or thought, her judgment remained sound, and, though she enjoyed life more than she had before, she was never euphoric or Pollyannaish. In mood and level of energy, she was "normal," but her place on the normal spectrum had changed, and that change, from "serious," as she put it, to vivacious, had profound consequences for her relationships to those around her.

As the stability of Tess's improvement became clear, my concern diminished, but it did not disappear. Just what did not sit right was hard to say. Might a severe critic find the new Tess a bit blander than the old? Perhaps her tortured intensity implied a complexity of personality that was now harder to locate. I wondered whether the medication had not ironed out too many character-giving wrinkles, like overly aggressive plastic surgery. I even asked myself whether Tess would now give up her work in the projects, as if I had administered her a pill to cure warmheartedness and progressive social beliefs. But in entertaining this thought I wondered whether I was clinging to an arbitrary valuation of temperament, as if the melancholy or saturnine humor were in some way morally superior to the sanguine. In the event, Tess did not forsake the projects, though she did make more time for herself.

Tess, too, found her transformation, marvelous though it was, somewhat unsettling. What was she to make of herself? Her past devotion to Jim, for instance—had it been a matter of biology, an addiction to which she was prone as her father had been to alcoholism? Was she, who defined herself in contrast to her father's fecklessness, in some uncomfortable way like him? What responsibility had she for those years of thralldom to degrading love? After a prolonged struggle to understand the self, to find the Gordian knot dissolved by medication is a mixed pleasure: we want some internal responsibility for our lives, want to find meaning in our errors. Tess was happy, but she talked of a mild, persistent sense of wonder and dislocation.

My discomfort with Tess's makeover had another component. It is all very well for drugs to do small things: to induce sleep, to allay anxiety, to ameliorate a well-recognized syndrome. But for a drug's effect to be so global—to extend to social popularity, business acumen, self-image, energy, flexibility, sexual appeal—touches too closely on fantasies about medication for the mind. Patients often have extreme fears about drugs, stemming from their apprehension that medication will take over in a way that cannot be reversed, that drugs will obliterate the self. For years, psychiatrists have reassured patients that medication merely combats illness: "If the pills work," I and others have said, "they will restore you to your former self. I expect you to walk in here in a few weeks and say, 'I'm myself again.' " Medication does not transform, it heals.

When faced with a medication that does transform, even in this friendly way, I became aware of my own irrational discomfort, my sense that for a drug to have such a pronounced effect is inherently unnatural, unsafe, uncanny.

I might have come to terms with this discomfort—the unexpected soon becomes routine in the world of pharmacology. But Tess's sense of dislocation did not disappear immediately, and her surprise at her altered self helped me to understand the more profound sources of my own concern. The changes in Tess, which I saw replicated in other patients given Prozac, raised unsettling issues.

Many of these were medical issues. How, for example, would Prozac affect the doctor's role? To ameliorate depression is all very well, but it was less clear how psychiatrists were to use a medication that could lend social ease, command, even brilliance. Nor was it entirely clear how the use of antidepressants for this purpose could be distinguished from, say, the street use of amphetamine as a way of overcoming inhibitions and inspiring zest.

Other questions seemed to transcend any profession, to bear directly on the way members of our culture see themselves and one another. How were we to reconcile what Prozac did for Tess with our notion of the continuous, autobiographical human self? And always there was the question of how society would be affected by our access to drugs that alter personality in desirable ways.

I wondered what I would have made of Tess had she been referred to me just before Jim broke up with her, before she had experienced acute depression. I might have recognized her as a woman with skills in many areas, one who had managed to make friends and sustain a career, and who had never suffered a mental illness; I might have seen her as a person who had examined her life with some thoroughness and made progress on many fronts but who remained frustrated socially. She and I might suspect the trouble stemmed from "who she is"—temperamentally serious or timid or cautious or pessimistic or emotionally unexpressive. If only she were a little livelier, a bit more carefree, we might conclude, everything else would fall into place.

Tess's family history—the depressed mother and alcoholic father—constitutes what psychiatrists call "affective loading." (Alcoholism in men seems genetically related to depression in women; or, put more cautiously, a family history of alcoholism is moderately predictive of depression in near relatives.) I might suspect that, in a socially stymied woman with a familial predisposition to depression, Prozac could prove peculiarly liberating. There I would sit, knowing I had in hand a drug that might give Tess just the disposition she needed to break out of her social paralysis.

Confronted with a patient who had never met criteria for any illness, what would I be free to do? If I did prescribe medication, how would we characterize this act?

For years, psychoanalysts were criticized for treating the "worried well," or for "enhancing growth" rather than curing illness. Who is not neurotic? Who is not a fit candidate for psychotherapy? This issue has been answered through an uneasy social consensus. We tolerate breadth in the scope of psychoanalysis, and of psychotherapy in general; few people today would remark on a patient's consulting a therapist over persistent problems with personality or social interactions, though some might object to seeing such treatments covered by insurance under the rubric of illness.

But I wondered whether we were ready for "cosmetic psychopharmacology." It was my musings about whether it would be kosher to medicate a patient like Tess in the absence of depression that led me to coin the phrase. Some people might prefer pharmacologic to psychologic self-actualization. Psychic steroids for mental gymnastics, medicinal attacks on the humors, antiwallflower compound—these might be hard to resist. Since you only live once, why not do it as a blonde? Why not as a peppy blonde? Now that questions of personality and social stance have entered the arena of medication, we as a society will have to decide how comfortable we are with using chemicals to modify personality in useful, attractive ways. We may mask the issue by defining less and less severe mood states as pathology, in effect saying, "If it responds to an antidepressant, it's depression." Already, it seems to me, psychiatric diagnosis had been subject to a sort of "diagnostic bracket creep"—the expansion of categories to match the scope of relevant medications.

How large a sphere of human problems we choose to define as

medical is an important social decision. But words like "choose" and "decision" perhaps misstate the process. It is easy to imagine that our role will be passive, that as a society we will in effect permit the material technology, medications, to define what is health and what is illness.

Tess's progress also seemed to blur the boundary between licit and illicit drug use. How does Prozac, in Tess's life, differ from amphetamine or cocaine or even alcohol? People take street drugs all the time in order to "feel normal." Certainly people use cocaine to enhance their energy and confidence. "I felt large. I mean, I felt huge," is how socially insecure people commonly explain why they abuse cocaine or amphetamine. Uppers make people socially attractive, obviously available. And when a gin drinker takes a risk, we are tempted to ask whether the newfound confidence is not mere "Dutch courage."

In fact, it is people from Tess's background—born poor to addicted and dependent parents, and then abused and neglected—who are most at risk to use street drugs. A cynic may wonder whether in Tess's case drug abuse has sneaked in through the back door, whether entering the middle class carries the privilege of access to socially sanctioned drugs that are safer and more specific in their effects than street drugs but are morally indistinguishable in terms of the reasons they are taken and the results they produce. I do not think it is possible to see transformations like Tess's without asking ourselves both whether street-drug abusers are self-medicating unrecognized illness and whether prescribed-drug users are, with their doctors' permission, stimulating and calming themselves in quite similar ways.

More unsettling to me than questions of definition—licit versus illicit—was an issue raised by Tess's renewed professional success: how might a substance like Prozac enter into the competitive world of American business? Psychiatrists have begun to recognize a normal or near-normal mental condition called "hyperthymia," which corresponds loosely to what the Greeks called the sanguine temperament.

Hyperthymia is distinct from mania and hypomania, the disorders in which people are grandiose, frenetic, distractible, and flawed in their judgment. Hyperthymics are merely optimistic, decisive, quick of thought, charismatic, energetic, and confident.

Hyperthymia can be an asset in business. Many top organizational and political leaders require little sleep, see crises as opportunities, let criticism roll off their backs, make decisions easily, exude confidence, and hurry through the day with energy to spare. These qualities help people succeed in complex social and work situations. They may be considered desirable or advantageous even by those who have quite normal levels of drive and optimism. How shall we respond to the complaint that a particular executive lacks decisiveness and vigor? By prescribing Prozac? In Tess's work, should the negotiators on the union side be offered Prozac, too? The effect of Prozac on Tess's style in her corporate work—and Sam's in his architectural practice—raises questions about how a drug that alters personality might be used in a competitive society.

Nor is it possible to witness Tess's transformation without fearing that a drug like Prozac might bolster other unfortunate tendencies in contemporary culture. Even Prozac's main effect in Tess's treatment—the relief it provided from social vulnerability—might, in societal terms, prove a mixed blessing. Tess had come for medication treatment only after a prolonged effort at self-understanding through psychotherapy. But I could imagine a less comfortable scenario: A woman much like Tess, abused and neglected in childhood, though not fully aware to what extent and to what effect, seeks treatment in a society that prefers to ignore victimization and that values economy over thoroughness in health care; the woman seems subdued and angry, is discontented for reasons she cannot easily put into words. By what means will her doctor attempt to help her? Would Prozac, alone, be enough?

But my central concern, as I watched Tess's story unfold, involved her personhood. Tess had every right, on the basis of both childhood experience and unhappiness in adult life, to be socially vulnerable in adulthood. But once she had taken Prozac, she—and those who knew her—had to explain her newfound social success on medication. If her self-destructiveness with men and her fragility at work disappeared in response to a biological treatment, they must have been biologically encoded. Her biological constitution seems to have determined her social failures. But how does the belief that a woman who was abused as a child and later remains stuck in abusive relationships largely because of her biologically encoded temperament affect our notions of responsibility, of free will, of unique and socially determinative individual development? Are we willing to allow medications to tell us how we are constituted?

When one pill at breakfast makes you a new person, or makes your patient, or relative, or neighbor a new person, it is difficult to resist the suggestion, the visceral certainty, that who people are is largely biologically determined. I don't mean that it is impossible to escape simplistic biological materialism, but the drama, the rapidity, the thoroughness of drug-induced transformation make simplicity tempting. Drug responses provide hard-to-ignore evidence for certain beliefs—concerning the influence of biology on personality, intellectual performance, and social success—that heretofore we as a society have resisted. When I saw the impact of medication on patients' self-concept, I came to believe that even if we tried to understand these matters complexly, new medications would redraw our map of those parts of the self that are biologically responsive, so that we would arrive, as a culture, at a new consensus about the human condition.

An indication of the power of medication to reshape a person's identity is contained in the sentence Tess used when, eight months after first stopping Prozac, she telephoned me to ask whether she might resume the medication. She said, "I am not myself."

I found this statement remarkable. After all, Tess had existed in one mental state for twenty or thirty years; she then briefly felt different on medication. Now that the old mental state was threatening to re-emerge—the one she had experienced almost all her adult life—her response was "I am not myself." But who had she been all those years if not herself? Had medication somehow removed a false self and replaced it with a true one? Might Tess, absent the invention of the modern antidepressant, have lived her whole life—a successful life, perhaps, by external standards—and never been herself?

When I asked her to expand on what she meant, Tess said she no longer felt like herself when certain aspects of her ailment—lack of confidence, feelings of vulnerability—returned, even to a small degree. Ordinarily, if we ask a person why she holds back socially, she may say, "That's just who I am," meaning shy or hesitant or melancholy or overly cautious. These characteristics often persist throughout life, and they have a strong influence on career, friendships, marriage, self-image.

Suddenly those intimate and consistent traits are not-me, they are alien, they are defect, they are illness—so that a certain habit of mind and body that links a person to his relatives and ancestors from generation to generation is now "other." Tess had come to understand herself—the person she had been for so many years—to be mildly ill. She understood this newfound illness, as it were, in her marrow. She did not feel herself when the medicine wore off and she was rechallenged by an external stress.

On imipramine, no longer depressed but still inhibited and subdued, Tess felt "myself again." But while on Prozac, she underwent a redefinition of self. Off Prozac, when she again became inhibited and subdued—perhaps the identical sensations she had experienced while on imipramine—she now felt "not myself." Prozac redefined Tess's understanding of what was essential to her and what was intrusive and pathological.

This recasting of self left Tess in an unusual relationship to medication. Off medication, she was aware that, if she returned to the old inhibited state, she might need Prozac in order to "feel herself." In this sense, she might have a lifelong relationship to medication, whether or not she was currently taking it. Patients who undergo the sort of deep change Tess experienced generally say they never want to feel the old way again and would take quite substantial risks—in terms, for instance, of medication side effects—in order not to regress. This is not a question of addiction or hedonism, at least not in the ordinary sense of those words, but of having located a self that feels true, normal, and whole, and of understanding medication to be an occasionally necessary adjunct to the maintenance of that self.

Beyond the effect on individual patients, Tess's redefinition of self led me to fantasize about a culture in which this biologically driven sort of self-understanding becomes widespread. Certain dispositions now considered awkward or endearing, depending on taste, might be seen as ailments to be pitied and, where possible, corrected. Tastes and judgments regarding personality styles do change. The romantic, decadent stance of Goethe's young Werther and Chateaubriand's René we now see as merely immature, overly depressive, perhaps in need of treatment. Might we not, in a culture where overseriousness is a medically correctable flaw, lose our taste for the melancholic or brooding artists—Schubert, or even Mozart in many of his moods?

These were my concerns on witnessing Tess's recovery. I was torn simultaneously by a sense that the medication was too far-reaching in its effects and a sense that my discomfort was arbitrary and aesthetic rather than doctorly. I wondered how the drug might influence my profession's definition of illness and its understanding of ordinary suffering. I wondered how Prozac's success would interact with certain unfortunate tendencies of the broader culture. And I asked just how far we—doctors, patients, the society at large—were likely to go in the direction of permitting drug responses to shape our understanding of the authentic self.

My concerns were imprecisely formulated. But it was not only the concerns that were vague: I had as yet only a sketchy impression of the drug whose effects were so troubling. To whom were my patients and I listening? On that question depended the answers to the list of social and ethical concerns; and the exploration of that question would entail attending to accounts of other patients who responded to Prozac.

My first meeting with Prozac had been heightened for me by the uncommon qualities of the patient who responded to the drug. I found it astonishing that a pill could do in a matter of days what psychiatrists hope, and often fail, to accomplish by other means over a course of years: to restore to a person robbed of it in childhood the capacity to play. Yes, there remained a disquieting element to this restoration. Were I scripting the story, I might have made Tess's metamorphosis more gradual, more humanly comprehensible, more in sync with the ordinary rhythm of growth. I might even have preferred if her play as an adult had been, for continuity's sake, more suffused with the memory of melancholy. But medicines do not work just as we wish. The way neurochemicals tell stories is not the way psychotherapy tells them. If Tess's fairy tale does not have the plot we expect, its ending is nonetheless happy.

By the time Tess's story had played itself out, I had seen perhaps a dozen people respond with comparable success to Prozac. Hers was not an isolated case, and the issues it raised would not go away. Charisma, courage, character, social competency—Prozac seemed to say that these and other concepts would need to be re-examined, that our sense of what is constant in the self and what is mutable, what is necessary and what contingent, would need, like our sense of the fable of transformation, to be revised.

Compulsion

As I was becoming acquainted with Prozac, I was consulted by a woman who I thought needed no medication at all but who, from the start, knew better. Julia telephoned because she had read a magazine article I had written about psychopharmacology. A patient described there, a woman who responded to Prozac, reminded Julia of herself. Would I see her and put her on the drug? As Julia elaborated, I was less impressed with any sign of mood disorder than with her frustration at work and home. I suggested that, rather than consider medication, she might speak to a psychotherapist. I referred Julia to a woman social worker who is reliable and charges modest fees.

In the course of the first two therapy sessions, the social worker came to believe that Julia's problems arose from a perfectionistic style. The evaluation took place just as stories about Anafranil, the first medicine approved for the treatment of obsessive-compulsive disorder, were appearing in the news. The social worker thought it might make sense for me to have a look at Julia after all.

When I met her, I was impressed, as I had been on the phone, with how well put together Julia seemed. She was pleasant and well spoken and appeared comfortable with herself. Her life had definite form to it: she had completed training as a registered nurse, married, had children, and taken a short-day job at a nursing home, a position that allowed her to be back at the house to greet her children on their return from school.

But there were problems on every front. She demanded extraordinary control in the household. The beds had to be made just so. The children had to be scrubbed and organized before leaving for school. Julia's husband was uncomfortable with her inflexibility, and she found herself raising her voice to him and the children more than was right. Also, the nursing-home job was beneath the level of her abilities. Julia was not challenged, but she saw no way out. How could she manage her tasks in the house and at the same time tackle a more demanding job?

These were the sorts of problems I had hoped might respond to a reassessment of her own or the family's needs in therapy. I certainly did not want to prescribe a "mother's little helper," a pill that would allow Julia to feel less frazzled in a domestic setup that, ideally, required better negotiating between spouses or a clearer understanding on Julia's part of her own anxieties over her competency as nurse, wife, or mother. I wanted, in short, to avoid medicating Julia for what looked like marital dissatisfaction.

I began with the most prosaic questions. Did the housework, child care, and job duties fall on Julia's shoulders in unfair ways? Had Julia considered hiring someone to help with the cleaning? Might she find after-school programs for the children? Would she feel relief if her husband took on additional responsibilities in the house? If he came home earlier, would she be freer to find fulfillment in her career?

Julia said her problems could not be solved in these mundane, operational ways. Her husband had made these suggestions and others, but she could not let go. She needed to be home in any event, because she disliked disorder. If she were not home, the straightening up would not be done to her satisfaction, and the children would not be neat and scrubbed in the way that pleased her.

And it was, she said, very much a matter of pleasing her, of her comfort. She was not absolutely compelled to perform any particular task; if there were sufficient reason, she could leave the house with chores unfinished, although she felt better if everything was done, and done according to her standards. I asked about explicit obsessions. Julia did not fear contamination, was not anxious over germs. In fact, she did not have any formed worrisome ideas; she just disliked it when things were left messy. But her style, her preferences, her sense of propriety, her perfectionism were so pronounced that she was continually angry at her children and husband and, given the impossibility of instilling her standards in them, stalemated in her career.

There are many ways of understanding Julia's dilemma, but perhaps it is most instructive to see how the problem was understood in the period before Julia telephoned to request medication.

Four years into her marriage, and some six years before I saw her, Julia and her husband visited a psychologist for couples counseling. The psychologist, the director of a university program here, found that Julia was unhappy in her marriage. She was not depressed, but she found her husband unresponsive to her needs. Things had to be "just so" to please her, and not only matters of household organization. The husband had to take her out a certain number of nights a month for her to feel loved. If he fell one night shy, she would fault him—but she might not have said openly how many was enough. The psychologist worked with the couple on "communication skills," and he believed they profited. He had never considered a formal diagnosis of depression or of obsessive-compulsive disorder for Julia, although he said she certainly was discontented and had a perfectionistic style.

Julia's internist also found her anxious and unhappy on occasion, conditions he attributed to her perfectionism and her sense that she was not getting enough attention from her husband. The doctor prescribed antianxiety medication for what he called a "situational reaction associated with depressive overtones," a label for a problem that does not quite rise to the level of illness but that nonetheless seems to call for treatment. Julia's gynecologist understood the same intercurrent problems as premenstrual syndrome, a condition he tried at various times to alleviate with diuretics ("water pills") and oil of primrose (a plant extract intended to raise prostaglandin-hormone levels), and more antianxiety medication, without apparent effect.

Julia, in sum, was a patient without a diagnosis, or with bits and pieces of many diagnoses. As a psychiatrist, I was in no better position to categorize Julia's problem than her psychologist, internist, and gynecologist had been. My preference, as I have said, was not to call her ill at all, but to focus on some intimate aspect of the self or the marriage. I wondered about her self-esteem. Where did her need for control, her ineffectiveness in marital negotiations, and her heightened frustration with the children arise, if not from a disorder in self-image? Her perfectionism, if I had to guess, might be a defense against the terrible feelings she anticipated if her imagined inadequacies were laid bare.

I also considered family pathology. Could the husband be undermining his wife, playing on her anxiety in some way that guaranteed she would tend to home and hearth rather than throw herself into her career? Frequently when an otherwise competent patient becomes dysfunctional in one limited sphere, the greater pathology is in the apparently more flexible spouse.

But, in order to consider biological treatment, it seemed important to capture Julia's waxing and waning symptoms in a diagnosis. Julia's other doctors had all on occasion noticed a depressive tendency. The current diagnostic system contains a category—"dysthymia"—for patients who do not quite meet the standards of major depression. But dysthymia applies to people who suffer depressed mood "for most of the day more days than not" for two or more years running, and who when depressed have disturbances of sleep, appetite, energy, concentration, and the like. Julia did not have that sort of disturbance, and her depression was not at all constant. What was constant was her perfectionism.

Perfectionism makes a psychiatrist think of two diagnoses, obsessive-compulsive disorder (OCD) and compulsive personality disorder. Julia did not meet the criteria for these, either, and she said as much in describing herself. She had read about OCD in the newspaper. "I'm a neat freak," she said, "but I am not at all like that— not that extreme."

OCD is among the most terrible of psychiatric disturbances. Anyone who has seen a man or woman whose skin is macerated from repeated scrubbings, or who cannot leave a room for fear of germs, or who spends long hours repeating meaningless calculations, or who cannot stop demanding reassurance over an unlikely but paralyzing source of dread, will have a sense of how distinctive and relentless OCD is. Personable, accomplished, interactive with friends, able to do any particular thing she chose—Julia bore little resemblance to the patients a psychiatrist ordinarily labels as having OCD, and she did not fit the standard definition.

That definition rests on two concepts, the obsession and the compulsion. Obsessions are "recurrent, persistent ideas, thoughts, images, or impulses that are experienced, at least initially, as intrusive and senseless." The example given in the official manual is a parent's impulse to kill a loved child. Julia had no such thoughts. Compulsions are "repetitive, purposeful, and intentional behaviors that are performed in response to an obsession" or in a stereotyped fashion and which are designed to neutralize the dreaded obsession or to prevent discomfort. Here Julia's behavior came closer to the mark, though her actions were more flexible and less strictly compelled than those the definition is meant to indicate.

Perhaps Julia almost met the criteria: there were weeks when she did two loads of laundry every day; if the floors were dirty, she might stay up late to wash them. But these behaviors appeared as compulsions only when her routine was disrupted. Most days, she was organized enough to do what felt right to her on a schedule she found acceptable. Julia's condition fell, let us say, in the penumbra of OCD.

Certainly she had a compulsive style. Extremes of style are called, in the insulting language of psychiatry, "personality disorders." Personality disorders have traditionally been thought not to respond to medication. In the case of compulsive personality disorder, the key elements are "restricted ability to express warm and tender emotions," "perfectionism that interferes with the ability to grasp 'the big picture,' " "excessive devotion to work," and indecisiveness—none of which Julia had—as well as "insistence that others submit to her or her way of doing things," which, along with a good many other people, she had to a fair degree.

I had seen many patients with compulsive personality disorder —the kind who threaten to bore you to death by perseverating on small details of topics whose emotional import is never made clear —and I found Julia entirely unlike them. She was engaging and able to focus well. This having been said, if we had to give a name to what ailed Julia, it would be hard to avoid reference to compulsiveness.

In making a referral to the social worker, I had attempted to define Julia's problem as one of either marital or inner conflict. Julia, however, experienced her disorder as medical. If she were made well, the turmoil in the family would disappear. And that is what happened.

By the time I met with Julia, reports had emerged that, like Anafranil, Prozac was effective in treating OCD, and it seldom caused the weight gain common with Anafranil. Julia was concerned about her weight, and she identified with the patient I had written about who responded to Prozac. We discussed the risks and benefits of different approaches, but in the end I gave her what she had come for. I wrote a prescription for Prozac and told Julia what I tell every patient, that antidepressants take about four weeks to work—two weeks to build up a good level in the brain, and then, for unknown reasons, two weeks to affect the illness.

The first week on medicine, Julia reported, was "like night and day." The children behaved more obediently, and when Julia remarked on the change, they told her she was yelling less. Her husband became more cooperative as Julia became more pleasant with him. Then she noticed she had markedly more energy. "I could not have imagined this" was her comment, meaning she did not want me to think she was experiencing a placebo effect.

I suspected Julia might be experiencing the lift of an amphetaminelike effect, the burst of energy that can arise early in the course of antidepressant treatment. I wrote in her chart, "Good early response," and asked her to return in three weeks.

By then, the early euphoria had worn off. Julia missed the sense of vitality she had felt in the first days, but she remained moderately improved, on better terms with her family. Obsessive-compulsive disorder often requires higher doses of medication than does depression. Though Julia's was at best a "penumbral" case of OCD, I raised the dose and marked her progress. She reported steady, modest improvement in her mood and in her ability to tolerate messiness. Antidepressants do work this way for some patients—a progressive amelioration of symptoms that does not plateau for months.

There were ups and downs. Some weeks, Julia reported having been nervous with her children and having yelled excessively. These fluctuations often correlated with particular stressors. For instance, being home on weekends was harder than responding to the structure of work.

And that structure was changing. First Julia quit her part-time job. She chose instead to do hospital shift work on an on-call basis —a particularly disruptive way to live, but, she felt, the best way for her to re-enter the career path of hospital nursing. She began to specialize in pediatric nursing and found she could enjoy the unpredictability of young children in a way that had been impossible for her in earlier years. She believed that without medicine she could never have taken this step, accompanied as it was by complex caretaking arrangements for her own children and a need often to overlook a degree of chaos in the home.

Julia felt—much as Tess had—that her life had been transformed. Her relations with her children and her husband were more easygoing, and she was able to tolerate a certain messiness in the structure of her life. Whatever intermittent anxiety and depression she had suffered had disappeared.

Once a patient has done well on an antidepressant for five or six months, I generally try to discontinue it. Julia reached that point early in the spring. She came in then to report she was "doing great—could not be better." She had requested and received a promotion at work and been offered regular hours. In the past, she had applied only for jobs for which she was overqualified: as a registered nurse, she had sought positions advertised for practical nurses. Now she was doing work normally done by nurses with master's degrees.

She proudly listed the indicators of her improvement. "I left for the hospital even though the beds were unmade! And I was not upset when the children got grease on their new pants. I didn't punish them or make them feel guilty." Then she told me the biggest news—she was getting a dog.

Before, the messiness of a dog had been repugnant to her, not to mention the effect on her schedule. Now she was ready. "I can't wait," she said, "even though I'm allergic." She had researched breeds whose fur she could tolerate. The children were ecstatic.

We lowered the dose of medicine, and two weeks later Julia called to say the bottom had fallen out: "I'm a witch again." She felt lousy—pessimistic, angry, demanding. She was up half the night cleaning. And there was no way she could consider getting a dog. "It's not just my imagination," she insisted, and then she used the very words Tess had used: "I don't feel myself."

I suggested we wait a bit longer to see whether Julia might be experiencing an odd effect related to medication withdrawal, or perhaps—this happened to be the timing—a premenstrual phenomenon of some sort. But the next week she saw the social worker, who called me to ask what I had in mind. Julia was back to square one, and none of the external circumstances of her life had changed.

Julia resumed taking the higher dose of Prozac. Within two weeks, she felt somewhat better; after five weeks, she was "almost there again," with many more good days than bad. She said work had been torture on the lower dose of medicine: "The patients drove me crazy." She had been unable to block out distractions and had been so aware of time pressure that she could never pause and enjoy the children she was tending.

And, at home, she had been unable to ignore her own children's failings. On the higher dose of medicine, she was once more tolerant. She was again ready to get the dog, and keenly aware that she could not have let a dog into the house when on the lower dose of Prozac. Julia went out of her way to impress on me how much more confident she was, how much more engaged in every facet of her life, when on an adequate dose.

Her husband had nothing but good things to say about the effect of the drug. Sometimes when she behaved in this more relaxed way, he wondered whether she was buttering him up, trying to get on his good side for an ulterior purpose, so unused had he been over the years to having a wife who could sit with him of an evening without being jumpy and critical.

By this point, Julia had stopped seeing the social worker entirely, and the social worker contacted me to express concern—not about Julia's well-being but about her own adequacy. I asked the social worker how she would have understood the case if medication were not available. As she saw it, Julia's story, and her needs, were not difficult to encapsulate.

When Julia first came to the office, her distress related to frustration over her stalled career and certain personal issues—unresolved family-of-origin conflicts that had re-emerged in her marriage. Julia's father, a businessman, had been a high-strung perfectionist; the son of a depressed mother, he was the more nurturant of her parents. Julia saw her mother as passive and distant. Julia's older sister seemed to stumble from failure to failure, and as a result, Julia was moved to care for her and to identify with her competent father.

The conflict in Julia's own marriage, as the social worker formulated the case, involved gender-role conflict. Identifying with her father, Julia secretly, or even unconsciously, felt herself to be more competent than her spouse. At the same time, not least for her own sense of security, she wanted to maintain the illusion that her husband was like her father, strong and decisive. The social worker saw Julia's obsessionality—and her paralysis in career and home life—as an expression of inner conflict over control in the family; she was torn by a wish to let her husband take the lead, opposed by repeated urges to barge in and do things right. These same conflicts emerged in her handling of the children, whom she pushed hard while telling herself she was giving them their head.

The social worker saw Prozac as having had an interesting effect on these conflicts. It had tipped the balance in favor of assertiveness, allowing Julia to make it clear to her husband what she needed and why; at the same time, it made her less urgent, which allowed her husband to do things at his own pace, a condition under which he appeared quite competent. Before she began her Prozac treatment, Julia had obsessed over which bedspread to buy her daughter. All were imperfect, because the real problem was that Julia disliked the paint color in her daughter's room, a subject she had been reluctant to raise with her husband. On medication, Julia simply asked her husband to repaint the room and then waited patiently for him to complete the task. Once the painting was under way, Julia had no trouble selecting a bedspread. In this interaction, both husband and wife were able to exert control in their different ways.

I asked the social worker why she felt guilty. The medication had done what she would have wished to accomplish with her psychotherapy: it had facilitated an improvement in the family dynamics. The problem, for the social worker, was that this change came about without any increased self-knowledge on Julia's part. I said that evidently insight had not been necessary. This comment did not allay the social worker's concern. She believed that medication-induced change, unaccompanied by growth in self-understanding, was inferior to what psychotherapy has to offer.

To Julia, the story was entirely different. As so often happens, the pill reified the illness. If there was a chance in the world that Julia might see her difficulty in adjusting to married life as anything but a result of a "biological disorder characterized by compulsiveness and depression," her relapse and rescue by the increased dose of medicine ended it. Once the drug kicked in, she had visited the social worker only infrequently, and then with skepticism. "If I had been on Prozac," she said, "I would not have needed to see the marriage counselor either."

I found I had little desire to cling to my earlier hypothesis of family pathology—the competent wife secretly undermined by the threatened husband. Even my sense of her perfectionism as a defense against low self-esteem was shaken, although I was beginning to wonder whether medication could perhaps provide self-esteem. Certainly on medication Julia was able to make major adjustments in her life with no sign of inner conflict. Her husband was enthusiastic when she moved on with her career. If anything, the response of Julia and her family to the medicine made the various scenarios conjured up by psychotherapy seem hypercritical and ungenerous.

But what did Julia "have"? Since her condition responded to a medication that can treat OCD, do we want to say she had OCD?

This decision is consequential. Large numbers of patients who visit doctors with psychological complaints are not "diagnosable." To make them diagnosable would mean expanding the current schema, and thus calling many more people mentally ill. Whether we want to change our view of mental illness and whether we want to make medication response a deciding criterion are interesting questions, with humane arguments available both for and against expansion.

If we do say that Julia has, say, an incompletely expressed case of OCD, we will be recapitulating in biological psychiatry the history of psychoanalysis. Once reserved for the most obviously ill patients, "obsessional" and its contrasting counterpart, "hysterical," came as the period of psychoanalytic dominance progressed to be applied to people's social styles. The advent of biological psychiatry originally resulted in a severe restriction of the use of such terms; but, with the discovery of new biological treatments, the operational definition of OCD is expanding once again, in part because what responds like OCD comes to be called OCD.

"Obsessionality" and "compulsiveness" are now used by those who treat illness with medication to encompass what in earlier days would have seemed mere personal idiosyncrasy. Increasingly, what was once the penumbra of OCD is fully in its shadow. But the expanded disease has its own penumbra. Now there will arise questions about how patients slightly less compulsive than Julia should be categorized and treated.

To see how far this new penumbra extends, I want to return to Julia's decision to contact me for treatment. Julia called because she identified with a patient I had described in a magazine article. That patient was Tess. I had described Tess as "a hard-working executive so attentive to detail in her professional life that she found little time to socialize. . . ." Those few words struck a chord with Julia, convinced her that she and Tess—very different women—might have something biologically in common.

And it's true that I had treated Tess for something rather like perfectionism. When Tess responded to imipramine but remained stuck in love and work, I began to wonder whether what held her back might bear some relationship to OCD.

Tess had no compulsions. She was, to be sure, obsessed with a hurtful lover; otherwise, she was not obsessional even in the colloquial sense. But she was *driven* to an unusual degree. What distinguished Tess was her success under impossible conditions, her determination, and her insistent and effective nurturance of others. She was, one might say, almost too giving. I don't know at what point I began looking at that goodness from the odd perspective of the biological diagnostician; I can only say that there are in pharmacology, as in psychotherapy, important moments when the clinician suddenly sees the patient afresh. In one such moment, I began to re-examine, to recategorize, those traits that made Tess special.

I have characterized clinical psychopharmacology as an impressionistic art. The doctor listens to a patient and, on the basis of the patient's story and the empathic response it evokes—bizarre biological probes, so qualitatively different from the usual blood, urine, and spinal-fluid tests—the doctor attempts to make an assessment of the state of the patient's neurons. The pharmacologist assumes that the complex constellation of behaviors and feelings a patient reveals reflects a simple physiological state. On the basis of the extraordinary, unique shape of a patient's life, the pharmacologist asks such questions as "Is this a disorder that is likely to respond to a drug that treats OCD?"

What an odd thought this is—"dedication to others less fortunate" as a form of aberrance that can lead a doctor to choose one medication over another. But, in the inexact process of extrapolating back from symptom and behavior to chemistry, the psychiatrist takes every bit of help he can get. We are not beyond grasping at straws, and I grasped at this one: I wondered whether Tess had a touch of the obsessional about her.

I began to ask Tess about her strengths as one might ask other patients about their weaknesses. How had she managed to raise her siblings so effectively? She answered, "You don't understand. I had no choice. The only other possibility was to disappoint everyone who counted on me, and I could not bear that."

We are accustomed to thinking of compulsiveness as a disorder or an annoying style of relating to the world, and it can be. But some of the characteristics of compulsiveness—the deep sense of responsibility, the vigilance, and the attention to detail—are also virtues. Sociobiologists have speculated that compulsiveness survived in the human species because it was a competitive advantage for our ancestors' tribes to contain one or two members who were prudent and driven in the extreme. Certainly Tess's family survived because of her inability to tolerate failure.

I am morally certain that I would not have had these ruminations if Prozac did not exist. Because an antidepressant likely to be useful for compulsive patients was available, it made sense to ask whether Tess's strength of character could be a manifestation of the same biological constellation that in other people shows itself as compulsiveness. Equally, it was because her dedication might be, in physical terms, something like OCD that—with so many tried and true medications available—I turned to a new and relatively untested drug for Tess.

In clinical pharmacology, contemporary technology plays a dominant role in shaping ideology. What we look for in patients depends to a great degree on the available medications. That Tess's depression was accompanied by what could be construed as compulsiveness was of interest only because this trait might be an indicator of something we could now treat.

Who Julia is—whether she is a fully functional woman with marital troubles or a slightly handicapped woman adjusting uncomfortably to reasonable constraints—is largely a function of drug development. We may decide on similar grounds whether Tess's dedication is a moral or a psychopathological trait. How we, as observers of our fellow men and women, look and listen, how we categorize, how we understand the tensions between people and their predicaments, is in part a product of the available means of influence. The interaction between a drug and cultural norms does not require the use of medication by the people we are assessing but can result from the mere availability of a substance that colors our beliefs about deviance and how it is produced.

Tess's self-understanding revolved around a quality she identified as seriousness. Once on medication, she explained her newfound success with men in simple terms: "I am less serious."

Seriousness covers a lot of ground. For most of her life, Tess did not allow herself to seek out pleasure. She focused on duty, and heeded the warning of a strong "superego," or conscience, that always put work before play. On medicine, her ability to attract men owed something to her increased flexibility, to a more generous sense of permission to enjoy. The problem earlier may have been as much one of unwillingness to attract men as inability. These traits, which might loosely be termed compulsive, disappeared when Tess took Prozac. And of course we may attribute her new ability to forget her married ex-boyfriend Jim to a true anticompulsive effect of drug treatment.

We have earlier considered Tess's transformation in terms of the alleviation of chronic depression. Here is a somewhat different way of conceptualizing her responses to medication: the imipramine had handled her acute depression. The Prozac cured her of a masked form, or variant manifestation, of compulsiveness.

Tess's recovery parallels Julia's. In both instances, the very traits targeted as compulsive disappeared on the appropriate medication. The question then becomes just how far we are willing to "listen to drugs." Will we want to expand the definition of OCD or compulsive personality disorder to include someone like Tess, who has no compulsions whatsoever and who meets none of the explicit criteria of illness except, perhaps, exaggerated devotion to work? Though we may resist it, the temptation is there. Surely, in a colloquial sense, part of what happened to Tess when she took Prozac was that she became less compulsive.

Facing someone like Tess, I think we are drawn in two directions.

One is to stretch the scope of illness to encompass her character traits. Another is to say we have found a medication that can affect personality, perhaps even in the absence of illness—only now, instead of restricting our powers to the depressive-to-manic continuum, we are considering whether we may not also be able to influence what we might call the obsessional-to-hysteric continuum.

Either way, we are edging toward what might be called the "medicalization of personality." Or perhaps, once we say that traits on both the depressive-to-manic and the obsessional-to-hysteric continua respond to medication, we are over the edge. Those two spectra cover a good deal of what makes different people distinctive. It is not only Tess's "seriousness" whose biological underpinnings are likely linked to compulsion or depression. If seriousness is subject to chemical influence, we can imagine a large collection of pairs of opposed traits that will be as well: contemplative/action-oriented, rigid/flexible, cautious/impulsive, risk-averse/risk-prone, masochistic/assertive, by-the-book/by-the-seat-of-the-pants, deferential/demanding, and many others. The first element in any of these pairs might equally be associated with depressive or obsessional leanings and might equally be a candidate for drug treatment.

The extension of our reach beyond depressed/manic to obsessive/hysteric is significant. The obsessional-to-hysteric continuum was once a mainstay of psychiatry. Toward the middle of this century, most relatively healthy patients, those with what was then called "neurosis," were discussed for treatment purposes in terms of whether they were more obsessional or more hysterical. Every person can be understood as sitting somewhere on this spectrum.

We recognize the flavor of compulsiveness even in the absence of a single symptom. Think about Bert and Ernie on "Sesame Street." They represent extremes in the diverse styles of healthy children. Bert has a fixed, serious, even worried look, and he is decidedly more reliable and less spontaneously playful than Ernie. Children identify with Bert because they love order; they identify with Ernie because they love mischief. Every child has mixed affinities for discipline and innovation, noise and quiet, group activity and solitude. I am hardly suggesting treatment for Bert or Ernie. But I suspect we would be near the truth if, putting aside such formal labels as "obsessional" and "hysterical," we were to say that what Prozac did for Tess was to shift her from a personality like Bert's to one more like Ernie's. Only Ernie would make or enjoy three dates a weekend; only Ernie would venture the gift of the red wagon.

This broad view of obsessionality, in which any affinity for the Apollonian virtues as opposed to the Dionysian suffices to make the diagnosis, gives some sense of what it might mean to introduce a medicine that can affect minor degrees of a trait that exists along a broad continuum, extending from illness to health.

We may not be convinced that Tess was compulsive. But even extending the definition of OCD to include Julia (and I think, especially taking into account the way her symptoms returned when her medication dose was lowered, many psychiatrists today would consider her to suffer from something like OCD) raises interesting questions for me. I recall, in my own childhood, having been specially scrubbed and warned against messy play before visiting certain demanding older relatives. Those relatives had grown up in Germany, where extremes of neatness and order were the cultural norm. Their homes were, every day, more tidy than any homes I have seen since even on special occasions. Julia reminded me of the wives in those families; perhaps my comfort with them explains my reluctance initially to accept Julia's behavior as symptomatic of medical illness.

Those wives, if my childhood perceptions are accurate, were not conflicted about their perfectionism, nor did their husbands seriously challenge it, though it was a matter for teasing and banter. I doubt the wives would have gone to bed with the floor or clothes dirty, but neither would their schedule often have required them to do so. There was in those families, I suspect, a certain male comfort in being the better-acculturated, more flexible spouse—the cock of the walk—while the wife assiduously tended the homefires. This arrangement inevitably led to a certain amount of marital unhappiness, but I would say that for the most part the couples managed to make their way through life contentedly.

Once Julia responded to medication, I found myself wondering whether those more contented perfectionists of years past would have responded to Prozac similarly. There are reasons for thinking not. To be neat in a culture that prizes neatness may bespeak a very different, less aberrant biological state than maintenance of the same behavior in a culture that has adopted different values. And if those perfectionistic housewives could have been relieved with medication of some of their need for order, their lives might not have been improved so much as made complicated in interesting ways. To say something less speculative: whether a particular behavioral style like perfectionism is deviant is very much a matter of cultural expectations, and that culture can be as broad as a nation and as narrow as a twosome.

This particular contrast—the contented and discontented perfectionist—gives rise to further thoughts about the notion of the "mother's little helper." Mother's little helpers were pills—Miltown, amphetamine, barbiturates, Librium, and Valium were the most popular and widely available in the fifties and early sixties—that were used to keep women in their place, to make them comfortable in a setting that should have been uncomfortable, to encourage them to focus on tasks that did not matter. I cannot think of the phrase even today without hearing it in Mick Jagger's sneering tones.

In Julia's story, the mother's-helper role is most clearly played by the various antianxiety pills given her over the years. Those medicines allowed her to perform her housekeeping tasks with a diminished, but still substantial, level of anxiety. The failing of those medicines was not that they did not work well enough but that they worked the wrong way altogether. The point, in retrospect, was not to make Julia less anxious but more bold.

Prozac's status in Julia's treatment is more complex. At the most obvious level, it was the opposite of a mother's little helper: it got Julia out of the house and into the workplace, where she was able to grow in competence and confidence. I see this result often. There is a sense in which antidepressants are feminist drugs, liberating and empowering. In this scenario, it is the failure to prescribe medication that keeps the wife trapped, apparently by her own proclivities. We may even want to say that nonbiological therapies, like the couples counseling, though apparently aimed at change through understanding, are in fact palliative and likely to lead only to a slightly more tolerable form of inertia.

It is hard not to see Prozac in these stories as the opposite of a mother's little helper. But the memory of my fastidious relatives makes me want to include a small caveat, a reminder that we might want to maintain awareness of how culture-bound this reading of events is. After all, should a person with a personality style that might succeed in a different social setting have to change her personality (by means of drugs!) in order to find fulfillment?

Even Tess's success falls under a similar caveat. I have in mind a recent remark by John Updike: "Masochism is as unfashionable now as aggressiveness was twenty years ago. . . ." If we see Tess's transformation as a victory, it's because of a change in mores, because we value the assertive woman and shake our heads over the long-suffering self-sacrificer. Perhaps medication now risks playing a role that psychotherapy was accused of playing in the past: it allows a person to achieve happiness through conformity to contemporary norms. This accusation is the "mother's-little-helper" label in modern colors.

We may have difficulty entertaining such a point of view, because cultural expectations have shifted so decisively. We can hardly imagine wanting to do anything other than relieve Tess's suffering by freeing her from her addiction to sadistic men. We can hardly imagine wishing for Julia that she find more fulfillment in her well-kept home. But to say this much is to excuse us as a society for failing to find a

satisfying, growth-enhancing niche for women with obviou
and two rather common forms of personality organizatio

Certainly our valuation of compulsiveness in men has
a change. One has only to consider Phileas Fogg, "the most punctual
man alive," who nonetheless had the spunk and resourcefulness to
travel around the world in eighty days. For decades, the eccentric
and fastidious Englishman was at once a figure of fun and of admiration—he ruled the Empire. It took the work of such writers as
Edmund Gosse and the Bloomsbury group to begin to make tenderness a male virtue, overattentiveness to work a failing, and eccentricity an aspect of fatherly tyranny rather than masculine charm.
(Indeed, from the 1930s through the 1960s, an influential critique
of capitalist society held that it created and rewarded the "anal
character"—compulsive, hoarding, and industrious—while repress-
ing sensuality and spontaneity.)

In the everyday practice of medicine, and in the everyday valuation
of human success and suffering, it is fruitless to try to maintain the
viewpoint of cultural relativism. Here is the physician's compulsion,
and perhaps society's as well: once we have seen Julia recover or Tess
become "better than well," we inevitably assess their personality styles
as handicapping forms of minor mood disorder. The operational definition of wellness must be in relation to the demands and goals of
our society, here and now. Once we have seen the joy on patients'
faces, we can only be grateful for the availability of more powerful
and specific medication. But the awareness that what we are altering
is a personal style that might have succeeded in a different, and not
especially distant, culture may make us wonder whether we are using
medication in the service of conformity to societal values. Indeed,
experience with medication may make us aware of how exigent our
culture is in its behavioral demands.

The reader may still be puzzling over a different question: whether
Tess and Julia and Sam had something "really" like compulsiveness

or "really" like depression. Not only do depression and OCD have penumbras and penumbras-of-penumbras, but these larger areas of shadow often overlap. People who are pessimistic tend to be cautious, and vice versa. Moreover, the effectiveness of Prozac for both conditions may lead us to wonder whether the conditions are related.

Here is another important aspect of listening to drugs: responsiveness to medication can influence our thoughts about which illnesses are distinct and which overlap. How doctors divide up mental illness may seem an issue merely internal to psychiatry, but for decades the debate over the continuity or separateness of mental illnesses has colored our understanding of the way human beings are related to one another.

The most basic diagnostic distinction in psychiatry is that between manic-depressive illness and schizophrenia, the disorders defined and declared to be separate by the father of modern diagnostic (or descriptive) psychiatry, Freud's contemporary Emil Kraepelin. At the turn of the century, Kraepelin showed that manic-depressives have a different course of illness from that of patients suffering from schizophrenia; he assumed that both diseases had a biological basis. By mid-century, many American psychiatrists were prepared to ignore Kraepelin's distinction and, indeed, to discard almost all diagnosis. As late as 1963, Karl Menninger wrote that "we tend today to think of all mental illness as being essentially the same in quality, although differing quantitatively and in external appearance."

This declaration was part of an egalitarian manifesto, the assertion that the well and the ill differ primarily in the degree of trauma they have suffered, and secondarily in the strength of their natural constitutions. This spectrum theory of mental illness arose from psychoanalysis. As Donald Klein, a formidable critic of the spectrum theory, put it, "The predominant American psychiatric theory was that all psychopathology was secondary to anxiety, which in turn was caused by intrapsychic conflict. Psychosis was considered the result of such an excess of anxiety that the ego crumbled and regressed, and neurosis, the result of a partially successful defense against anxiety that led to symptom formation." The well and the mentally ill differed only in the degree of anxiety they bore; and therefore the same treatment, the diminution of inner conflict via psychotherapy, was applicable to all ailments and all people. The spectrum theory was part of a broader psychology that emphasized the qualities people have in common.

Disregard for diagnosis was an American phenomenon. Though admirable in its demand that people be seen and treated similarly, it led to peculiar contrasts with observations in Europe. Considering diagnosis a mere administrative requirement, American psychiatrists had begun calling all seriously ill patients schizophrenic, a practice Menninger encouraged. The result was international data showing that New York had more schizophrenics and fewer manic-depressives than did London. This discrepancy was then treated as reflective of real phenomena, and theories were generated to explain it: perhaps urban violence in New York caused schizophrenia, whereas the calm and dull life of London was conducive to mood disorders. Racial theories were also advanced.

At last an epidemiological study was conducted, using uniform criteria (the British criteria, based on Kraepelin's distinction) to diagnose patients in the two cities. The landmark "U.S.-U.K. study," published in 1972, concluded that, "In spite of the gross differences in the diagnostic statistics produced by the hospitals of the two cities, in spite of the profound social and cultural differences between the cities themselves . . . when uniform diagnostic criteria are employed the diagnostic distributions of patients entering hospital in New York and London are to all intents and purposes identical." The apparent differences in proportions of illness were due entirely to differences in doctors' diagnostic practices. But which diagnostic system was superior? That question would be answered by a drug, lithium.

The story of lithium has the quality of legend. Lithium is an element of the periodic table, where it sits just below sodium. Like sodium, lithium readily forms salts. Early in the century, lithium bromide had been used as a sedating tranquilizer (hence our term "bromide" for a commonplace saying), but lithium fell out of favor in the 1940s, when it was used in an uncontrolled way as a sodium substitute for cardiac patients, some of whom died. At just this inauspicious time, in 1949, the Australian John F. J. Cade, "an unknown psychiatrist, working alone in a small chronic hospital with no research training, primitive techniques and negligible equipment," discovered that lithium salts were a remarkable specific treatment for manic depression.

Cade's discovery is often characterized as serendipitous. Cade had found that the urine of manic patients was especially toxic to guinea pigs, and he was looking for the responsible substances. He thought one might be uric acid, and he began experimenting with lithium urate, not because of any psychiatric properties of lithium, but because lithium urate was the most soluble salt of uric acid. To Cade's surprise, far from being toxic, the salt protected guinea pigs against the urine of manics, and it also sedated the animals, effects Cade found were due to the lithium. He immediately tried other lithium salts on himself and, when they proved safe, on ten hospitalized manic patients, all of whom recovered, some almost miraculously. The discovery of lithium as an antimanic agent resulted from one man's curiosity and powers of observation and deduction.

Because of the cardiac deaths, as well as Cade's lack of renown in the profession, the use of lithium for mania spread slowly. But by the late 1960s, doctors once more considered lithium to be a reasonably safe drug. It was also understood that lithium can treat and prevent recurrences of manic-depressive illness but is only rarely effective for schizophrenia. Once lithium's safety and specific efficacy for manic depression were accepted, diagnostic distinctions mattered in a way they had not before. At the same time, pharmacologic outcome could guide diagnosis.

This reasoning was precisely circular: since diagnosis was needed to predict medication response, medication response should determine diagnosis. It seemed, for the most part, that lithium treated all manic-depressive illness and nothing else; and no other medication treated manic depression. That is, lithium conformed to a one-drug/one-disease model of pharmacology, a model so aesthetically pleasing as to be irresistible. Lithium responsiveness confirmed the Kraepelinian model of manic depression and caused American psychiatrists to expand their use of the diagnosis. Lithium had performed an extraordinary "pharmacological dissection," defining for all the world the boundaries of a particular disorder.

The success of lithium set off an explosion of precise psychiatric diagnosis. In a few decades, American psychiatrists went from using only two diagnoses, neurosis and schizophrenia, to using hundreds.

Lithium and the one-drug/one-disease model had an enormous influence on the minds of physicians. Lithium made it look as if medications would be splitters—definers of illness. But, sadly, there has never been another lithium. Most subsequent medications have been lumpers, and none more so than Prozac. Within a couple of years of its introduction, Prozac was shown to be useful in depression, OCD, panic anxiety, eating disorders, premenstrual syndrome, substance abuse, attention-deficit disorder, and a number of other conditions.

The firm link between one drug and one diagnosis has become an ideal model which even lithium no longer fits. With an effective medication available, American psychiatrists became such enthusiastic diagnosers of manic depression that today only half of the patients who receive that diagnosis respond to lithium, and two or three other drugs are in common use for the illness. And lithium is now being used to treat other forms of disturbance.

Medications, it is increasingly understood, alter neurochemical systems. They do not treat specific illnesses. And the proliferation of illnesses has become so disturbing that the cutting edge of research involves attempts to elucidate links between them.

OCD and dysthymia, for example, are classified in contemporary psychiatry as discrete entities, one related to anxiety and the other to depression; but a countervailing movement, based in part on observations of drug effects, characterizes them as related disorders. Our confusion over just what the medication is working on in Sam, Tess, and Julia suggests that diagnostic specificity may have its limitations. Especially in mildly disturbed or near-normal patients, syndromes that should be distinct overlap. As a drug prescribed for these fairly healthy patients, Prozac casts a spotlight on the indeterminateness of diagnosis. This boundary-blurring constitutes an unanticipated—humanistic—effect of listening to drugs: like psychoanalysis, drug response can emphasize commonality, and the futility of attempts at mechanistic categorization. Tess and Julia and Sam share something very much like "neurosis," psychoanalysis's umbrella term for the mildly disturbed, the near-normal, and those with very little wrong at all.

What is especially noteworthy about the blurring of boundaries is its source. For decades, the thrust of biological psychiatry—not only because of lithium, but in response to evidence from brain scanners, genetic studies, and research on neurotransmitters—has been to bolster the discrete-disease model of mental deviance and to undermine the spectrum concept. Thoughtful people may have anticipated that the pendulum would some day swing the other way, but not, perhaps, that the new challenge to distinctions among illnesses, and between health and illness, would come from one of the fruits of biological psychiatry, the psychotherapeutic drug.

Antidepressants

Though the reception accorded Prozac is unique, it is not unprecedented. The first modern antidepressant, iproniazid, enjoyed its own meteoric career.

Iproniazid was developed as an antitubercular drug in the early 1950s and at first it appeared successful. Not only did it decrease the number of tubercule bacilli in the sputum, it also stimulated patients' appetites, gave them energy, and restored to them a general sense of well-being. Iproniazid was immortalized in an Associated Press photograph of 1953 that shows residents of the Sea View Sanatorium on Staten Island, attractive black women in ankle-length cotton print skirts and white blouses, smiling and clapping in a semicircle while two of their number do what looks like the Lindy Hop. "A few months ago," the caption read, "only the sound of TB victims coughing their lives away could be heard here."

Iproniazid did suppress the replication of bacteria, but the patients' inclination to dance did not derive entirely from the remission of their illness. Iproniazid was discovered to be a "psychic energizer," to use the phrase of Nathan Kline, the psychiatrist who investigated the drug's effects on the mind. Kline hoped an increase in a patient's vital energy would reverse depression. Using the language of psychoanalysis, then the dominant theory of mind, Kline wrote: "The plethora of id energy would make large amounts of energy easily available to the ego so that there would be more than enough energy available for all tasks. Such a situation would result in a sense of joyousness and optimism."

The drug's manufacturer was unenthusiastic. Iproniazid had been superseded by other antituberculars, and the company was ready to stop production. But in April 1957, *The New York Times* reported the contents of papers to be given at a research conference in Syracuse indicating preliminary successes in treating depression with iproniazid. Years later, Kline wrote: "Probably no drug in history was so widely used so soon after the announcement of its application in the treatment of a specific disease."

Approximately four hundred thousand depressed patients were treated in the first year. Unfortunately, 127 of these patients developed jaundice. Given the prevalence of viral hepatitis, this was probably a small number of cases for the population involved, but the manufacturer thought (wrongly) that it had a more potent antidepressant coming to market, so, rather than fight the bad publicity, it withdrew iproniazid. Iproniazid's reputation had been fatally tainted by the report of side effects, and it was never heard from again.

The extraordinary initial reception of iproniazid had been due to two factors. First, it had already been used in the treatment of tuberculosis. As a result, doctors were comfortable with it, and when the research results were announced, it was already on the market, ready for use. Second, the pent-up demand was enormous. Depression is an extraordinarily prevalent affliction, and there was at the time no acceptable way to treat it biologically. It was well understood among physicians that, though certain medications could alleviate one or another symptom of depression, short of such extreme interventions as inducing a seizure through administering high doses of insulin or through shocking the patient's brain electrically, there were no physical treatments that gave relief from the whole spectrum of symptoms and ended the episode of depression.

While Nathan Kline was on the lookout for energizing drugs, a leading researcher in Switzerland, Ronald Kuhn, was pursuing a different line of reasoning. At the time of the discovery of iproniazid, the most effective drug treatment for depression was opium. Opium was recognized as an odd substance. It caused some of the symptoms of melancholy in healthy subjects and alleviated symptoms in the depressed. Kuhn thought opium presented the proper model for a true antidepressant.

For unknown reasons, rare depressed patients even today will respond to no medicine except opiates, and a few researchers into depression have become newly interested in these substances. Fifty years ago, most patients who felt better on opium probably valued it for its ability to ameliorate scattered symptoms, such as sleeplessness, anxiety, and a general sense of malaise. Perhaps for mistaken reasons, Kuhn took the occasional success of opium to set the standard in the search for antidepressants. The hallmark of opium was that it restored energy in the depressed without being inherently energizing. Kuhn set out "to find a drug acting in some specific manner against melancholy that is better than opium"—that is, a nonstimulating antidepressant.

Iproniazid met only part of the standard. In some patients, it ameliorated all the symptoms. But it also seemed to have the ability to stimulate a variety of people—witness the dancing tubercular women—so it was not clear at first whether its effects came from reversing a basic process of depression.

In his search for a nonstimulating antidepressant, Kuhn began by looking at antihistamines. Antihistamines are the drugs, like Benadryl, used to treat allergies. Many antihistamines are sedating—indeed, the active ingredient in Sominex, the over-the-counter sleeping pill, is the same as the active ingredient in Benadryl. Kuhn was interested in sedation because opium is sedating, and he was interested in the antihistamines because the first modern psychotherapeutic medicine, chlorpromazine, was an antihistamine.

Chlorpromazine (Thorazine), introduced in 1952, constituted a breakthrough in the treatment of schizophrenia—it is known as the drug that emptied the state mental hospitals. Chlorpromazine had some efficacy in depression, calming agitated patients. Kuhn had already tested new antihistamines to see whether they were effective as sleeping pills. He now returned to the sedating antihistamines, especially those whose structure resembled that of chlorpromazine, to see how they affected depression.

In September 1957, less than half a year after the reports regarding iproniazid's initial success, Kuhn announced that he had found a substance that sedated normal people but relieved depression. As Kuhn put it: "We have achieved a specific treatment of depressive states, not ideal, but already going far in that direction. I emphasize 'specific' because the drug largely or completely restores what illness has impaired—namely the mental functions and capacity and what is of prime importance, the power to experience."

Kuhn's new drug was called imipramine. The theoretical importance of imipramine (Tofranil), the first nonstimulating antidepressant, is underscored in a memoir by Donald Klein, the pharmacologic researcher who so eloquently opposed the spectrum theory of mental illness. Klein worked with imipramine on an experimental basis in 1959. He later wrote:

> We knew that amphetamine was ineffective in the treatment of severe depressions, but we hoped this new agent would be much more stimulating and blow the patients out of their pit.
>
> Imagine our surprise when we found that giving imipramine to severe depressives first resulted in sedation, and shortly after that in an increase in appetite, hardly stimulant effects. Further, marked mood improvement was usually

not evident for several weeks. At that point many patients' moods returned to normal but they rarely became overstimulated. . . .

Therefore this drug was certainly not a stimulant. Further, when given to normals it did not cause stimulation or elevation of mood, but rather sedation. So, whatever the drug was doing was the result of an interaction between the medication and the pathophysiological dysregulation that produced the pathological state. In this sense the drug seemed a normalizer, not a stimulant.

In other words, imipramine was the grail—the true antidepressant, a substance of more conceptual importance even than iproniazid.

Despite the enthusiasm of isolated researchers, the announcement of the efficacy of imipramine was mostly met with skepticism. An entirely new medicine with no other indication than the treatment of depression, imipramine took some years to catch on. Though slower out of the blocks, imipramine was to enjoy a fate happier than that of iproniazid; but it turned out both drugs were antidepressants. The nearly simultaneous demonstration of the efficacy of imipramine and iproniazid signaled the opening of the modern era of research into human emotion. The two medications still set the terms for our contemporary understanding of the biology of mood.

In discussing patients' responses, and my own, to the success of psychotherapeutic medication, I have alluded to the tendency to "listen to drugs" as if they could tell us something about how human beings are constituted. (If Julia's fastidiousness diminishes in response to Prozac, then it "really" was a penumbral form of OCD; Sam's prurience, similarly, is revealed as a biological obsession. Tess has "really" been depressed all her life, and her social failures are a consequence of that depression.) Listening to drugs is not merely a popular phenomenon. For the last half-century, scientists have relied on medication response to infer the cause of disease.

"Pneumonia is not caused by a lack of penicillin" is the sort of statement used to ridicule such reasoning. But, in the absence of other easy approaches to the human brain, researchers have tended to use drugs as probes and to try to understand mental disorder in terms of the mechanism of action of effective medication. The great result, in terms of our theoretical understanding of mental functioning, has been the biogenic-amine theory of depression.

Stated simply, the theory holds that mood is determined in the brain by biogenic amines—complex chemicals a part of whose structure resembles that of ammonia. Even before the discovery of antidepressants, amines were known to be involved in the regulation of a variety of functions, from heart rate and gut motility to alertness and sleep. The discovery of iproniazid and imipramine led scientists to conclude that these amines also regulate mood.

Shortly after the drugs were introduced, it was shown that both iproniazid and imipramine influence the way nerve cells terminate messages. Nerves communicate by releasing "transmitter" substances—in this case amines—into the space, or synapse, between cells. The message is then ended by a two-stage process in which the amines are taken back up into the transmitting cell and inactivated by "janitorial" enzymes. Imipramine slows the reuptake of amines from the synapse into the transmitting cell, thus leaving the amines active in the synapse for a longer period of time. Iproniazid poisons the janitorial enzyme that digests the amines. Poisoning the enzyme makes more amine available for use in transmission. Thus, both known antidepressants (imipramine and iproniazid), by different mechanisms, made biogenic amines more available in relevant parts of the brain. This finding was taken as strong support for the hypothesis that depression is caused by a deficiency of amines.

If the amine theory held true, then (by somewhat circular reasoning) iproniazid and imipramine acted on the core biological problem in depression. They were increasing the efficacy of necessary, naturally occurring bodily substances. The amine theory was a very attractive model of mood regulation, because it made depression look like illnesses whose causes were well known. A person who has too little insulin suffers from diabetes; an excess of insulin causes low blood sugar (hypoglycemia). Thyroid hormone can be too high (hyperthyroidism, as in Graves' disease, suffered by President and Mrs. Bush); or it can be too low (causing hypothyroidism, or myxedema). Under the amine hypothesis, mood disorders now looked like those ordinary illnesses. An excess of amines was thought to cause mania (not least because an overdose of iproniazid could sometimes precipitate mania), and a deficiency, depression. For technical reasons, it was impossible to deliver biogenic amines directly to the relevant part of the brain. But the deficiency state could be ameliorated by slowing the breakdown or reuptake of the amines.

The amine hypothesis is perhaps false and at least incomplete. Like the evidence supporting the amine hypothesis of depression the evidence against it came from drug effects. For one thing, researchers identified antidepressants (not in use in this country) that have no direct effect on the amines. For another, there is a curious time lag in the onset of action of antidepressants. Imipramine can block the reuptake of neurotransmitters in a matter of minutes or hours. But it takes about four weeks for patients on imipramine to begin to feel less depressed. Why should a patient with effective levels of the relevant neurotransmitters not experience an immediate change in mood? Why do some depressed patients not respond at all? The amine hypothesis cannot answer these questions.

A particular line of evidence made it clear early on that the biogenic-amine hypothesis was imperfect. There are drugs that deplete the brain of complex amines, in effect doing the opposite of what antidepressants do. (One of these drugs, reserpine, has been used for many years to lower blood pressure.) Depleting the brain of amines should cause depression, and it does—but only in about 20 percent of patients. People who get depressed in response to amine depletion tend to be those who have already been depressed in the past or who are under stress in their lives. Depletion of amines is not enough in itself to cause depression.

From the time it was propounded, researchers understood that the amine hypothesis could not be the whole story. Indeed, the amine hypothesis is, in a sense, a self-deceptive form of listening to drugs. Most drug development takes place by homology. If one drug is effective, researchers will create physically similar substances, chemicals structured with what some cynics call the "least patentable difference" from the already successful medication. Scientists synthesized a host of substances similar in chemical structure to imipramine, and the success of these medications in treating depression strengthened the hold of the amine hypothesis. Almost all drugs on the market could be shown to affect amines—not surprising, given the modes for their development. The second popular way of developing drugs is through analogy: if one chemical that works as an antidepressant affects amines, then researchers will look for antidepressants among structurally different substances also known to affect amines. The potential for circular reasoning in this case is even more evident.

Only 5 percent of neurotransmission in the brain occurs via amines, but amines are the lighted streetlamps under which the secret of depression is most often searched for. The amine hypothesis may some day be superseded. In the meantime, its usefulness in predicting the effectiveness of compounds for the treatment of depression, and its heuristic power to explain their mechanism of action, have led it to dominate the scientific landscape. That these compounds were developed by analogy or homology with other compounds that affect amines is the irony embedded in the amine hypothesis.

Imipramine is a highly effective antidepressant. Perhaps 60 or 70 percent of classically depressed patients—those with insomnia, depressed appetite, low mood, and low energy—will improve on imipramine, as will certain patients with a variety of other disorders. But imipramine has serious limitations. One is side effects.

When Ronald Kuhn chose to look at antihistamines as a source for antidepressants, he created a complication the field did not overcome until the advent of Prozac. The antihistamines known in the 1950s, as well as most developed thereafter, tend pharmacologically to bring on the body's fight-or-flight response. They do this by interfering with a neurotransmitter called acetylcholine. When acetylcholine-related nerve transmission is diminished (as imipramine causes it to be), the body is ready for action. The heart beats rapidly, and energy is withdrawn from functions that can be postponed, like evacuation of bodily wastes. As a result, imipramine can cause a host of side effects—sweating, heart palpitations, dry mouth, constipation, and urinary retention among them.

Iproniazid and its relatives arouse the fight-or-flight response somewhat less often. This advantage alone might have made them popular. But an unexpected effect on blood pressure emerged in those drugs, a complication that pushed them to the sidelines, at least in the United States, and left the field to imipramine.

The drugs related to iproniazid are of particular interest because, although they are chemically quite distinct from Prozac, they can be seen, in terms of their effect on patients, as Prozac's predecessors. Like Prozac, they seem to reach aspects of depression that imipramine does not. In particular, it was recognized as early as the 1960s that they can be especially effective in patients who may not suffer classic depression but whose chronic vulnerability to depressed mood has a global effect on their personality.

The relatives of iproniazid are called monoamine-oxidase inhibitors, or MAOIs. Monoamine oxidase is the janitorial enzyme that oxidizes (burns, or inactivates) certain amines. By inhibiting monoamine oxidase, MAOIs prolong the effective life of those amines in the brain. In the years before Prozac was available, a doctor might have considered putting a patient like Tess on an MAOI, especially after she experienced an incomplete response to imipramine; but the doctor likely would have hesitated, because of concern over what else an MAOI might do: in the 1960s, a rash of deaths from brain hemorrhage was reported among patients taking MAOIs; other patients, though they did not die, experienced severe headache on the basis of extremely high blood pressure, an odd occurrence because the MAOIs were used to *lower* blood pressure in people with hypertension.

The means by which MAOIs make blood pressure skyrocket was elucidated in an interesting way. A British pharmacist who read a description of patients' headaches wrote a seemingly naïve letter noting that they resembled those his wife suffered when she consumed cheese, but not butter or milk. He asked whether the reaction might not be related to an interaction between MAOIs and some substance in cheese. Barry Blackwell, the doctor to whom the pharmacist had written, at first dismissed the suggestion—no drugs were known to interact with food substances in this way. But then he began to observe a series of patients on MAOIs who suffered headache and even extremely high blood pressure upon eating cheese.

Convinced that the "cheese reaction" was real, Blackwell set out to identify the offending ingredient. It turned out to be a chemical, ordinarily broken down by MAO, that causes nerve cells to release complex amines. Aged cheeses contain large amounts of this substance—so much that, when the janitorial enzyme is poisoned, a cheese eater on MAOIs will be flooded with biologically active amines, including ones that raise blood pressure.

Once the problem had been explained, it was a simple matter to advise patients to avoid foods that interact dangerously with MAOIs. But sticking to a restricted diet is constraining—the list of proscribed foods has grown over the years, and includes such disparate items as Chianti wine, fava beans, and ripe figs—and the requirement is dangerous for impulsive patients who "don't care if they live or die." MAOIs remained in widespread use in England, where they have been mainstay antidepressants for over thirty years. But in America the drugs were withdrawn from use, and even though they were later reintroduced, American doctors remained wary of them. Imipramine and related compounds dominated the medical treatment of depression.

Imipramine, however, is a "dirty" drug—a drug that affects many systems at once. Not only are its side effects wide-ranging—the result of its action on nerves using such chemicals as histamine and acetylcholine—but imipramine's main effects are also nonspecific.

From the time antidepressants were developed, two different amines were understood to influence mood: *norepinephrine,* a substance that was familiar to pharmacologists because of its close relationship to adrenaline, and *serotonin,* another substance that is active throughout the body but about which less was known. Imipramine is "dirty" in its main effects and its side effects because it affects both norepinephrine and serotonin. Once imipramine's mechanism of action was understood, pharmacologists set out to synthesize a "clean" antidepressant—one as effective as imipramine but more specific in its action.

This goal proved unexpectedly elusive. In the three decades after imipramine's introduction, pharmacologists synthesized and tested many chemicals similar to it in form. Like imipramine, the better known among these drugs, such as the antidepressants Elavil (amitriptyline) and Norpramin (desipramine), had three carbon rings in their chemical structure, and thus the group came to be called "tricyclics." Each new tricyclic antidepressant, as it was introduced, was said to have fewer side effects than imipramine—to have less effect on the acetylcholine or histamine pathways—or to act faster on depression. Some of these claims held up marginally. But most of the purported advantages evaporated as the drugs came into general use. None of the tricyclics is more effective than imipramine, probably none has a different time course of action, and all are "dirty" in the sense of influencing pathways involving both histamine and acetylcholine.

The only increase in specificity was the development of drugs that affected norepinephrine (and histamine and acetylcholine) without affecting serotonin. Desipramine, for example, is perhaps fifteen hundred times more active on norepinephrine than on serotonin pathways, and as a result a good deal of modern research has been done using this drug. But two goals eluded researchers: finding an antidepressant without side effects related to histamine and acetylcholine, and finding an antidepressant that preferentially affects serotonin.

This last goal was especially enticing. As the years passed, it seemed a number of conditions, ranging from atypical forms of depression to OCD and eating disorders, might involve derangements of serotonin. Here the MAOIs sometimes played a role. The MAOIs were very dirty. They affected not only norepinephrine and serotonin but a third amine, dopamine, the substance implicated in schizophrenia and Parkinson's disease. But the MAOIs were often more effective than the tricyclics for the disorders thought to be related to a lack of serotonin. Pharmacologists came to believe that the MAOIs' distinct efficacy might have to do with a strong effect on serotonin pathways, and that the tricyclics' limitations related to their lack of potency in raising serotonin levels. The new grail, pursued throughout the 1960s and 1970s and well into the 1980s, was a drug that would be like imipramine but that would selectively influence serotonin.

In its search for a clean analogue of imipramine and for an analogue that would strongly alter serotonin levels, psychopharmacology treaded water for over thirty years. This stalemate was frustrating to clinical psychiatrists. I remember as a medical student, and then again as a psychiatry resident, struggling to memorize charts regarding the characteristics of the tricyclic antidepressants. Generally, these charts would have a list of drugs running down the left-hand side and a list of neurotransmitters across the top. In each cell where the drug and a neurotransmitter intersected would be a series of plus or minus marks. Thus, a given drug would be $+ + + +$ for norepinephrine, $+ +$ for serotonin, $- -$ for histamine, and $- - -$ for acetylcholine. Medical students and residents for the most part do not mind this sort of chart; it makes demands on familiar skills and helps psychiatry seem like the rest of medicine. But the charts for antidepressants had no reliable relation to patients' responses.

The embarrassing truth about clinical work with antidepressants was that it was all art and no science. Various combinations of symptoms were said to be more serotonin- or norepinephrine-related, and various strategies were advanced for trying medications in logical order for particular sorts of patients. But these strategies varied from year to year, and even from one part of the country to another. It was true that a given patient might respond to one antidepressant after having failed to respond to another, but the doctor would have to manufacture a reason to explain why.

Psychiatrists were reduced to the expedient of choosing antidepressants on the basis of side effects. A patient whose depression was characterized by restlessness would be given a sedating antidepressant to be taken at night; a similar patient who complained of lack of energy would be given a stimulating antidepressant to be taken in the morning. But these choices said nothing about how the medications acted on depression: in all probability, both drugs amplified the effect of norepinephrine. It was as if, after discovering penicillin, researchers had synthesized a series of antibiotics, some of which incidentally made patients weary and some hyperalert—and then, when treating pneumonias, clinicians chose between these antibiotics not according to the susceptibilities of the infecting bacteria but according to whether the patient was agitated or prostrated by the illness.

Hopes that a more specific agent would make a difference were dampened by the advent of Desyrel (trazodone) in the early 1980s. Desyrel worked via serotonin, but its effects were difficult to distinguish from those of earlier antidepressants. Much of the problem, again, was side effects. Desyrel was so sedating that it had been marketed first in Europe as an antianxiety drug. You could do with Desyrel what you had been able to do with the tricyclics—treat a fair percentage of seriously depressed patients—but patients would tend to become tired or dizzy before you could get them on doses that radically changed the functioning of nerves that use serotonin.

This was the stage onto which Prozac walked: thirty years of stasis. The tricyclic antidepressants were wonderful drugs, but in practical terms they were all more or less the same. And it was not clear whether a drug that was pharmacologically distinctive would be any different in clinical usage from the many antidepressants that were already available.

Prozac was made to be distinctive. In the history of therapeutics, the development of Prozac belongs in a different chapter from the stories of lithium, imipramine, and iproniazid. Prozac was not so much discovered as planfully created, through the efforts of a large pharmaceutical firm, using state-of-the-art animal and cellular models and drawing on the skills of scientists from diverse disciplines. And yet, as was true in the cases of lithium and iproniazid, the development of Prozac required serendipity.

The story begins in the 1960s, with Bryan Molloy, a Scots-born organic chemist who had been synthesizing cardiac drugs for the pharmaceutical firm Eli Lilly. Molloy was interested in acetylcholine as a regulator of heart action. In the 1960s, a pharmacologist, Ray Fuller, came to Lilly to test potential new antidepressants. Fuller had worked with a method, using rats as test animals, for measuring drugs' effects on serotonin pathways; he tried to convince Molloy that the availability of this method made the time ripe for research in brain chemistry. Fuller proposed that Molloy leave his heart research to look for a substance that could affect amines in the brain without acting on nerves that use acetylcholine.

Like prior researchers, Molloy thought the right place to start in looking for an antidepressant was the antihistamines. He did not know whether he could develop an antidepressant without antihistaminic properties, but he thought he might have a tool that would allow him to minimize the acetylcholine-related side effects—dry mouth, urine retention, and rapid heartbeat—that so limited the use of the tricyclics.

In his cardiac research, Molloy had hooked up with Robert Rathbun, a member of the group at Lilly called the "mouse-behavior team." Rathbun was working with a model in which mice were given an opium variant, apomorphine, which lowers the body temperature in mice. Antihistamines block this response—except for antihistamines that also affect acetylcholine. Using Rathbun's model, Molloy hoped to be able to distinguish drugs that work purely on the histamine pathways from ones that affect acetylcholine as well.

Molloy synthesized compounds to test. He began with Benadryl, the antihistamine in common use as a remedy for stuffy noses and allergic rashes. He played with the Benadryl molecule, substituting one or another chemical group at one or another spot in its structure. Molloy developed dozens of compounds, including several that were good at blocking the effect of apomorphine on body temperature in mice. He thought he might be on the path toward eliminating acetylcholine-related side effects.

Meanwhile, a fourth researcher at Lilly, David Wong, had become dissatisfied with his area of work. Wong had been looking at mechanisms within the cell that allow antibiotics to combat infection, but to date all his research had led to medications for agricultural uses. He wanted to make drugs for humans, not animals, and in 1971 he began moonlighting in the area of neurochemistry. A particular book had caught Wong's attention, a newly published summary of what was known about the chemistry of mental disorder. Whereas by 1970 most research in America was focused on norepinephrine as the key chemical in mood regulation, this book summarized findings, better appreciated in Europe, that pointed to a role for serotonin.

The paths of Wong and Molloy crossed at a lecture by Solomon Snyder of Johns Hopkins University. Snyder is one of the great minds in modern biological psychiatry, a man whose name is often mentioned for the Nobel Prize. Most major developments in American biological psychiatry rely to some degree on an element of Snyder's work. Snyder had been invited to Lilly's laboratories in 1971 to receive an award and deliver a lecture. As his topic, Snyder chose his research into neurotransmission.

Snyder had been trying to isolate the nerve endings that handle biogenic amines. He found that, by grinding up rat brains and using various techniques to divide the ground-up products, he could produce a collection of nerve endings that still functioned chemically. This preparation he called a "synaptosome."

The synaptosome promised to be immensely useful in neurobiological research. You might, for example, pretreat a rat with imipramine, allowing the drug time to bind to nerve endings. Then you could kill the rat, grind up its brain, centrifuge and separate out the nerve endings, and produce an extract that was still active —still worked like the terminals of living nerve cells. You could then expose this extract (the imipramine-treated synaptosomes) to a neurotransmitter, such as norepinephrine or serotonin, and see how much of the neurotransmitter was taken up. This procedure almost defied belief—you could more or less blenderize a brain and then divide out a portion that worked the way live nerve endings work— but in Snyder's hands the technique succeeded. Not only did Snyder lecture on synaptosomes, he also instructed the Lilly team on the fine points of what neurochemists call "binding and grinding."

Wong immediately set about applying the bind-and-grind technology to Molloy's series of promising antidepressants. It turned out that the compounds on which Molloy was focused, those that worked in Rathbun's apomorphine-mouse model, were, like drugs already on the market, potent blockers of norepinephrine uptake in rat synaptosomes. But Wong did not stop there. His research showed that the rat synaptosome, and presumably the human brain, treated very similar drugs differently. If one chemical blocked the uptake of norepinephrine, a structurally similar chemical might block the uptake of serotonin. So Wong decided to look also at chemicals in Molloy's series that had failed in the apomorphine test.

One of those compounds, labeled 82816, blocked the uptake of serotonin and very little else. In all, Wong quickly tested over 250 compounds, but none looked as selective in its effect on serotonin as did 82816. The chemical was then tested in Fuller's rat system, the one that had initially sparked Molloy's interest in brain chemistry. There and elsewhere, 82816 selectively blocked the reuptake of serotonin into transmitting cells. Compound 82816 was fluoxetine oxalate; it turned out to be easier to work with a related preparation, fluoxetine hydrochloride. Fluoxetine hydrochloride is Prozac.

In June 1974, David Wong's laboratory and Bryan Molloy publicly reported that fluoxetine is a selective inhibitor of serotonin uptake into synaptosomes of rat brain. Fluoxetine was two hundred times more active in inhibiting the uptake of serotonin than of norepinephrine—and it did not affect the histamine or acetylcholine systems either. Fluoxetine was a clean drug. Wong and Molloy understood they had a new powerful research tool with which to study the functioning of serotonin, as well as a potential new type of antidepressant. Later research showed that the drug was suitable for the treatment of depression in humans.

The research that produced Prozac succeeded despite a number of mistaken beliefs early on. At the time Molloy was developing his series of compounds, no one knew what Rathbun's apomorphine-mouse model really did. It turns out the model is a reasonable test of a drug's ability to block norepinephrine reuptake; that is why a substance that had no activity in Rathbun's model proved to be of such interest.

Molloy's series of compounds paid off for an unanticipated reason: the molecule in the nerve-cell membrane that transports norepinephrine (in the reuptake process) is similar to the molecule that transports serotonin; so drugs that block the transport of serotonin can be quite similar structurally to those that block the transport of norepinephrine. In a series of related drugs, many of which block norepinephrine reuptake, there may well be a few that block serotonin reuptake. In other words, Molloy played with antihistamines and tested them in a system that measured action on norepinephrine neurons—and he ended up producing a drug that is not an antihistamine and has minimal effect on norepinephrine activity.

Also, the model that signaled Molloy that the time was ripe to study neurotransmission, Fuller's rats, turned out to be tangential to drug development. Molloy and Fuller were right about timing because of an unrelated breakthrough, Snyder's work with synaptosomes. A key element in the story is Wong's appreciation of the potential of bind-and-grind methods and his persistence in testing compounds in Molloy's series of molecules that had failed to block the effects of apomorphine on mouse body temperature.

The Prozac story represents a typical sequence in modern drug development. The medication resulted from an expensive and profitable process, the collaborative efforts of scientists working at the limits of the technology of their time.

Prozac stands in marked contrast to lithium. Whereas lithium is the simplest of chemicals, an element, unpatentable, its usage discovered by a solitary practicing doctor with no eye toward profit, Prozac is a designed drug, sleek and high-tech. It comes from a world even most doctors do not understand. I sometimes wonder whether this "feel" of Prozac—so different from that of lithium—has had some subtle influence on its reception, as regards both the sense of wonder and the sense of discomfort at its (alien) power.

The story of Prozac is typical in another way as well. Chemists working today to develop drugs for the mind start not so much with diseased patients as with models of nerve transmission, and they tailor molecules to affect that basic process. The goal is clean drugs—drugs that are ever more potent and specific in their effects on nerve transmission. The likely result of this form of research is not medicines that correct particular illnesses but medicines that affect clusters of functions in the human brain, often both in well and ill persons.

When Prozac was released in December 1987, no one knew whether potency and specificity would make a practical difference. There was some reason to think not. Psychiatrists were aware that Anafranil (clomipramine), a relative of imipramine that had achieved wide usage in Europe and Canada, was about to be introduced in the United States. Though as dirty a drug as any—it alters serotonin transmission the most but, like its cousin compounds, also affects norepinephrine, histamine, and acetylcholine pathways—Anafranil seemed to have a special efficacy in a hard-to-treat, serotonin-related condition, OCD. Also, psychiatrists had become newly accustomed to admixing medications for difficult-to-treat depressions—for instance, adding lithium to imipramine—and thus making a dirty drug dirtier. Perhaps antidepressants worked best when a variety of pathways were affected. Now that a clean drug had been found, no one knew whether it would prove superior to the many dirty ones.

Professional complacency about what, on theoretical grounds, promised to be a breakthrough antidepressant had also to do with the way new drugs are tested for marketing. To get approval from the Food and Drug Administration, a drug company has to show that a new substance is safe and effective for a given indication. With antidepressants, this standard means, in effect, that a drug is shown to be as safe and effective as imipramine for major depression. So Prozac had been tested on patients with typical major depression, the kind in which decreased sleep and appetite lead the way in the whole picture of severe mental slowing. In these patients, Prozac was only barely as effective as imipramine. This testing—combined with the repeated failure of scientists since the middle of the century to produce a drug that remained distinctive once it entered the doctor's office or patients' lives—led to muted expectations.

What no one appreciated in advance of Prozac's widespread clinical use was how different from its predecessors it really was.

The relative lack of side effects allowed Prozac to be used freely. A psychoanalyst colleague told me he almost never prescribed antidepressants before Prozac. Merely listing the side effects of the tricyclics interfered too much with the analysis. Patients would accuse him of hostility, of unconsciously wanting to poison them. If they did take the medicine, patients would spend long sessions on the couch complaining about how the analyst had made them constipated. MAOIs, with their requirement of a restricted diet and risk of strokes and death, mixed even less well with psychoanalysis.

Prozac did not interfere with the psychotherapeutic relationship as other antidepressants had. Also, Prozac was safer in the hands of potentially suicidal patients who might attempt to overdose on the drug. Because of the reduced likelihood of effects on the heart, Prozac overdoses are relatively benign. The lack of effect on acetylcholine proved to be enormously important as well. Patients do not feel "drugged" on Prozac, as they do on tricyclics or MAOIs. Because both patients and doctors were comfortable with Prozac's side-effect profile, the medication came to be prescribed both for less ill patients—those heretofore treated with psychotherapy alone—and for more impulsive patients with depressive symptoms. These are people in the penumbra of major depression. In other words, the group for whom Prozac was prescribed was different from the group on whom it had been tested. Before Prozac, drugs were dirty, but the disorder for which they were indicated was clean; here was a drug that was clean, but its field of action was, if not dirty, then at least amorphous in shape.

Prozac turned out to be remarkably effective for certain "penumbral" patients. Indeed, it may be these patients, who are not densely depressed, for whom Prozac is most helpful, so that Prozac's side-effect profile led it to be prescribed for just those people it could benefit most.

Prozac's lack of side effects and its ability to ameliorate disorders in which tricyclics often fail have led to changes in the way psychiatrists see patients and the way patients see themselves. In particular, Prozac has occasioned a heightened awareness of a phenomenon that occurs commonly in people who have never had a mental illness— indeed, a phenomenon so ordinary that it may seem intrinsic to the human condition: sensitivity to rejection or loss.

Sensitivity

A young woman comes to the office complaining she is boy-crazy. Last week, she found herself walking through a dangerous part of town at two in the morning in the cold and dark. She had a crush on a certain young man, and she knew he liked a rock band that was playing a one-night stand at a small club. So she showed up at this club in a godforsaken neighborhood to hear music that did not even appeal to her. Heading home alone in the small hours, she thought, "I really ought to talk to someone about what I am doing."

She says her focus on this young man and others like him—they are all dismissive of her and a bit wild—is disconnected from the way she ordinarily sees herself. She is a quiet and self-effacing young woman, dressed in a way that plays down her femininity, devoid in her manner of any hint of seductiveness.

Her history is dominated by one event. When Lucy was ten and living in a third-world country where her father was stationed, she came home to find her mother dead, shot by a young manservant—a beloved and trusted member of the household—who had become crazed and violent. Lucy showed no immediate reaction to this ghastly occurrence. She remained a productive, well-liked girl. As the oldest child, she assumed additional responsibilities, helping her father raise the other children. For his part, the father, though concerned and loving, had always been focused on his work, and became even more so as he felt the family responsibilities on his shoulders alone. In supporting him, Lucy delayed meeting her own needs until she could leave home. Her father's attention to his work hurt her repeatedly; she often felt he was not there when she needed him.

How we see a person is a function of the categories we recognize—of our private diagnostic system. A psychotherapist may see Lucy, wandering through the darkened city, as suffering from father hunger, mother hunger, adolescent rebellion, repetition compulsion, or a delayed grief reaction. Each of these very different frames is historical: to "understand" Lucy's behavior is to place it in relation to her traumatic past.

She is a young woman with a damaged self-image, a tendency to place men first, and a willingness to put herself at risk. To the part of her that every moment remembers her mother's murder, the world is so fraught with danger that to exercise caution seems derisory self-delusion. Lucy is, in her tolerance for danger, re-enacting an aspect of her childhood, seeing whether in her young-adult life she can control fate. We may find there is some urgency to the matter, a need to save her from a compulsive association between men and violence. We may also wonder about the love object she has chosen—is he too much like the hard-to-reach father, too much like the murderous servant? Lucy herself, when asked to explain her boy-craziness, puts forth a theory related to deprivation: she had to postpone her adolescence, and she yearned for warmth and closeness, so now she is sacrificing everything to the quest for love.

Psychotherapy—talk—calms things down. Lucy, an Ivy League undergraduate, sublimates her morbid impulses to her studies, writing papers on abnormal psychology, the sociology of violence, and other topics obviously related to the central questions of her history. And she begins dating a classmate who has none of the openly frightening qualities of the young men she has tended to pursue.

But though the form is more subdued, the boy-craziness persists.

Lucy begins to notice a disturbing tendency in herself. She cannot bear it when her boyfriend looks away for a moment. If he turns his back on her to glance at the television screen, her heart sinks. She experiences terrible feelings of worthlessness if he shows up five minutes late for a date. If he says "I" instead of "we" in talking about something they have done together, or if he says goodbye in the wrong way, Lucy may experience pain for days. When she sees her boyfriend talking to another girl, Lucy becomes listless for the better part of a week, and no amount of reassurance can break the spell of demoralization. These moods are often deep and protracted. She is disorganized, paralyzed, hopelessly sad, overtaken by unfocused feelings of urgency.

Lucy understands this sensitivity, too, as originating in the apprehension that she will lose anyone she loves. But she cannot shake it—it has a life of its own. The smallest slight throws her into a tailspin. Although she may start the day optimistic and focused, she knows she may at any moment be swamped by despondency. She finds herself putting her boyfriend to little tests: If I set my book down, will he set his down as well? Will he notice the pin I am wearing? The day is full of these tests, some of them magical: He must look at me before the light turns green; he must place the keepsake I gave him at the front of the dresser. When her boyfriend fails to act as Lucy hopes, confusion or sadness sweeps over her. She does small things to get his attention—and at the same time she understands that the dependency she communicates may doom their relationship.

Lucy's craving for attention has deep roots. She remembers feelings of desperation on nights when her father came home late, tells of recurrent pain in response to his focus on work rather than on her. She remembers as a child playing sick—heating the thermometer under a light bulb—to elicit her father's concern. She would often do more than her father expected, would, even as a fairly young child, set the table at night for the following day's breakfast, in hopes of winning his approval. Sometimes she feels she is addicted to attention.

Lucy's neediness, like her sensitivity and her flirtations with violence, is rooted in her history. But her hunger for approval and the disorganizing pain she feels on rejection will bring to mind, for psychiatrists of a certain ilk, a particular understanding of what ails Lucy, one that all but divorces the present from the past.

This other approach entails taking Lucy's hunger for attention and her fear of rejection very much at face value, as discrete symptoms, in the way that insomnia and loss of appetite are symptoms. More broadly, this ahistorical viewpoint sees the combination of applause hunger and rejection-sensitivity as an autonomous syndrome, a category of human behavior that might respond to treatment with medication. If Lucy can be spared the pain that rejection causes her, she will not need to behave in a dependent or self-injurious way. Examination of history, even of so evocative a history as Lucy's, will be superfluous, an interesting enterprise in its own right, perhaps, but not crucial to the patient's healing.

· · ·

We all react to disappointments, even minor ones. A date stands us up. A colleague makes a cutting remark. A bad grade or a critical review arrives unexpectedly. The business proposal, the grant submission, the application for promotion is rejected. A friend announces he is moving away. A phone call is not returned; an expected invitation fails to arrive. We are ridiculed, scorned, slighted, given the cold shoulder. Always there is a visceral response: the sinking in the stomach, a feeling of weakness, confusion of thought, a momentary sense of sadness and world-weariness. It will pass, we know, this leaden dullness, but for the moment we are deeply affected.

For some this pain is worse than for others—lasts longer, paralyzes more thoroughly. They are not depressed, but they are vulnerable. "Sensitive" is what we call such people, as in: "Oh, don't be so sensitive," or "She's just overly sensitive." It is not only what a person feels but also how he or she shows it that makes for sensitivity.

Someone who displays a slight wound too insistently, or who too assiduously avoids the risk of disappointment, is most liable to the charge. "Oversensitivity," in this use of the word, is a personality trait, sometimes annoying, sometimes endearing.

What lies behind oversensitivity? Is it a manipulative style, a form of self-pity, or one among many reasonable ways of addressing the complexities of the social world? For the most part, psychiatry has ignored sensitivity as unremarkable—not a category of analysis. In the standard diagnostic manual, there is no category labeled "sensitive."

But the standard manual is a mere matter of consensus. There are many unofficial ways of mapping human variation, charts highlighting colorful byways that, though they have never made it into the conventional guidebook, promise rewarding vistas. One such conceptual route, a diagnosis that under various names has intrigued biological researchers for decades, may be, with the help of Prozac, on its way to becoming a major thoroughfare. The idea underlying this diagnosis is that certain people are physiologically wired to be deeply sensitive to rejection. On experiencing a loss, these people feel more pain or come closer to depression than do most men and women. According to this theory, a variety of personality styles, typical behaviors, and even mental illnesses can be traced to the complex adaptations oversensitive people make to the abnormality in their emotional thermostat.

Rejection-sensitivity as a psychological category is a contribution of the psychopharmacologic pioneer Donald Klein, a conceptualizer of great originality. This is the same Donald Klein who was an early opponent of the spectrum theory of mental illness and an early proponent of imipramine. He is director of research at the New York Psychiatric Institute and a professor at Columbia University. Although he has long held positions of leadership in psychiatry, the field has always treated Klein as a maverick, a man whose thinking, even if difficult to refute, is almost too creative.

Klein started looking at antidepressants in the late 1950s. He began with an idiosyncratic approach to research, one shaped by the diagnostic sloppiness of American psychiatry in those years. In most pharmacologic studies, a researcher looks at patients with a single, strictly defined diagnosis and attempts to treat them with one or two particular medications. But when Klein was doing his early work, no one knew which diagnostic distinctions were relevant to medication choices, and, moreover, there were few medications to try. Klein worked at Hillside Hospital (now part of the Long Island Jewish Medical Center), a typical psychotherapy-oriented mental hospital of its day. His method was to take whatever inpatients he could get colleagues to refer him—generally patients not responsive to psychotherapy, most of whom were diagnosed as schizophrenic by the ward staff—and to medicate them with whatever was at hand, often matching medication to patient on the basis of one or another small clue. He then worked backward from drug response to diagnosis, sometimes creating a new diagnostic category to fit his observations. In other words, he took on all comers and tried to say something about them based on their response to the medication.

To Klein, a number of hospitalized patients labeled schizophrenic, borderline psychotic, or hysterical seemed at base to have not so much an abnormality of thought or personality as a nasty disorder of mood. To these hidden mood disorders, Klein gave a variety of names depending on the form of the affliction. Two such categories are of particular interest: atypical depression (in which patients increase rather than decrease their eating and sleeping when depressed) and hysteroid dysphoria. This latter category expressed Klein's notion of pathological vulnerability to loss.

To appreciate the originality of Klein's contribution, one has to understand the central place in psychotherapy of the hysterical patient. Freud's first psychoanalytic patients, those around whose treatment the new science of psychoanalysis developed, were hysterics. Hysterics in the nineteenth century had physical symptoms, such as seizures and paralyses, and were (incorrectly) understood to suffer from neurological illness. One of Freud's early, legendarily controversial contributions was the assertion that hysteria is a disease of the mind and that the seeming neurologic symptoms are actually a metaphorical, almost poetic expression of repressed psychological conflicts.

For half a century or more, when Freudian thinking dominated in America, hysteria was considered the easiest disorder to treat with psychoanalysis. Hysterics' symptoms bore exploration and interpretation, and the patients were responsive to the charm of the psychotherapeutic relationship. Training institutes saw to it that the first patient of almost every psychoanalytic candidate was a hysteric.

But in time there developed two problems with the diagnosis. First, the term "hysteric" spread far beyond those with unexplained neurological symptoms to cover almost any patient who was emotional, unresponsive to reason, or seductive, particularly if the sufferer was a woman. And, second, many hysterics proved refractory to psychotherapy. In the therapy, as in their lives outside the psychoanalyst's office, these hard-to-treat patients were emotionally volatile. They often seemed more intent on winning the therapist's attention than on recovery, and might become desperately seductive or otherwise self-destructive if the therapeutic relationship appeared to be coming to an end. Characterizing the hysteric's potential in the psychoanalytic setting, the renowned analyst Elizabeth Zetzel began a generative essay with the nursery rhyme lines "When she was good she was very, very good, but when she was bad she was horrid."

In considering how to medicate horrid hysterics, Klein took into account their eating and sleeping habits. Although they generally did not suffer true, protracted depressions, these flamboyant patients tended, when upset, to overeat and oversleep, just like atypical depressives. Privy to the work of British researchers who made the case that atypical depression responds better to MAOIs (relatives of iproniazid) than to tricyclic antidepressants like imipramine, Klein tried an MAOI on the difficult hysterics referred him by his psychotherapeutic colleagues. He found that it sometimes smoothed the course of the patients' lives. Klein tried to encompass these medication-responsive patients descriptively, thereby—and herein was the apostasy—carving out a group of hysterics whose disorder was after all not so much of the mind as of the brain. The patients looked hysterical, but the underlying disorder was a problem in biological regulation of mood. These were the patients Klein called "hysteroid dysphorics."

Klein tried to distinguish such antidepressant-responsive hysterics according to their behavior. They were not, for instance, hysterics with unexplained seizures or paralyses; nor were they the most irritable, impulsive ones. What distinguished the hysteroid dysphorics was an extreme appetite for attention and a marked fear of rejection, a desperate emotional state that resulted in a constellation of behaviors amounting to a caricature of femininity. Here is a typical, brutally clear description by Klein of hysteroid dysphorics:

> These patients are usually females whose general psychopathological state is an extremely brittle and shallow mood ranging from giddy elation to desperate unhappiness. Their mood level is markedly responsive to external sources of admiration and approval. Such a patient may feel hopelessly bereft when a love affair terminates, then meet a new attentive man and feel perfectly fine and even slightly elated within a few days. Their emotionality markedly affects their judgment. When euphoric, they minimize and deny the shortcomings of a situation or personal relationship, idealizing all love objects. When they are at the opposite emotional pole, feelings of desperation are expressed very disproportionately to actual circumstances.
>
> They are fickle, emotionally labile, irresponsible, shallow, love-intoxicated, giddy, and short-sighted. They tend to be egocentric, narcissistic, exhibitionistic, vain, and clothes-crazy. They are seductive, manipulative, exploitative, sexually

provocative, and think emotionally and illogically. They are easy prey to flattery and compliments. Their general manner is histrionic and flamboyant. In their sexual relations they are possessive, grasping, demanding, romantic, and foreplay centered. When frustrated or disappointed, they become reproachful, tearful, abusive and vindictive, and often resort to alcohol.

Klein's second paragraph may sound less like a neutral syndromal description than a misogynist's picture of womankind. But it probably does not differ much from a psychoanalyst's behavioral characterization of what by mid-century had become the prototypical hysteric—a woman seeking desperately for the attentions of an idealized version of the father who in reality had disappointed her. Klein contended that these symptoms arose not from persisting inner conflict (such as emotional ambivalence about the father) but from the effects in her contemporary, adult life of the patient's recurrent, intense, abnormally painful experience of loss.

Klein did not at first enter the debate over whether hysterics had one or another sort of childhood experience; presumably a person might come to rejection-sensitivity through any number of genetic or environmental pathways. It hardly mattered what set the sensitivity in motion. For hysteroid dysphorics, the pain of rejection was so extreme, and the elation following approval so (fleetingly) intense, that it made sense for seduction to become a full-time imperative. The phrase Klein selected to deal with questions of causation was "functional autonomy." In Klein's words, "a cause engenders an adaptive response (function) that persists after the termination of the cause (autonomy)." Regardless of its origins, the vulnerability to loss had a life of its own in adulthood.

The concept of functional autonomy makes biological treatment attractive. The great claim of psychoanalysis is that it removes the causes of neurosis. To a psychoanalyst, every hysterical symptom has hidden within it, in secret code, its cause—both the historical cause (early emotional trauma) and the ongoing, active cause (unconscious conflict, resulting in the mind's attempt to repress the memory of that trauma and the mixed emotions it arouses). A similar assumption has long predominated in the popular consciousness as well, and it is this model that makes Lucy's boy-craziness so naturally understandable. For psychoanalysis, the route to recovery is bringing the unconscious struggle into consciousness. Psychoanalysis is often called a pessimistic discipline, but it revolves around an appealing, humane view of symptoms and the people who carry them: that the truth can set men free. Functional autonomy implies that symptoms become unmoored from their origins, so there is no longer any special reason to imagine that truth will have the power to heal.

Klein saw symptoms—in this case histrionic behavior—as being fully explained by patients' expectable reactions to instability of mood. Where the unstable mood came from was irrelevant. Such concepts as conflict, the unconscious, trauma, and truth were superfluous. Klein described his relationship to psychoanalytic hypotheses of causation in proudly agnostic terms: "It is hard to prove a negative—that is, that there is no case in which intrapsychic conflict plays a necessary role. . . . [But] like Laplace, I have no need for these hypotheses."

What Klein felt need of was a tool to reregulate hysteroid-dysphoric patients' emotional thermostats—to decrease the pain they felt when rejected. We have already noted that hysteroid-dysphoric patients were not, in the classical sense, depressed. Their mood, unlike that of people in a dense depression, tended to be quite responsive—too responsive—to external events. There was no *a priori* reason to believe that antidepressants would help these patients; as we have seen, one of the heuristically appealing aspects of antidepressants was that the medications did not, on the whole, help people unless they were in the midst of a depressive episode. But Klein found that MAOIs acted to prevent the brief terrible mood downturns of hysteroid dysphorics.

The medicine set a floor beneath patients; it prevented the bottom from falling out.

Klein wrote, "A crucial consequence of putting these patients on MAO inhibitors is that they do not become dysphoric upon loss of admiration. This affective modification makes it no longer necessary for them to fling themselves into self-destructive or unrewarding romantic involvements." At the heart of Klein's formulation is the notion of a simple psychobiological defect (heightened pain in response to loss) elaborated by the patient into a complex adaptive behavior (the caricature of femininity). The treatment for the disorder is to restabilize the affective regulator and then to help the patient learn that she no longer needs her self-injurious character style.

• • •

Klein's model of emotion and behavior—the elaboration of simple mood disregulation into complex symptoms and even personality traits—found widespread acceptance, not with regard to hysteroid dysphoria, which remained an obscure diagnosis, but in relation to a quite different condition, panic anxiety.

Panic anxiety is a commonplace, understood by everyone. It is the condition in which a person is subject to panic attacks, those awful moments in which the pulse races, each breath is hard to come by, nausea and dizziness threaten, and it feels as if death were imminent, although—so awful is the foreboding—death may seem almost preferable to the terror at hand. Panic anxiety has been shown in surveys to be among the most prevalent of psychiatric disorders. The term "panic attack" has transcended psychiatry and entered everyday speech. We find it unremarkable if in a shopping mall we hear one person say to another, "I was so shocked I almost had a panic attack."

It is hard to recall that fifteen or twenty years ago there was no such concept. Neither in medical school nor psychiatry residency, both in the 1970s, did I ever meet a patient with "panic anxiety." Only toward the end of residency did I hear of research into the panic attack. Although it is now among the most common diagnoses in psychiatrists' offices, in the recent past panic anxiety prevailed neither in the clinic nor in the popular consciousness.

That blindness to what is now a ubiquitous phenomenon may seem all the more remarkable when we learn that, unlike hysteroid dysphoria, panic anxiety is not a newly described entity. In 1895, when he stood on the cusp between neurology and the discipline he was to create, psychoanalysis, Sigmund Freud wrote a monograph about what we now call panic. Though it contains no case vignettes, the monograph is fascinating. It attempts to carve out of neurasthenia, the nineteenth century's broad category of mental weakness and distress, a particular entity, "anxiety neurosis."

As always, Freud was an exquisite observer. In characterizing anxiety neurosis, he listed every symptom we now ascribe to panic anxiety: rapid or irregular heartbeat, disturbances of breathing, perspiration and night sweats, tremor and shivering, vertigo, diarrhea, night terrors, and what he calls "anxious expectations." Freud also recognized incomplete forms of the disorder, which he called "rudimentary anxiety attacks," "equivalents of anxiety attacks," and "larval anxiety-states." He also understood anxiety neurosis sometimes to be associated with agoraphobia, the fear of leaving the home.

Freud considered anxiety neurosis to be entirely biological. Throughout the monograph, he insisted that the anxiety "does not originate in a repressed idea, but turns out to be *not further reducible by psychological analysis, nor amenable to psychotherapy*." Anxiety neurosis was either congenital or caused, directly and physiologically, by the pressure of undischarged sexual excitation, as in virginity, abstinence, or, most notoriously, *coitus interruptus*. Women whose husbands were sexually inadequate or subject to premature ejaculation were at risk.

Freud's assertion that anxiety neurosis is biological sounds firm. But in his clinical reports he had begun undermining that position even before he stated it. One of my favorite footnotes in Freud appears in the *Studies in Hysteria* (1893–95). It concerns a case that looks for all the world like anxiety neurosis—except that the symptoms arise from repressed conflict. Freud begins: "I was treating a woman of thirty-eight, suffering from anxiety neurosis (agoraphobia, attacks of fear of death, etc.)." Though at first the patient indicates the attacks are of recent onset, Freud finds they began in her teenage years as episodic "dizziness, anxiety, and feelings of faintness." He traces their onset to a particular moment, when she was shopping in preparation for a ball. The patient remembers little more, and Freud presses his hand on her head to make a recollection appear. She thinks of two girls who had just died—one a close friend—and remembers that with the dizziness she thought, "I am the third." What had been driven from consciousness was shame at preparing for a ball in the wake of a friend's death, and fear that the frivolity would result in divine punishment. Moreover, the attack occurred near the dead friend's house. And—deeply important, from Freud's point of view—the patient was having her first menstrual period (presumably a shameful event) just at the time, so that the attack, and all subsequent attacks, become understandable as the expression of ongoing conflictual feelings. Freud does not name the conflict explicitly; presumably, awakening sexuality and perhaps even satisfaction at a rival's death are counterbalanced by fear and shame.

This understanding of anxiety in terms of personal history and inner turmoil began as the exception but soon became the rule. During Freud's lifetime, the discrete category of anxiety neurosis—an irreducible somatic disorder—was swallowed by a broader category, "neurosis," a catchall term for minor mental disturbances rooted in the psyche. By the 1960s, "neurosis" even encompassed conditions in which the patient was unaware of feeling anxious. The specific diagnosis "anxiety neurosis" was applied loosely. Any fairly healthy psychotherapy patient typically had an anxiety neurosis, a usage that corresponds closely to the ordinary-language term "neurotic."

This declawing of anxiety neurosis resulted from the growth in importance of the concept of anxiety in Freud's work. As Freud focused on the unconscious, he relied increasingly on meaningful anxiety as a motive force. At first, he merely expanded his original formulation, so that the notion of undischarged sexual drive became ever more symbolic and less biological. But as the theory grew in scope, Freud, and especially his followers, came to see meaningful anxiety—the result of conflict between repressed drives and defenses (this is the "dynamic" in "psychodynamic psychotherapy")—as underlying a broad spectrum of illness. Such terms as "castration anxiety," a key element in the Oedipus complex and the Oedipal period in normal male development, moved into common speech. It was this reliance on anxiety as virtually the sole motive force in the development of mental illness that led Klein to make his remarks regarding the spectrum theory of mental illness: "The predominant American psychiatric theory was that all psychopathology was secondary to anxiety, which in turn was caused by intrapsychic conflict."

Klein began to focus on anxiety because of a discrepancy between the prevailing theory and the results of pharmacotherapy. By 1959, when Klein was studying imipramine, it had been established that Thorazine was helpful to many people suffering from schizophrenia, generally considered the most severe mental illness. If all mental illness lay on a spectrum—the major disorders differing from the minor ones merely in terms of the degree of anxiety involved—then a medicine that works for schizophrenics should work all the more powerfully for patients who merely suffer from overt anxiety but are not psychotic. Klein knew Thorazine did little for these less ill patients; indeed, it often made them worse. This result spoke against the spectrum theory of illness.

So Klein took on anxiety, a concept as central as hysteria to the theory of psychoanalysis. Just as he had asked whether there were forms of hysteria unrelated to intrapsychic conflict, Klein asked whether there were different varieties of anxiety. He was attempting to use pharmacology as an investigative tool to unearth flaws in psychoanalytic theory and practice.

Klein focused on the most insistently anxious patients on the hospital ward—the ones who constantly ran to the nurses for help. Because there was no other solution to their problems, Klein persuaded a group of these patients to try imipramine. For the first couple of weeks—and remember that imipramine takes a few weeks to work—patients and staff were in agreement that imipramine was of no help. But, as Klein recalls:

> By the third week, although both patients and psychotherapist insisted that no gains had been made, the ward staff had a different, more positive view. When pressed to stipulate exactly how the patients had improved, the staff was at a loss. Finally, some keen clinical observer pointed out that for the past 10 months the patients had been running to the nursing station three times a day, every day, proclaiming that they were about to die and needed instant succor. The nurses would hold the patients' hands, reassure them and sit with them for about 20 minutes. The patients would finally walk away, their acute, overwhelming distress somewhat alleviated. A few hours later, however, they would be back again. The nurses pointed out that for the past week or so the patients had not been doing this.
>
> When we suggested to the patients that they were feeling better, they vociferously denied any improvement and accused the staff of obtuseness concerning the degree of their distress. When I asked them, "Why have you stopped running to the nurses' station?" their answer was that they had finally learned that the nurses could not do anything for them.
>
> "You mean that after 10 months you learned that just this week?"
>
> "Well," said the patient, "you have to learn some time."

Klein came to a different conclusion. In taking patients' histories, he had found that they typically recalled a series of what are now called panic attacks that came out of the blue. Klein hypothesized that the patients' disorder began with these spontaneous instances of overwhelming terror. It is a terrible thing constantly to be liable to debilitating panic. Around the attacks, patients would elaborate secondary fears: they might fear driving over bridges because being enclosed in a car with no route of escape while suffering panic anxiety is worse than suffering anxiety when apparent escape is possible. But there was no special symbolic significance to the bridge, no meaning traceable to childhood trauma or current ambivalence; the only significance of the bridge was as an unpleasant place in which to suffer spontaneous panic. In general, Klein considered agoraphobia a secondary elaboration of spontaneous panic attacks.

The difference between what patients reported and what nurses observed was easily explained. The imipramine had cured the patients of their spontaneous attacks, but the patients did not yet know they had been cured. Since they still bore all the anticipatory anxiety— the fear of having panic attacks—they continued to feel anxious even in the absence of the underlying disease. The patients had to be taught over time that panic anxiety would not return, and the elaborated secondary or anticipatory anxiety would fade.

Klein published his results and hypotheses in 1962 and again in 1964. "These reports were received like the proverbial lead balloon," Klein recalls, and for a number of reasons. Imipramine was believed to be an antidepressant, and therefore it ought not to be effective in treating anxiety. According to the spectrum theory, it especially should not cure severe anxiety, since it was known to have no effect on mild anxiety. And, of course, Klein was striking at the heart of psychoanalysis, anxiety, without talking the language of psychoanalysis. Klein recalls that the simplest prevailing response was that he had misdiagnosed depression as anxiety.

As a side note, Klein did hypothesize about the origin of panic anxiety. From the early months of life, human infants—and ape and monkey infants, too—exhibit separation anxiety. In infants mature enough to have a mental schema of "mother," the mother's absence will elicit squalling, presumably in order to allow or even compel the mother to relocate her young. Separation anxiety later disappears, as primitive brain functions in the developing primate are suppressed by more complex ones. Klein thought spontaneous panic attacks might be a recrudescence of separation anxiety—an atavism or form of neurological disinhibition.

The separation-anxiety hypothesis goes a distance toward explaining anxious patients' greater comfort when at home or in the presence of relatives—the patients feel "separated" only when cut off from home or family. But the theory has problems, too, among them that separation anxiety and panic anxiety seem to involve different neurotransmitters.

Klein and others have put forth alternative models of panic, including a much-studied hypothesis called the "false-suffocation alarm." The healthy brain and body rely on a variety of mechanisms to prevent suffocation. If a person begins to asphyxiate, physiological monitors detect the problem and cause intense arousal, gasping for breath, and the urge to flee. The false-suffocation-alarm theory holds that, in a person with panic anxiety, defective monitors fire even when he or she has enough oxygen. Common to both the separation-anxiety theory and the false-suffocation-alarm theory is the absence of any need for causation rooted in the subtle psychological experiences of the anxious person. Faulty wiring is enough to elicit the panic; the complex psychological elaboration then evolves in response to the random bouts of anxiety.

By 1980, Klein (and the many other biological psychiatrists who researched this issue) had prevailed, at least in terms of the diagnostic manual. Panic anxiety became a recognized disorder, distinct from what was by then called "generalized anxiety." But what appeared in the manual was not yet universally accepted by practitioners. When

Klein presented his most fully elaborated discussion of panic anxiety, also in 1980, his paper was followed by a lecture by an eminent psychoanalyst who made the case for panic anxiety having a psychodynamic root. The analytic talk very much echoed the argument Freud had made in his footnote of the previous century.

Even among biological psychiatrists, there remained doubt as to whether imipramine in agoraphobic patients was acting directly on the syndrome or was making a nonspecific contribution through lessening coincident depression. In fact, it is anxious patients who are not simultaneously depressed on whom imipramine works best. But those in the field were for a long time uncomfortable with the idea that what had been called an "antidepressant" might also be an anxiolytic (as the antianxiety drugs are called). The most acceptable model for a medicine was still the use of one drug for one disease.

On the theoretical level, Klein had achieved a breakthrough—a "pharmacological dissection." That is, he had carved out panic anxiety from the sort of nonspecific anxiety that underlies "neurosis," using response to imipramine as the crucial test. (Pharmacologic dissection is a high-level form of "listening to drugs"—that is, of allowing drug response to inform or even dominate our sense of how human behavior is best categorized.) But, for various reasons, Klein's achievement did not have the overwhelming impact of the work John Cade, the Australian physician, had done with lithium in manic depression. Klein did not discover the therapeutic use of imipramine, as Cade had discovered that of lithium. Imipramine was already in use, though not for anxiety disorders. And whereas there was a clear pool of manic-depressive patients waiting to be treated, psychiatrists had by 1980 lost touch with panic anxiety—they had to be educated before they could see the problem. Also, imipramine was a confusing drug for this indication. It had many side effects; despite Klein's early success, the necessary dosage turned out to be difficult to determine; and the drug made some patients worse before it made them better, so inexperienced office psychiatrists had trouble convincing themselves that imipramine worked. The real explosion in diagnoses of panic anxiety awaited the marketing in 1981 of a new medicine—Xanax.

Xanax is an unusual compound. The molecule looks a great deal like a benzodiazepine—the class of medication that includes Librium, Valium, Dalmane, Halcion, and most of the other currently popular anxiolytics and sedatives—although part of the Xanax molecule looks like an antidepressant. The great benefit of Xanax is that it lowers anxiety without, for the most part, making people sleepy as Librium and Valium do. In other words, Xanax is more specific for anxiety than is Valium, and for certain indications, like panic anxiety, it may also be more potent. (Some pharmacologists believe Valium would be as good for panic anxiety as Xanax if you could give it in high enough doses, but at those doses most patients are asleep.)

Although the FDA did not make this use a specific "indication" for ten more years, it was recognized by the time Xanax was first released that the new drug was an extraordinary treatment for panic anxiety. Unlike imipramine, Xanax made patients with panic anxiety feel better from the first dose. And Xanax has very few side effects.

With a convenient, effective drug available, doctors saw panic anxiety everywhere. Patients told one another about the drug, and the mass media spread the news. Panic anxiety and panic attack became bywords.

The newly rediscovered panic anxiety looked pretty much the way Klein said it would. It was of no use to get patients a little better. You had to medicate them to the point where they got no more attacks at all, and then you had to use a crowbar to get them back out into the world to conquer their anticipatory anxiety.

Not only did the full syndrome of panic anxiety respond to Xanax; many of the partial syndromes Freud had observed responded, too. If a patient had bouts of unexplained diarrhea or dizziness, or feelings of dread without palpitations or perspiration, or even if he just seemed inexplicably timid about making forays from the home, doctors would press for a more complete story and might prescribe Xanax whether or not a full picture of panic emerged. The underlying dynamic for a broad range of symptoms and behaviors is now understood to be incompletely expressed panic anxiety rather than unconscious conflict.

The profession, and then the public, had listened to drugs in two stages: imipramine, through its success in Klein's studies, re-created panic anxiety in theoretical terms; Xanax made it ubiquitous. But then Xanax proved to be a fiercely addicting drug; it is also short-acting, so certain patients are constantly chasing their anxiety, and their withdrawal from Xanax, with another pill, around the clock. Probably imipramine, if patients can tolerate it, is a better long-term treatment for panic anxiety than is Xanax. But in terms of social impact—translating an esoteric theoretical concept into a new public understanding of how people's emotions work—Xanax will have had a lasting effect even if, as is likely, it is superseded by longer-acting, less addictive compounds.

● ● ●

Donald Klein's model of panic anxiety now prevails. When it comes to anxiety, clinicians accept the concept of a complex behavioral syndrome rooted in simple dysregulation of emotion.

That the same did not happen for rejection-sensitivity and its elaboration into hysterical personality is perhaps due, as much as anything, to the absence of the right drug to act as a popularizer, in the way that Xanax popularized panic anxiety. As long as MAOIs remained the drug of choice to "set the floor" under rejection-sensitive patients, the concept of hysteroid dysphoria was unlikely to take hold. Patients who eat or drink the wrong foods can have strokes or die on MAOIs. Few physicians were willing to take a flamboyant, self-absorbed woman prone to brief catastrophic depressions and put her on a pill that would allow her to commit suicide by drinking a glass or two of Chianti or eating a piece of Stilton. A similar line of thought inhibited the widespread use of medication in less disturbed "hysteroid" patients. It is difficult to justify putting a relatively healthy person at risk of stroke. Besides, healthier histrionic patients were still thought to be among the most responsive to psychotherapy. For forty years, Klein's formulation of hysteroid dysphoria remained a stimulating concept without widespread application.

Prozac may change all that. Regarding hysteroid dysphoria, Prozac may be to the MAOIs what, in the case of panic anxiety, Xanax was to imipramine.

This assertion may sound odd. MAOIs affect many transmitter systems, whereas Prozac affects mainly nerves that use serotonin. Nevertheless, converging evidence of diverse sorts suggests that Prozac has a good deal in common with the MAO inhibitors.

One experiment, performed recently by a group at Yale, is so simple and elegant that it is remarkable it was not done long ago on the early antidepressants. It is based on an old technology used by scientists studying human dietary requirements. Besides vitamins, we need amino acids—"the building blocks of protein"—in our diet. Some amino acids the body can manufacture, but others are "essential"; that is, we need to eat foods that already contain them. L-tryptophan is an essential amino acid, and it is the substance from which the body makes serotonin.

When testing amino-acid requirements on army recruits, researchers developed a low-tryptophan diet, one whose protein content is supplied by foods such as gelatin that do not contain L-tryptophan. The researchers could then stress the body by giving the recruits a drink made of amino acids but omitting L-tryptophan. The sudden supply of amino acids induces the body to manufacture proteins, thus depleting it of what little tryptophan remains. This tryptophan-starving amino-acid drink results in rapid serotonin depletion in the brain. In normal people, the results of this dietary stress are not dramatic, although certain subjects may become tired or irritable or blue.

The Yale researchers applied the old technology to patients who had been depressed, had recently recovered on antidepressants, and were still taking the medication. The results were striking. Patients who had recovered on a selective serotonin-reuptake inhibitor (similar to Prozac) became depressed *within hours* of taking the amino-acid drink, and in just the way they had been before taking the SSRI, with precisely the same constellation of symptoms coming on in the same order. Upon their return to a normal diet, the depression once more remitted, within a day. This result makes sense. If the SSRI is working through maintaining effective serotonin levels, serotonin depletion should result in a return of the depression, and refeeding should allow the drug once again to take effect.

The same dietary regimen was applied to patients who had recovered from depression on desipramine, a tricyclic antidepressant that affects norepinephrine (but not serotonin) pathways. These patients did not relapse when given the amino-acid drink.

In the same test situation, patients who had responded to MAOIs relapsed within hours, just as the SSRI-treated patients had, taking on all the aspects of the depressive syndrome from which they had recently recovered. Thus, even though MAOIs are known to act on a number of neurotransmitter pathways, it seems their effect in depressed patients depends on serotonin.

Research at the level of the cell supports this conclusion. The way in which serotonergic cells respond to MAOIs has a similar time course to the response of depression to the medication; cells that use norepinephrine respond also, but changes in norepinephrine levels do not seem to occur at the same time as changes in mood.

At the level of anatomy, the effects of Prozac and the MAOIs also look similar. Psychotherapeutic medications tend to be anatomically selective—to affect circuits only in certain parts of the brain. If you look at changes in receptors on nerve cells, you find that certain MAOIs and Prozac are active in similar parts of the brain, whereas medications like desipramine present a very different pattern of local action.

Cellular research, anatomical studies of brain function, and the dietary challenges all suggest that Prozac and the MAOIs share common sites and mechanisms of action on depression. There is also early work indicating that Prozac and MAOIs are effective in similar subgroups of depressed patients. Small studies first from England and more recently from the University of Michigan show that Prozac, like the MAOIs, may be especially effective in atypical depression, the kind characterized by weight gain and excessive sleep.

Such preliminary data, as well as experience with patients, have led practicing doctors to suspect that Prozac will turn out to be a clinically acceptable alternative to the MAO inhibitor. This speculation extends beyond atypical depression to the issue of sensitivity to rejection and loss. Prozac's relatively benign side-effect profile is especially important here: if you can "set a floor" under emotionally brittle patients—consistently spare them the terrible pain and disorganization that follow losses—without putting their health and safety at risk, then the concept of rejection-sensitivity becomes useful in practical terms. Because of experience with panic anxiety, psychiatrists are quite comfortable with the idea of using medication to head off affective crises in the hope of "breaking the back" of a more complex problem of behavior and self-image. Thus, within psychiatry, the availability of Prozac has reawakened interest in hysteroid dysphoria.

If hysteroid dysphoria were the whole story, Prozac's specificity and potency would be of limited interest: after all, to how many women does Klein's description apply? I don't see many hysteroid dysphorics. Nor, I suspect, do other psychiatrists. Partly this is due to a change in vision. Because of the derogatory implications of hysteria, we prefer to see patients' problems in other terms—depression, anxiety, post-traumatic stress syndromes, multiple personality, borderline personality disorder. The diagnosis that succeeded hysteria, "histrionic personality disorder," is used infrequently.

But I do see people who are highly sensitive to loss or rejection. A few have a flamboyant style; many more are controlled, self-effacing, focused, and driven. Lucy is a good example of a person whose interpersonal style is shaped by her extreme sensitivity to rejection but who is clearly different from the women Klein described. It seems rejection-sensitivity may be a much broader category than hysteroid dysphoria.

To understand how the broad category of rejection-sensitivity came to be represented by hysteroid dysphoria, we must return to Donald Klein's early work. Klein was not merely dissecting out diagnoses but also wielding his scalpel on the prevailing hidebound, pseudo-Freudian, antibiological form of psychoanalysis. Because Klein cured with drugs rather than with interpretations, it was harder to discern that he, like Freud, was as much invested in theory as in clinical results. Imipramine for panic and MAOIs for dysphoria were primarily test cases for the accounts of psychic causation inherent in the psychoanalytic concepts of anxiety and hysteria. This focus on theory helps explain why, among all possible forms of rejection-sensitivity, Klein focused on hysteroid dysphoria. The question is whether the concept needs to be so narrowly restricted. Why should all emotionally vulnerable women become *femmes fatales,* or *femmes fatales manquées?*

Klein tried to explain why rejection-sensitive women become "hysteroid." He believes, as do many theorists, that the appetite for social approval is a direct reinforcer, or a primary, innate drive, for humans. To satisfy that drive, both boys and girls learn early in life to use the interpersonal skills valued in them by their families and society at large. Because sex typing occurs early, and because certain forms of charm are valued in females, girls may be drawn to exhibitionistic and seductive social tactics to win admiration and approval. Most learn to use "feminine" social skills effectively and discreetly. But a girl with a wider range of moods—keener pleasure and pain in response to others' attention and inattention—may become overtrained, an "applause addict." This pattern will be particularly marked in the daughter of narcissistic parents who neglect the child unless she provides the sort of performance they require for their own stimulation and gratification.

Klein's account can be seen as a biological behaviorist's version of the Electra complex. The great difference is that in the psychoanalytic account the family trauma is primary—the competition for the father produces the emotional instability, and therefore merely treating moods will miss the mark—whereas in Klein's version "the interpersonal tactics and . . . relationships are secondary reverberations of the basic affective difficulty."

Working backward from instances of difficult-to-treat pathology, Klein explained plausibly how hysteria might be grounded in a mood disorder. But is hysteria the only possible outcome of rejection-sensitivity? Klein's metapsychology shows how rejection-sensitivity can cause hysteria, but it does not explain why hysteria should be the unique consequence of mood instability. Surely for every rejection-sensitive person who evolves into a caricature of femininity there must be a dozen who adapt and cope in other ways.

Once we focus on rejection-sensitivity apart from hysteria, all sorts of people come to mind to whom the label might apply. There are people who feed their applause addiction through competition at work, and people who respond to unmet needs with withdrawal, self-pity, and excessive caution. Klein, in his academic writings, never moved past the early battle with psychoanalysis. But, in response to his own discomfort with the widespread misuse of "hysteria," Klein did twice rename his syndrome, first as "chronic overreactive dysphoria" and then as "rejection-sensitive dysphoria." Implicitly, these new labels de-emphasize hysterical traits and focus on the underlying inner state—the disordered affective regulator. Indeed, Klein has written that his major contribution in this area has not been the identification of a group of hysterics who respond to medication but, rather, the highlighting of responsiveness to loss as a critical factor in shaping personality, self-image, habitual behaviors, and symptom complexes.

•   •   •

Rejection-sensitivity is a powerful concept. Looking once again at Tess and Julia, we may see the overly controlled quality of their lives as due in part to an apprehension that minor failure can bring catastrophic sensations of loss and inadequacy. Perhaps rejection-sensitivity looks different in risk-avoiders like Tess and Julia than in stimulus-seekers like Klein's hysteroid dysphorics.

As is true of compulsiveness, rejection-sensitivity occurs in quite healthy people, where its effect can nonetheless be pervasive. I am thinking of an accomplished woman who came to see me. Gail had had an uneventful childhood. She grew up in the 1940s, in a warm, supportive family, which she described in stereotypical, sit-com terms: the blustery, warmhearted father, and the driven and directed mother who ruled the roost. Gail attended a one-sex parochial school where girls naturally assumed positions of leadership. With her mother's encouragement, she went on to become a physician at a time when few women did so. She married her teenage sweetheart, Frank, also a doctor; they were two of only a handful of children who emerged as professionals from their working-class ethnic community.

Gail and Frank successfully raised twin daughters, but in time the marriage became unsatisfying, and when Frank was offered a job at a university some hours away, he took it, leaving Gail alone except on weekends. She preferred this arrangement, because it allowed her greater control at home. She had been reluctant to fight with her husband, fearing his sharp tongue—she could not stand mockery—and she felt she had let him dominate for years.

Frank was constantly angry because he could not control Gail's spending. To Gail, her professional status justified her shopping. She was always dressed in the latest fashions—not in a seductive way, but with the sort of "drop-dead" effect of perfectly matched outfits and exclusive accessories. I often had trouble scheduling a session with Gail, not because of her busy practice or academic obligations but because of her hair and nail appointments, which were frequent and inviolable. By her own, certainly conservative estimate, clothes purchases consumed 20 percent of her pretax income.

Gail consulted me because she realized she was "taking too many pills for a woman who has nothing wrong with her." She was more or less addicted to Fiorinal for headaches (Fiorinal is aspirin plus caffeine and a barbiturate), even though she was already taking another medication, Inderal, to prevent migraines. She took Restoril to sleep and BuSpar for anxiety and Xanax for the anxiety the BuSpar and Restoril did not handle.

As we talked, I formed the impression that, between shopping and medicating, Gail was almost constantly rushing to treat or head off a succession of ill-defined bad feelings. The fuller story took time to emerge, as is sometimes the case with people who have compensated for emotional shakiness with extraordinary social skill. Gail found little pleasure in life and was very vulnerable to attacks on her self-esteem. Minor insults or oversights would leave her feeling incapacitated for days and might even result in weeks of minor depression. She did not so much choose as need to be well dressed, perfectly dressed, for fear someone would find fault with her. When Frank decided to change jobs, Gail did not resist in part because she suffered so badly when he mocked or teased her—which he did often, in response to threats to his own sense of self-worth. Spending money made her feel valuable and independent, reassurance she craved because she so often felt worthless and needy.

Imipramine can sometimes prevent migraines, and I suggested that Gail try it; my hope was to be able to wean her off Fiorinal, which can be a fiercely addicting drug. It is always difficult to stop taking barbiturates, harder if you anticipate debilitating headaches as the price. Imipramine was fairly successful, not just as an anti-migraine drug but as an anxiolytic. On imipramine, Gail was able to stop taking Inderal, Restoril, BuSpar, Xanax, and most of the Fiorinal. But the success of imipramine had a paradoxical effect. Imipramine lifted her heretofore unrecognized depression enough for

Gail to feel half-treated—more aware of her vulnerable emotional state than she had been before taking medicine, or perhaps newly aware that the condition could be altered. After she had spent eight rather good months on imipramine, I switched her to Prozac.

Gail was a good responder. Like Tess, she felt newly confident on Prozac, able to make public presentations without notes, able to engage in confrontations without breaking down. Gail was one of the patients who made me understand that Prozac might have a role in the treatment of rejection-sensitivity. I had not given it to her precisely for that indication (although the emphasis on dress brought the diagnosis to mind), but as soon as the drug kicked in, she began to report an unusual change in attitude: her sensitivity to social slights had diminished. A friend had often remarked, "You never ask for anything." Gail said she had always dreaded being refused. Now she asked for more.

One thing she wanted was a hospital-department chairmanship that had opened up. Friends had urged her to apply for the post, but she had feared being turned down and had transformed that fear into a belief that the job was beyond her skills and status. On medication, she believed that she could do the job—that any sentiment on the part of others to the contrary was prejudice against women. But it was still hard for her to put her hat in the ring. She asked whether I could raise the dose of Prozac so she would feel comfortable applying for the post. I did not know whether a different dose would have a different effect, but I saw no reason not to try. She took extra Prozac, and she applied for the promotion. She was eventually turned down, but was able to take the rebuff in stride. She put her response in words of the sort I have heard from other patients: "I can stand disappointment. I feel confident. I don't tear myself down."

Perhaps the most interesting medication effects were those evident in the marriage. Gail now found her husband more affectionate and less hostile. I understood this change in perception as stemming from Gail's greater tolerance for teasing—that is, a diminished sense of vulnerability. Of course, her husband might have modified his behavior, but it seemed that the initial change was one in the way she experienced him—and a change in the way a wife experiences her husband can influence the way he responds to her, and vice versa. To the extent that this understanding of events is right, we can see medication as having broken a marital stalemate.

In time, both spouses were able to contemplate living together again. In Gail's case, this newfound tolerance was linked to an enhanced sense of independence. Before, she had felt the urge to turn to her husband during each episode of upset, and the resulting feeling of dependency had made her want to keep her distance. Now that she was less desperate, she could allow him back home.

On Prozac, Gail had little use for Fiorinal. It would be convenient to report that she also did without shopping sprees, but though Gail's need to dress perfectly may have diminished, she held on to her right to spend money on herself as a badge and an instrument of independence, and as a bargaining chip in the marriage. If anything, she enjoyed shopping more. "I don't feel guilty about spending," she said. "My husband can say what he wants."

●　　●　　●

Gail, a well-adjusted woman who sits more at the inhibited than the histrionic end of the behavioral spectrum, nonetheless suffered limitations in her life as a result of a heightened emotional responsiveness to disapproval. She was not totally without the symptoms Klein uses to characterize hysteroid dysphoria: she was focused on clothes, and she turned to medication for self-stabilization. But she otherwise had nothing in common with the impulsive, flamboyant, desperately self-centered women Klein studied. It can also be argued that Gail—a decisive physician, able to choose to live apart from her husband— had little in common with people we ordinarily call "sensitive." To understand Gail as suffering from rejection-sensitivity is to enlarge the scope of what we mean when we say someone is sensitive.

It is the effect of Prozac on patients like Gail that leads me to believe our understanding of sensitivity will undergo a sea change. Like panic, sensitivity will become reified, I suspect, so that when we call a person "sensitive" we will come to mean that the person we are discussing has a slight biological derangement, one that must be taken into account in assessing his behavior or opinions. Prozac's ability to decrease rejection-sensitivity suggests that how people respond to loss is a function of the state of their serotonergic neurons.

Once we think about it—and I believe that one of the effects of medication is to make us think about it—we will find reasons why the set point for sensitivity should be biologically regulated. We are an affiliative species. The idea that depression serves to maintain social stability is an old one: the threat of depression keeps primates bonded. But major depression is an infrequent event. It seems much more likely that pair-bonding is maintained through small experiences of loss—that is, through rejection-sensitivity.

The psychiatrist Ronald Winchel has even suggested that primates' affiliative needs are constantly spurred by what he calls the "aloneness affect," a dysphoric feeling that is present unless inhibited by association with others. Winchel suggests that people differ in the responsiveness of this system to successful bonding. In some people, bonding suffices to suppress the aloneness affect; others remain always hungry for more affiliation, and they run through many mates, scratching an itch that will not go away. Winchel suggests that the relevant neurotransmitter in this system is serotonin.

For the moment, it may be enough to say that one of the unanticipated benefits of Prozac's potency and specificity is its ability to act as an acceptable substitute for MAOIs. This function makes hysteroid dysphoria a workable diagnosis and, more broadly, makes rejection-sensitivity a distinct phenomenon worth looking for. The efficacy of medication for rejection-sensitivity makes interesting a whole body of speculative literature that emphasizes the physiological underpinnings of human nature. The medicine likewise draws attention away from the causes of sensitivity—whether inborn or acquired, a person's level of sensitivity is presumed to be encoded as a particular state of the neurons—and refocuses it on the effects of what is now presumed to be a functionally autonomous trait.

Rejection-sensitivity is not a diagnosis—neither an illness nor a personality disorder. It is a personality trait, one that plays differing roles even in the few patients we have met. Sometimes, as in Lucy's case or perhaps Tess's, it appears to be the result of trauma; at other times, as in Gail's case or Julia's, its cause is unclear. Rejection-sensitivity is both a manifestation of difficulties and a pathogen, causing further difficulties of its own.

Rejection-sensitivity is the sort of category we would expect to arise in a discussion of psychotherapy, like "narcissism" or "low self-worth." And this is exactly the point: it is now sometimes possible to use medication to do what once only psychotherapy did—to reach into a person and alter a particular element of personality. In deciding whether to do so, the psychopharmacologist must rely on skills we ordinarily associate with psychotherapy.

Treatment of rejection-sensitivity reveals a new wrinkle in "cosmetic psychopharmacology." It is one thing for a doctor to be able to transform a patient with medication, quite another for the doctor to be able to sculpt the patient's personality trait by trait. Psychotherapists have sometimes been demonized as Svengalis, but at least psychotherapy requires extensive collaboration on the part of the patient. How much more uneasy will we be if doctors can reshape patients' social behavior in detail, through chemicals?

•　•　•

Once you have reason to look for rejection-sensitivity, you see it everywhere.

For instance, I treated a case of homesickness with Prozac, on the grounds that at root it was an instance of rejection-sensitivity. The patient was a young man from a prominent European family. He had come to do graduate work in this country because the best training in his field of study was to be found here. After meeting an American colleague he might want to marry, he considered settling in the United States, but he felt a constant pull to return home to Europe. What tugged at him, he was aware, was the hope of hearing words of approval from a strong mother who was, by the son's account, stinting in her attention to her children. Though his girlfriend was somewhat warmer, her occasional failure to act empathically could send the young man into a severe tailspin. The patient understood his plan to return home as a way of resisting the urge to display undue dependency on his girlfriend, as well as an attempt to gain his mother's attention. On Prozac—along with focused psychotherapy—he settled in and made progress with both career and relationship.

A very different patient, a claims processor in a large insurance company, complained bitterly of social isolation. She pursued men but never enjoyed more than the briefest relationships with them; she said her hunger for approval frightened men off. She felt mired in her job but, because she had invested almost enough time to achieve a good pension, she saw no way out. Her rejection-sensitivity was most evident in the details of her life. For example, she said, "If I get a letter I think may contain criticism or anger at me, I put it aside for a year; even then, I may be afraid to open it, so sometimes I just throw letters out." Hearing statements of this sort made me ask further about her isolation and career paralysis. It turned out that she cut off social contact whenever she felt she might become close enough to be injured by loss or disappointment. She complained she was overlooked at work, but in fact she had never applied for a promotion, because she feared the pain she would suffer on being turned down. Prozac allowed her to date a variety of men calmly, and to settle into a long-term relationship with one. She also was able to tolerate applying for and accepting a promotion.

I perceived rejection-sensitivity in a private banker who, despite enjoying his marriage, needed a series of mistresses in order to feel emotional security. The problem, as he put it, was that he could not feel close to his wife because he was so much more affected by fear of her criticism than by the experience of her support. (Though both applause hunger and fear of humiliation may be present in rejection-sensitivity, the latter is generally far stronger than the former.) He suffered for days when he lost an account, even if the reason had nothing to do with his competency—for instance if a client moved out of state. Attainment of an equivalent new account would not restore his peace of mind. Tellingly, he said, "I cannot engage in banter. If I am strong with someone, he may be strong back, and I can't stand it."

One patient showed a sort of sensitivity that seemed periodic—and therefore all the more strongly biological. She was the daughter of parents both of whom had suffered recurrent depression as well as a degree of social isolation. Productive, considerate, socially mature, the young woman ordinarily liked to spar with her boyfriend, teasing and being teased. But there were also weeks when for no apparent reason she felt infinitely vulnerable, threatened, and often thrown into brief episodes of depression by jokes that involved barely perceptible threats of loss of love. These intervals appeared—came over her, so that she was aware she was "in a state"—in a way that seemed unrelated to external stressors.

Having seen Prozac in action, I now look for signs of rejection-sensitivity in any patient with marked social difficulties. Consider two quite common problems: first, the young man or woman, well into the usual age of courtship, who has never had an adult romantic relationship, and, second, the man or woman stuck in an abusive relationship. These patterns—on the one hand, social avoidance, inhibition, or phobia; on the other, social masochism or the sort of disregard for self associated with low self-worth—can be understood in a variety of ways. But socially isolated or injured patients will commonly describe themselves as exquisitely sensitive to slights, and often attending to that part of their makeup will afford them relief and allow some behavioral flexibility. In instances where I see a combination of rejection-sensitivity, lack of social flexibility, and continuous or recurrent minor depression—and this is by no means a rare grouping—I often find antidepressants to be helpful.

Rejection-sensitivity is not limited to people with social difficulties early in life. When a spouse dies, the remaining partner may reveal a long history of vulnerability, just barely buffered throughout adulthood by the constant attentions of a supportive mate. This lifelong rejection-sensitivity will sometimes respond to medication, resulting in a quite confident widow (or widower), surprised by a newfound competence.

The mitigation of rejection-sensitivity has, like some of the other uses of Prozac, both its welcome and its uncomfortable aspects, not least because the target of treatment has ill-defined boundaries. My own sense of discomfort in this regard is strongest in my work with college students. Late adolescence is a time in which it is normal for rapidly changing moods to accompany an unstable sense of self. Identity, which includes sensitivity to approval and rejection, is a central developmental issue. Still, some undergraduates seem more sensitive than others.

Some of these more vulnerable students have sustained a loss in childhood, perhaps the death of a parent or a divorce. Others have a history of temperamental sensitivity; they have always been "easy blushers," keenly aware of their appearance in social interchanges. In either case, these students' hunger for attention may have been gratified through the response of teachers in grammar and high school —I have in mind children who are bright, or artistically talented, or perhaps just "prematurely mature" and therefore especially charming to adults. Social challenges may have been delayed, particularly if the child went through school with an unchanging cohort of classmates, so that the task of making new friends arose rarely.

Arriving at college, such students may become suddenly unconfident. Meeting with an adult in an intimate setting such as the psychiatrist's consulting room, they appear composed and well spoken. But, though they may have friends on campus, these vulnerable students lack the social skills to elicit the high degree of attention and approval they require. They may respond to their inner sense of urgency by becoming withdrawn and studious or, on the contrary, wild and exhibitionistic. In either case, it is hard for them to act constructively or to feel comfortable unless their drive for approval is addressed.

One student I treated said she became disorganized as soon as she realized a boyfriend was sexually experienced: "If he has a past, he is more likely to leave me, and I feel terrible as soon as I have that thought, long before he has any chance to leave." Another said, "I can't stand to see anyone lose at tennis. I have too vivid an imagination." That is, he imagines people feel as devastated when they lose as he does. Most often, a student may say, "My lover can do nothing right with me, because when the least thing goes wrong I get too deeply hurt."

Shall we medicate these students? They are just the people for whom certain forms of short-term psychotherapy were developed. Probably we will go that route first. And then? For reasons that probably have less to do with objective clinical judgment than with a cultural mistrust of psychotherapeutic medication, I am reluctant to prescribe for patients this young. But if there is any additional reason to prescribe—if, for example, the student undergoes a depression of any duration, or if it is evident that, whatever the prospect for psychotherapy in the long run, the student's vulnerability is creating too much immediate damage to his or her sense of self-worth, social standing with peers, or ability to function—I may go ahead and try a course of medication, and often the student will do substantially better in all areas. An incidental consequence of this success is that it reinforces my tendency to see "functionally autonomous rejection-sensitivity" everywhere.

●　　●　　●

Lucy, the boy-crazy college student who as a child had discovered her mother's murder, continued to suffer emotional turmoil, despite psychotherapy. During a period of particularly disorganizing upset for Lucy, I started her on Prozac. Lucy never met Klein's criteria for hysteroid dysphoria: she was not "egocentric, narcissistic, exhibitionistic, vain, and clothes-crazy," nor was she "seductive, manipulative, exploitative, sexually provocative" or "histrionic and flamboyant." She was, to the contrary, quiet, cautious, self-protective, and self-effacing. But I thought she was nonetheless rejection-sensitive.

Lucy's initial response to Prozac was promising. The medication interrupted her downward spiral. She reported a newfound ability to "back off" in her relationship with her boyfriend. The medication may have allowed her to stay at school, and to preserve the romance. These effects were of some importance; they stabilized her life. Lucy's brief, strong response to Prozac allowed me to consider the possibility that a good deal of her behavior, despite its obvious roots in her reaction to the murder of her mother, was now grounded in a functionally autonomous emotional sensitivity whose biological encoding had something to do with serotonergic neurons.

It was not possible to keep Lucy on Prozac. She reported an increase in her sense of undirected urgency. Overcome with cravings, she did not know what she craved. She had to do something, yet she did not know what. Case reports had emerged of Prozac's causing patients to experience suicidal ruminations, and I thought that Lucy's agitation resembled aspects of incidents in those reports. I lowered the medication dose, but Lucy had one more episode of agitation, so I stopped the Prozac. I might have tried medicating her with another antidepressant, or perhaps even restarted the Prozac, if her sense of bleakness had deepened. But without any medication Lucy began gradually to feel better.

One factor was, I think, her heightened awareness of her response to subtle slights. The brief period, on medicine, of relative invulnerability to loss allowed Lucy to understand her social behavior as stemming from exaggerated apprehensiveness. (We might say the medication acted like an interpretation in psychotherapy: it gave Lucy a new perspective.) Or perhaps having been prescribed medication in itself gave Lucy a sort of dual vision—an ability to see how her behavior looked, say, to her boyfriend. She became more open to examining her responses to rejection. When she found herself too acquiescent in her relationship, she was able to ask herself whether she was holding back out of fear of a catastrophic emotional response. Merely labeling the problem allowed Lucy to act more assertively. She felt more in control, and her confidence elicited attentive behavior from her boyfriend.

There was a change in my psychotherapy, too. I remained interested in Lucy's memories of her childhood. But Lucy's hunger for attention and her pain in response to rejection were also at the forefront of my thinking, and this constant awareness, on both our parts, of her social behavior seemed to hasten her progress. Or perhaps a biological effect of Prozac—the calming of an overexcited system—had something to do with Lucy's ability to change.

Sigmund Freud's granddaughter, the social worker Sophie Lowenstein Freud, made a thoughtful comment at a hospital academic conference where I presented an aspect of Lucy's case. Sophie Freud suggested that all people are rejection-sensitive, in the sense that rejection hurts them, but that Lucy might be more skilled than most at *perceiving* rejection. That is, her boyfriend really is spurning her (perhaps even half-knowingly, sadistically) when he turns to the television, and Lucy differs from others only in being aware of that truth. It follows that a therapy based on treating rejection-sensitivity is asking Lucy to decrease her accurate perceptual acuity. The goal is to blind her partially.

The comment is a wise one. It recognizes two factors we have already discussed, the ubiquity of rejection-sensitivity and the enhanced perceptiveness of those who have had to contend with certain special childhood circumstances. But Sophie Freud's comment goes further. It is grounded in the belief that all people—if they perceive themselves to be rejected—feel the same pain internally. They differ only according to how small a cue they need to recognize rejection. This reading of sensitivity is very much in line with the traditional psychoanalytic belief that people differ mainly in the way their history has shaped the cognitive processes by which they integrate, interpret, distort, and screen out current experience. If all people are similar in how they translate loss into pain, then the instrument we are adjusting is not the internal amplifier but the external receiver—we are asking the person to create an artificial attentional deficit, to ignore loss. Sophie Freud, in her brief comment, went on to say that in some therapies we do have to teach people to be less sensitive—less perceptive.

The alternative view—one that seems more likely—is that sensitive people, when they perceive rejection, feel it more keenly. I take this to be Klein's position. The primary deficit is increased amplification, but a person who is vulnerable to extreme pain will become, secondarily, hypervigilant, and therefore more aware of hints of rejection. A medicine capable of treating major depression is probably, even in the realm of minor depression, altering an internal mechanism concerned with such things as mood stabilization and resilience in response to stress.

For the most part, I do not believe that either medicine or psychotherapy makes people less perceptive. But people come as wholes. You cannot tinker with one part and expect others to remain unchanged. Once we turn down the amplification, small slights, even if they are noticed for a moment, may pass without being registered into memory. If they are not remembered, it is as if they never happened. In this sense, a secondary effect of reduced amplification is reduced perception. If the recurrent pain can be muted, a sensitive person ought to become less apprehensive, and perhaps less apprehending as well. He or she might go on in time to ignore small cues that portend minor rejection. The slight blandness apparent in some cheerful, formerly sensitive patients may reflect this loss of subtlety.

Lucy did not become bland. But I think it is true that she moved from being confusingly perceptive—able to see people doing things to her that not even they knew they intended—to being perceptive in a way that allowed a less painful interaction with friends and strangers.

Off medicine, Lucy plateaued at a certain level—better but not well. I was aware of an irony in her treatment. Even though Lucy had been unable to tolerate Prozac, the concept of rejection-sensitivity continued to dominate the psychotherapy. She and I now saw rejection-sensitivity as a central problem for her, even though Prozac had failed to cure her. The persistence of our focus on rejection-sensitivity, in the absence of the drug response that would have justified it, underlined for me the remarkable imperialism of the biological.

In thinking about medication for Lucy, I had begun with evidence that a well-defined disorder, hysteroid dysphoria, responds to a given type of medication, the MAOI. From there, by a series of leaps, I devised the untested hypothesis of rejection-sensitivity in people who are by no means hysterical. Another chain of reasoning justified the use of a quite different type of medication, one that selectively blocks serotonin reuptake. I then applied this weakly supported model to a particular case, Lucy's, in which psychological causes of social discomfort were vividly apparent. The medication did little for Lucy. And still the medication had the power to shape my understanding of how Lucy functioned.

Now Lucy *had* a particular treatable thing, vulnerability to loss. I was continually amazed that I could look at a woman with such a distinct history—such clear psychological cause for suffering and self-injurious social behavior—and, even some of the time, see a quasi-biological quasi-entity, "sensitivity."

Even if medication fails, the patient and the therapist alike may tend to think not that the model is wrong but, rather, that the biological problem persists, untreated. In Lucy's case, I turned to medication a second time when, toward the end of a semester, she became irritable with her roommates. She felt constantly hurt by them and desperate about the self-isolation she created by her demands on their attention. She began to complain of panicky feelings as well as a lack of interest in her work, and she became afraid her mood state would damage her relationship with her boyfriend.

By this time, a new antidepressant was available that, like Prozac, inhibits serotonin reuptake without directly affecting other neurotransmitter systems. Lucy began taking Zoloft, the new selective serotonin-reuptake inhibitor (SSRI), and after four weeks she reported a striking change. She no longer worried about whether her boyfriend called on time: "I don't freak out."

As weeks passed, this change only increased. Lucy began to prefer space and time to work alone. She reconciled with her roommates and expanded her circle of friends, no longer isolating herself with her boyfriend. She decided to take on junior teaching responsibilities in her department at school, and she found herself able to plan ahead. In general, she said, she was less fearful, better able to count on herself, more open to others' points of view, and at the same time more confident in her own responses. And in the therapy, Lucy found herself—this is after over two years of meeting at least once a week—newly able to discuss aspects of private feelings, in relation to both the past and the present. She was altogether less fragile and more available. These changes were of the sort that psychotherapy had produced, but with the medication there was a sense of a leap forward, of communication with aspects of the self that had been closed off for half of Lucy's young life.

After a few weeks on Zoloft, as on Prozac, Lucy experienced an intensification of her objectless cravings. These cravings ended in an interesting way. Lucy had occasion to visit with her boyfriend's mother, a woman who heretofore had seemed cool and judgmental. This weekend went much better, and Lucy felt her cravings disappear. They had been, she reported, a form of longing for her own mother, a feeling Lucy believed had enveloped her from time to time and that had always seemed too overwhelming to face. She decided in retrospect that the sense of urgency had not been a side effect of medication but, rather, part of its restorative function: on medication, her emotions and memories were more available to her. The medication seemed to have weakened inhibitory barriers to a visceral yearning stemming from the loss of her mother. It was impossible to know whether Lucy's understanding of the phenomenon was correct. But if it was, as a psychotherapist I had once more been misled by my attention to the biological. My focus on medication side effects had blinded me to the obvious psychological meaning of this young woman's sense of urgent intentionality.

I don't imagine Lucy would have done as well as she did without psychotherapy. At the same time, Lucy's response to the SSRI was decided and convincing. "I have the feeling if I fall I won't crack," she said. "Nothing can stop me now." And these declarations came only weeks after a period of marked fragility.

Lucy had harbored a kernel of vulnerability that the psychotherapy did not touch. It was as if psychological trauma—the mother's death, and then the years of struggle for Lucy and her father—had produced physiological consequences for which the most direct remedy was a physiological intervention. But how does psychic trauma become translated into a functionally autonomous, biologically encoded personality trait? How can a mother's death become a change in serotonergic pathways? Lucy's response to medication raises those questions. We are in a speculative realm, but there are answers to be had.

5

Stress

The stories of transformation we have considered so far have involved people with mild degrees of impairment: minor depression, minor compulsiveness, sensitivity to loss, personality styles fallen from favor. In order to understand how painful experiences can lead to conditions that respond to medication, we must look further afield, because in psychiatry biological research is rarely done on healthy people. It is done on nerve cells, on rats and monkeys, and on patients with serious levels of illness.

What is probably the dominant theory regarding the influence of experience on mood is grounded in observations of the gravest mood disorder, "rapid cycling." In discussing rejection-sensitivity, we encountered the notion that the social style of certain people represents less a response to inner conflict than an attempt to cope with vulnerability to painful emotions. Now to take a further step: there are people in whom mood seems to have lost its attachment to any psychological stimulus whatsoever, in whom affect has become utterly dissociated from their experience of the everyday world.

These people may shift back and forth from deep depression to startling euphoria or to extreme irritability, sometimes in a matter of days or even hours. The radical swings may occur in response to very slight provocation, such as a minor disruption of sleep. Or the cycling may be entirely autonomous—that is, the shift from mania to depression or vice versa may occur out of the blue, or even at fixed time intervals.

These rapidly cycling patients are notoriously hard to treat, so they tend to collect at institutions of last resort. Robert Post, a psychiatrist who has devoted his professional life to the elucidation of manic-depressive illness (or "bipolar affective disorder," as it is now properly called), decided to study a series of rapid cyclers on the clinical wards of the National Institute of Mental Health in Bethesda, Maryland. Though a biologist trained to work at the level of chemical processes within the single neuron, Post has always remained interested in the experience of the patient. Since the start of his career, he has been curious about the time course of manic depression. Through painstaking interviews with patients and their families, Post compiled time-line charts of the onset, termination, and severity of manic and depressive episodes in the lives of bipolar patients. He found that rapid cycling was the end stage of a chronic recurrent illness. Sufferers would typically experience a single episode, usually of depression, in early life. Three to five years later, they might have a second episode. Two years later, an outbreak of depression would blend into subsequent mania. The later recurrences would typically include all the symptoms of earlier episodes, plus additional symptoms. The general pattern was a decrease in the interval between episodes and an increase in the severity and complexity of the episodes, until finally rapid cycling set in.

Post also tried to determine whether a given episode of mania or depression could be related to a trauma, such as loss or disappointment. In general, he found that, as time passed, it required ever smaller stimuli to trigger an episode. In a summary by Post of his own studies and those by other researchers, a psychosocial trauma could be found to precede 60 percent of first episodes of depression or mania, but only 30 percent of second episodes, and so on out to rapid cycling, where only 6 percent of episodes could be linked to discrete stressors.

Like Donald Klein in the case of panic anxiety, Post was redocumenting in the modern era a finding that had been noted at the turn of the century and then neglected. Emil Kraepelin, the contemporary of Freud who differentiated manic depression from schizophrenia, had noted that a severe mood disorder typically began with trauma, was later reactivated, and finally took an "independent course."

Post defined the progression of rapid-cycling bipolar affective disorder: decreasing intervals between episodes ("increasing cyclicity"); increasing complexity and severity of episodes; and an ever-diminishing requirement for external stimuli to set off overt illness. He then searched for a biological model. How do you create an illness characterized by increasing cyclicity and decreasing requirements for trauma? Most processes in biology look just the opposite. They operate according to a "negative feedback loop" in which a system requires ever-increasing stimulus to elicit a response. For example, an addict of street drugs may require progressively larger fixes to obtain the same "high."

But there are a few examples in biology of conditions in which the organism becomes sensitized to, instead of tolerant of, stimuli. One that attracted Post's interest was the "kindling" of seizures, a concept developed in the 1960s by neurosurgeons interested in an animal model for epilepsy. Seizures are "kindled" in an experimental animal—usually a rat or a monkey—by applying an electrode to a relevant part of the brain and passing current. If you pass a small amount of current, at first nothing observable will happen. After a series of intermittent small stimuli, the animal will have a limited seizure. If after an interval you again stimulate the sensitized site, less electricity will be required. With enough intermittent stimulation, the animal will exhibit more widespread seizures: first it will chew and nod its head, then one forepaw will go in and out of spasm, then both forepaws, and so on. In time, the animal will start to seize spontaneously, with no stimulus at all. Eventually, the interval between these seizures will decrease, with spontaneous seizures occurring in ever more rapid succession and with greater symptomatic complexity.

To Post, the kindling model of epilepsy looked highly analogous to what he was seeing in the life charts of rapid-cycling bipolar patients. The limitation to Post's model was that it was "nonhomologous." That is, although the progression over time of induced epilepsy in animals resembled that of manic depression in humans, no one was suggesting that bipolar patients had epilepsy. Kindling merely provided a way of thinking about possible biological mechanisms in recurrent affective illness.

If Post had restricted his work to theoretical modeling, it might have gained a following among laboratory researchers only. But Post was faced with a distressing clinical population, the rapid cyclers. Some of these patients responded to lithium, the standard medication for manic depression, but many did not. Post decided to try these patients on Tegretol, a medicine heretofore used mainly to control seizures in outright epilepsy but bearing a chemical resemblance to the antidepressants. (Among other things, as with the tubercular patients on iproniazid, Tegretol seemed a promising drug because of a sort of "experiment of nature": epileptics on Tegretol were observed to experience improvements in mood.) Psychiatrists were wary of Tegretol. Like MAOIs, it has a rare, severe side effect: Tegretol can cause an irreversible drop in the production of white blood cells, which are needed to fight infection. But Post was dealing with such terrible illnesses that he and his patients were willing to take a risk. Post had marked success. Tegretol turned out to be a better medication for rapid cycling than lithium; indeed, Tegretol has turned out to be useful in other types of manic depression that do not respond to lithium.

Nothing drives the interest of practicing doctors like success with medication. Here was a new treatment for a refractory disorder. And the fact that Tegretol is a neurologist's drug, an anticonvulsant (anti-epileptic), made it even more intriguing. If rapid cycling and epilepsy are connected, beyond analogy and their responsiveness to Tegretol, it is in a complex, still-undiscovered way. Both do often occur in the same part of the brain, and both probably involve a disorder in the transmission of signals, but there was still a good degree of serendipity involved in the discovery that two possibly "kindled" illnesses respond to the same medicine. The kindling model was not necessarily any more intellectually compelling after the application of Tegretol to rapid cycling than before. Nonetheless, once they began successfully treating bipolar patients with an anticonvulsant, clinicians found Post's nonhomologous model, kindling, hard to ignore.

Researchers soon turned from the time course of kindling to an examination of the physical processes that underlie it. Kindling has dramatic effects on nerve pathways. Applying current to relevant cells in the rat's brain causes "downstream" cells (those receiving signals from the electrically stimulated cells) to change *anatomically*, and these changes can occur early on, before the animal develops seizures. Cellular biologists are right now studying the process in detail, and they are already speculating about the general picture. It looks as if a series of chemical reactions in the downstream cell reach right to the nucleus and affect the way the cell's DNA and RNA produce complex chemical substances. These substances include hormones that determine whether the cell makes new connections with other neurons or allows old connections to wither. Some cells die; others "sprout," or change shape. Kindling rewires the brain.

Changes in "hard wiring" become apparent long before a kindled animal has its first seizure—the brain reshapes itself anatomically in response to small noxious stimuli. If kindled epilepsy is an accurate model for the development of mood disorders, then we would expect anatomical changes in the brains of traumatized people—perhaps children with the sorts of experiences Tess or Lucy suffered—even before any symptoms of depression appear. It is important to emphasize that we are reasoning by analogy: kindled rats suffer physical trauma, whereas the histories of most depressed people reveal psychological trauma. But the similarity in pattern of illness between depressed patients as they progress to rapid cycling and kindled rats as they progress to epilepsy allows researchers to speculate that, for certain brain cells, physical and psychological trauma may be quite similar in their effects.

Here, then, is a biological image of "functional autonomy": trauma is translated into anatomical changes in the brain, even before any major illness becomes evident. Under the kindling model, rats become sensitive to ever more subtle stimuli. This model reflects some of what we see in certain rejection-sensitive patients: Symptoms become "unmoored" from their historical antecedents, and people who have suffered serious trauma later find themselves vulnerable to what for others would be minor losses or threats of loss.

The kindled-epilepsy model also resembles models of how animals learn to see. At first, animals have to scan a visual field painstakingly; in time, they presumably make hard neural connections that allow certain complex shapes (or rules about perspective) to be processed simply and rapidly. In both cases, kindled epilepsy and perceptual learning, a repeated stimulus results in an anatomical change in the brain. Kindling appears to be a kind of learning, but a learning that can occur independent of cognition.

Researchers have used the kindling model to study treatment and prevention, as well as causation, of illness. They have given kindled rats various medications and discovered two interesting things: First, medication can normalize chemical production in the brain cells of kindled animals; that is, it can prevent the production of hormones that reshape the brain's wiring. And, second, different drugs are effective at different stages of the disorder.

Early in the development of kindled epilepsy, Valium will prevent seizures; but once the seizures become spontaneous—independent of external stimuli—Valium is ineffective. Dilantin (another anticonvulsant) is ineffectual against early seizures but effective in preventing spontaneous seizures in the end-stage disorder. This latter observation parallels experience with manic-depressive patients. Lithium tends to be most effective when a patient has had three or fewer episodes of mania. Thereafter, antiepileptic drugs, such as Tegretol, are more likely to work.

The kindling model has led researchers to fear that, in progressive manic depression, drugs appropriate to the early stages of illness become ineffective as the illness worsens, because of structural changes in the sufferer's brain. Most researchers now recommend medicating manic depression early and keeping patients for extended periods of time on the drugs that treat the initial stages of the disorder. Increasing evidence that depression alone, in the absence of mania, can have the form of a progressive, kindled illness is causing psychiatrists to apply these same rules broadly to all mood disorders. The goal is to prevent the hard-to-reverse deterioration that occurs as the illness progresses.

If we accept the analogy between mood disorders and kindled epilepsy, this is how we will see manic depression, and perhaps all depression: It is a progressive, probably lifelong disorder. It can be induced in normals. The induction can take place through a series of small stimuli, none of which at first causes overt symptoms. The latency to fully expressed illness can be long, and the absence of overt symptoms is no guarantee that the underlying process is not under way. Illness, once expressed, can become responsive to ever smaller stimuli and, in time, independent of stimuli altogether. The expression of the disorder becomes more complex over time. Even the early stimuli are translated into anatomical, difficult-to-reverse changes in the brain. Different treatments are appropriate to different stages of the illness. Early and prolonged intervention is crucial.

• • •

Kindling mimics the time course of mood disorders, but the stress to which animals are subjected, electrical current, is not the same as the stress that depresses humans. Researchers have tried to bridge the gap through experiments in which rats are exposed instead to various forms of physical and psychosocial stress.

Biochemical responses to stress have been of interest to researchers for decades. By the middle of this century, scientists were focused on the functions of the adrenal glands, small organs sitting atop the kidneys (therefore ad-renal). The adrenals were known to produce hormones that set the body's tone in response to stress. One such hormone is adrenaline, a fight-or-flight substance named after the gland that produces it in greatest quantity. "Adrenalin" is actually a proprietary name for the chemical that scientists, using Greek rather than Latin roots, call "epinephrine." Parsimoniously, nature often uses the same substance as a hormone in the body and a transmitter in the brain. It was the role of epinephrine or adrenalin in the body's handling of stress that led scientists studying depression to look at epinephrine and its close relative, norepinephrine, in their role as brain neurotransmitters.

For an equally long time, psychiatric researchers have been interested in another hormone produced by the adrenal gland, cortisol. Cortisol is the hormone that is abnormal in Addison's disease and Cushing's disease. Its effects on healing and inflammation are taken advantage of in creams, pills, and inhalants containing synthetic analogues of cortisol, such as hydrocortisone. The body's own cortisol, when released into the bloodstream, affects mood, food intake, the sleep-wake cycle, and level of locomotor activity—all factors altered in depression—and cortisol is known to be released in response to stress; so close is the connection that cortisol and related substances are sometimes called "stress hormones." Scientists have long wondered whether cortisol will turn out to be the biochemical factor that connects stress to resultant depression.

A host of observations associate depression with abnormalities in stress hormones. Many depressed patients, if given a substance that ordinarily causes the body to decrease its output of cortisol, fail to suppress—that is, the system is so revved up that it no longer responds to ordinary forms of regulation. Cortisol levels (the amount of hormone in the blood) are high in many acutely depressed adults. Autopsies often show the adrenal gland to be enlarged in adults who have died by suicide. The gland is also enlarged, according to imaging studies, in about a third of depressed patients. Put briefly, elevated, nonsuppressible cortisol levels can be a marker of depression. Elevated cortisol may even account for certain symptoms of depression.

The adrenals are far from the brain, and most of what interests researchers is not so much cortisol produced by the adrenals as the substances in the brain that stimulate the adrenals. There is a cascade of such hormones; one brain center stimulates another, and so on down the line until a hormone is released that causes the adrenals to produce and release cortisol. At the top of the cascade is a substance produced in the brain called corticotropin-releasing factor (CRF). Elevated CRF levels can be measured in the brains of rats subjected to stress—and here is where a more homologous model of stress and depression emerges.

Rats can be stressed in a variety of ways—through pain (such as electric shock to the foot pads or pinching of the tail), through exposure to cold, through switching of cage-mates, or through close confinement in a small cage. There are also more complex forms of stress, one of which, "learned helplessness," is the basis for a variety of research. In the learned-helplessness model, a rat may be trained to avoid a foot shock by pressing a lever; later, shocks are administered randomly. The rats from whom control has been withdrawn evince symptoms, such as social isolation and passivity, that look like depression. As in humans who commit suicide, chronically stressed rats have enlarged adrenal glands. Moreover, stressed rats produce excess CRF in regions of the brain that parallel those known to affect mood in humans.

As in the case of kindling, repeated stress "sensitizes" rats to produce ever higher levels of CRF. The mediating substances within the receptor cells look very similar in stressed and in kindled rats; that is, the same sorts of substances lead to the changes in what the cell's genetic material, the DNA and RNA, produces. Like electrical current, stress can cause cell death and changes in the neural architecture—the hard wiring—of the brain. For instance, one study has shown that rats restrained in small cages for part of each day will experience localized brain-cell death within three weeks. As in kindling, medications (in fact, antidepressants) can prevent neural damage in stressed rats. The anticonvulsant Dilantin blocks cell loss in stressed rats, just as it blocks kindling.

It is harder to work with stress than with kindling (for instance, it is easy to measure the number and frequency of seizures in rats, but harder to assess the time course of depression), so researchers know less about the cellular effects of stress than they do about the results of electrical stimulation. But the parallels between rats' responses to electrical current and to psychic stress make it tempting to combine the two models conceptually. Together, they give weight to the conclusion that psychosocial stressors like pain, isolation, confinement, and lack of control can lead to structural changes in the brain and can kindle progressively more autonomous acute symptoms.

Lest the stressors to which rats are subjected seem too simple to relate to the influences that might cause depression or behavioral inhibition in humans, we should note that researchers have found that a variety of psychological "stressors" can cause cell death in the nerves affected by the cortisol system. Entirely nonpsychological stressors can have the same effect: chronically diminished blood flow to the brain causes comparable brain-cell death, and so does normal aging. The "stress-hormone" system seems vulnerable to a variety of noxious influences.

One psychological stress that has been looked at in humans is sexual abuse. An important study in progress appears to be pointing to a marked effect of childhood sexual abuse on the stress-hormone system. The National Institute of Mental Health has been following

160 girls, aged six to fifteen when the research began, who had in the prior six months been subjected to legally documented sexual abuse by a family member. Over a four-to-five-year follow-up period, these girls (as opposed to a group of girls matched for age, social class, presence of one or two parents in the home, and other factors) were found to have consistently higher-than-normal cortisol levels, disruption of the normal daily pattern of the rise and fall of cortisol levels, and exaggerated cortisol responses to stimulation. These disruptions of the stress-hormone system were correlated with high levels of depression in the abused girls, generally some years after the episodes of abuse. Early results indicate that abuse may even affect physical maturational changes in the abused girls.

This and other studies seem to make the rat model of "stress-hormone" dysfunction relevant to our understanding of human mood regulation. Taken together, the rat studies indicate that a variety of stressors can cause chemical and anatomical changes whose behavioral effects may not be apparent for some time.

● ● ●

The credibility of the kindling model has been further strengthened by studies of nonhuman primates, such as rhesus monkeys. Rhesus monkeys are of particular interest because they are our near neighbors genetically and they bond socially. Underappreciated for many years, research on mood in rhesus monkeys has attracted widespread attention recently, not least because monkeys manifest disturbances parallel to those that in humans respond to antidepressants.

The rhesus monkey (a type of macaque) shares over 90 percent —perhaps as high as 94 percent—of its unique segments of DNA with humans. Rhesus monkeys are, after humans, the most successful of the primates, in terms of their numbers, their distribution over the globe, and their ability to thrive in a host of settings from the jungle to the city. Highly social, rhesus monkeys travel in troops of twenty to one hundred or more members. Monkeys identify and interact on an individual basis with all other members of the troop. Infants are tied closely to their mothers in the first year, and they also rapidly become attached to their peers.

In the wild, rhesus monkeys are seasonal breeders who court and mate intensively over the same two-month period each year, so that babies are born in clusters; for the same reason, young monkeys are routinely deserted by their mothers at seven months, when breeding females again focus on courtship. The young monkeys respond to this separation with increased activity (perhaps searching for the mother) and what are called "coo" vocalizations. Some temporarily abandoned monkeys are "adopted" by older siblings. Others go on to display signs of distress, withdrawing and clasping themselves. No one looking at a photograph of such a monkey can miss the blank, defeated, hopeless look around the eyes. It seems rhesus monkeys are a species in which a particular stressor, separation, routinely, and in the natural setting, causes something very much like depression.

The best-known study of the effects of separation on monkey social development is an experiment by the pioneer animal ethologist Harry Harlow involving monkey infants separated from their mothers and exposed to wire-and-cloth "mother surrogates." Harlow demonstrated that warmth—a soft place to cling—is more crucial even than feeding in determining what an infant monkey will treat as a mother. In subsequent years, researchers have taken advantage of the social nature of rhesus monkeys to devise ever more complex observations of the effects of separation. Harlow's student and colleague, the psychologist Stephen J. Suomi, now director of the Laboratory of Comparative Ethology of the National Institute of Child Health and Human Development in Bethesda, Maryland, has extended Harlow's work in ways that bear directly on contemporary models of human depression.

It has long been known that rhesus infants reared apart from other monkeys for six months ("isolation-reared") will later exhibit pathological behavior, such as failure to explore or to affiliate socially when returned to the troop. As adults, isolation-reared monkeys may be inappropriately aggressive toward other monkeys; if they bear children, the females are likely to be neglectful or even abusive mothers, especially toward their firstborn. (To a psychiatrist who has seen a number of abused or neglected firstborn children, these findings have an eerie resonance.) It is clear that severe stress in infancy and childhood can produce major changes in monkeys' adult social behavior. But isolation-reared monkeys may seem too grossly disturbed to illuminate the more common minor disorders we see in humans.

Suomi has studied ever more subtle forms of separation stress. In particular, he has observed monkeys who were "hand-reared" (reared by humans, in the presence of inanimate surrogate "mothers") for the first thirty days of life. The hand-reared monkeys are then united with age-mates and later with a larger mixed troop. Such "peer-reared" monkeys look behaviorally normal throughout. Except for thumb-sucking, they show none of the abnormal behavior of infants raised in isolation. Peer-reared monkeys engage in normal social activities at every age, except that they cling to their peers longer than mother-reared monkeys cling to their mothers. The peer-reared monkeys are also somewhat more timid and slow to explore than are mother-reared monkeys. None of these differences is dramatic. Compared with isolation-reared monkeys, peer-reared monkeys have been only relatively deprived, and their behavior overlaps generously with the behavior of normals. Such aberrant behavior as exists tends to disappear with time. Peer-reared monkeys are, in effect, near-normal monkeys with a history of moderate trauma.

In Suomi's critical experiments, both peer-reared and mother-reared monkeys are subjected yearly to repeated social separation—housing in individual cages for four four-day periods—at a variety of ages (six, eighteen, and thirty months, and so on). When peer- and mother-reared monkeys who have lived in the same social group are separated from that group, they behave differently, the peer-reared monkeys showing more signs of distress and withdrawal. These include signs generally assumed to be related to depression (passivity, distress vocalizations, and such self-directed behaviors as huddling and rocking) and signs more related to compulsiveness or anxiety (self-directed behaviors such as excessive grooming and picking, as well as other repetitive stereotyped behaviors). Even though peer-reared monkeys act normal between separations, each subsequent separation elicits a greater variety and intensity of depression-related behavior.

The monkeys' biochemical reactions also show progressive deterioration over time. At the age of six months, the peer-reared monkeys, on separation, show higher levels of cortisol and more abnormal indicators of norepinephrine activity than do monkeys reared by their own mothers. At eighteen months, the biochemical distress indicators are more pronounced, and now markers for serotonin activity, which had previously been the same between the two groups, are abnormal in the peer-reared monkeys. "Moreover, the same basic pattern of more extreme behavioral and physiological response to separation in peer-reared monkeys was continued during subsequent annual separations," Suomi writes, though "there were few, if any, significant rearing condition differences during periods of stable group housing as the monkeys passed through puberty and into early adulthood."

Suomi's experiment produces in young rhesus monkeys a phenomenon that has a good deal in common with rejection-sensitivity, kindling, and the stress model of depression. Suomi's peer-raised monkeys are, under ordinary circumstances, not depressed. They may at first appear a bit more timid and clinging than mother-reared monkeys, but even that behavior is within the normal range and short-lived. However, upon subsequent separation, these monkeys are more likely than mother-raised troop-mates to show behavioral signs of mood disorder and biological changes in the relevant hormone and neurotransmitter systems. Moreover, as in Post's rapid-cycling patients and kindled rats, each "depressive" episode is more complex, both behaviorally and biologically, than the preceding one. This kindled rejection-sensitivity occurs in response not to externally applied electric current but, rather, to the sort of stressor we know affects humans—disruption of important social bonds.

What happens to monkeys who are stressed early and then not restressed for a substantial time? It turns out that discrete trauma can sensitize animals for long periods, even in the absence of repeated challenges. A brief separation from the mother early in life—one or two six-day periods at thirty to thirty-two weeks of age—followed by a reunion and normal parenting predisposes young monkeys to an enhanced response to separation *two to three years later,* even in the absence of intervening abnormal stressors. Like the repeatedly separated monkeys, monkeys who have been subjected only to a brief separation from their mothers look largely normal in subsequent months, except for subtle evidence of social inhibition. (Though they are as ready as other monkeys to approach strange objects in a familiar environment, they will approach strange objects less readily in a strange environment.) But their protest and despair responses to later separation are heightened. What would appear to be a modest social stress, albeit at a critical period, produces a minor but long-standing change in personality style, and a vulnerability to separation that is highly reminiscent of rejection-sensitivity in humans.

The three models we have discussed interconnect. The kindling model implies that at least one sort of depression is a progressive condition, biologically encoded long before it manifests itself in the form of overt episodes. The stress research in rats implies that a variety of psychosocial stressors can serve as triggers for this insidious encoding. And the monkey-separation studies show what animals look like early in the course of stress-induced kindling: except for transient, minor social inhibition (anxiety in the face of novelty), they appear normal in ordinary social circumstances; but they have a heightened sensitivity to loss.

•   •   •

It is possible to argue that animal models should not influence the way we see mood patterns in humans, but there is no denying that the response of monkeys to early trauma bears a striking resemblance to patterns of behavior in certain patients we have met. The patients are normal in their everyday behavior and feeling states. They are, however, prone to extreme discomfort—minor variants of depression, anxiety, and compulsiveness—in response to social stressors. These patients may also be socially inhibited (just as the monkeys are timid or anxious in the face of novelty), perhaps not in an extreme fashion that is obvious to others, but enough so that their private social dealings are affected. Some of these patients have experienced social disruption early in life; others have not. Certainly the notion of functional autonomy—of a biologically sustained disorder of mood reactivity—in people who have suffered dramatic losses early in life gains credibility from analogous animal models that extend from the level of social behavior to that of chemical functioning within the individual brain cell.

The animal models seem to say that pain has its price, even for those in whom trauma does not produce major depression. The victim carries his scars. Indeed, the vagaries of life being what they are, we all bear scars. We should not expect any clear line of division, then, between health and the early stages of illness. Very likely, a good many of us are in the early stages of kindled depression. The only question is whether good fortune or ongoing processes of protection or repair will save us from suffering a full-blown course of illness.

What distinguishes this view of depression from, say, traditional psychoanalytic models is the recognition that the scars are not, or not only, in cognitive memory. It is not merely a question of inner conflict or of "growing up": "Stop fussing over what your parents did to you!" as skeptics command patients in therapy. The scar consists of changed anatomy and chemistry within the brain. Some of that brain change *is* memory: presumably recollected thought and emotion are encoded in ways that bear resemblance to the kindling model. But another part of that change is "functionally autonomous" emotional sensitivity, even vulnerability to quite serious emotional disorder.

Psychological theories have long held that personality is largely the expression of "defenses"—that is, characteristic ways of avoiding awareness of inner conflict. By adding the concept of functional autonomy, we are saying that defenses, and therefore the whole array of character armor, are not mobilized only against inner conflict but also against the likelihood of further pain from injury in the social world, a type of pain to which certain people have been biologically sensitized. And part of what we consider personality—the part corresponding to traumatized monkeys' reluctance to explore—may be directly encoded by trauma.

A parsimonious, though not entirely comfortable, way of describing these events is to expand our concept of memory. We readily accept the notion of cognitive and emotional, or at least emotion-laden, memory. But perhaps sensitivity is memory as well—"the memory of the body," as we might say "the wisdom of the body." In this sense, social inhibition and rejection-sensitivity are both memory. That is, they do not *stem from* a (cognitive, emotion-laden, conflicted) memory of trauma; they represent or just *are* memories of trauma. According to this way of thinking, much of who Lucy is— her neural pathways, her social needs—constitutes a biological memory of her mother's murder, just as Tess's social style is a memory of her precociously responsible childhood.

The separation, stress, and kindling models have pronounced implications for treatment of a variety of psychological conditions. If minor depression is an early stage of a kindled disorder—the period of latency between a sensitizing injury and overt illness—then continued depression, not to mention further stress or loss, will be dangerous to mental health. It is possible that minor depression can lead to mood disorders, like recurrent depression, manic depression, and even rapid cycling, that are difficult to influence. People to whom medication has been prescribed often express concern over unknown side effects, and this concern is understandable. There are instances in which taking medication has had terrible unanticipated consequences. What is less appreciated, especially in the case of mental health, are the unanticipatable consequences of failure to treat. Living with rejection-sensitivity and inevitably sustaining a series of perceived losses may lead to continued and worsening injury, further enhanced sensitivity, and even severe depression. Living with the sort of personality style that leads to repeated social failure may, beyond the pain caused to self and others, entail health risks.

Kindling studies have already affected the way some psychiatrists treat recurrent depression. Rather than take patients off medication as each episode of depression or mania ends, psychiatrists tend more and more to maintain patients on medication, sometimes indefinitely, once they have experienced a certain number of episodes within a brief period of time. This new method of treating recurrent depression is becoming widespread even in the face of evidence that antidepressants can set off episodes of mania in vulnerable people. The kindling model of recurrent depression as a dangerous progressive illness is coming to dominate within the profession.

•   •   •

Our interest here is in chronic low-level unhappiness or recurrent minor periods of demoralization, rather than in major depression. Just how the kindling, stress, and separation models ought to influence treatment of these near-normal conditions is not yet clear. No one advocates long-term antidepressant treatment for people who have had a single episode of major depression. But the question of how vigorously to treat low-level depression has suddenly been made more pertinent with the availability of new medicine that has more tolerable side effects.

A small body of evidence indicates that selective serotonin-reuptake inhibitors such as Prozac may be particularly effective for mild chronic and recurrent depression—the sort of depression that looks like the early stages of a kindled disorder. SSRIs may even be to depression what Valium is to kindled epilepsy, a specific treatment for the early stage of a kindled disorder.

Some of the evidence is indirect: SSRIs look just about as effective as tricyclics, like imipramine, in treating mildly depressed patients, primarily outpatients; but studies of severe depression—for instance, a large series of patients treated at a consortium of universities in Denmark—show that for *hospitalized* depressed patients SSRIs are substantially *less* effective than tricyclics.

It is difficult to show medication effect in minor mental illness, because so many subjects will improve spontaneously over the course of any study. A group at Indiana University has approached this problem by looking beyond response rates to the *pattern* of recovery of mildly depressed patients given either Prozac or a placebo. A sizable number of patients given placebo improved, as did a larger number of patients given Prozac. What distinguished the groups was the quality of response. The Prozac-treated group included many more patients who got *very substantially better* and *maintained* their improvement. The researchers concluded that, even if mildly depressed patients improve early in treatment (say, with psychotherapy), those whose improvement is not dramatic or does not persist should be considered for medication with an SSRI.

Finally, there is evidence that the type of depression being treated makes a difference. Psychiatrists at the University of Utah looked at a series of moderately depressed patients treated with antidepressants. The groups treated with imipramine and Prozac did about equally well. But those in the imipramine group who recovered tended to be patients with a clear-cut first episode of major depression. Those who did well in the Prozac-treated group were people with a chronic low-level course of depression or with "mixed chronic and episodic histories."

Taken together, these studies suggest that, whereas drugs like imipramine are more effective in major depression, drugs like Prozac have a special role in the treatment of minor depressive illness. If this sort of research holds up, we may find that SSRIs can help prevent the progression of early mood disorder into florid illness. It is at least possible that we will some day advocate early detection of depression the way we now advocate early detection of cancer or hypertension, and that treatment of nearly normal conditions will become standard preventive medicine.

• • •

Of course, the appropriate treatment for these normal or near-normal depressive states might be psychotherapy. Perhaps what is learned one way can be relearned another, and the memories created by psychotherapy will affect neural structure as well.

There is only a small literature on animal recovery from injury, most of it involving medication. Antidepressants or anticonvulsants can block the deleterious effects of the various sorts of stress we have discussed, from electric shock to separation, but whether they can induce or permit healing is not known.

The most influential animal study of social healing concerns separation-reared monkeys, the monkeys raised apart from troop and mother for six months, who typically grow into aggressive, abusive, socially isolative adults. The effects of separation from the mother can be lessened by exposing separation-reared young monkeys to other young monkeys, in a variety of formats. For instance, if separation-reared young monkeys are exposed to "therapists"—younger (because the isolated monkeys would fight with age-mates), troop-reared monkeys—they will within weeks accept invitations to play, then initiate play, and subsequently engage in normal social behavior whether or not the "therapist" monkeys are present. Indeed, the "rehabilitated" monkeys will display normal behavior through adolescence and adulthood, except when stressed. When stressed, the rehabilitated monkeys will briefly show abnormal self-directed behavior (for instance, clasping or sucking themselves), even if they have not shown such behavior for months—a sign of residual effects

127

of early deprivation in these otherwise behaviorally normal adults.

These various animal studies depict mood disorder as a direct consequence of trauma. The precise nature of the trauma seems unimportant. In rats, a variety of stressors will reliably raise cortisol levels. In rhesus monkeys, separation, especially early in life, is a special stressor, regardless of the details of the separation experience. The resultant disorder presumably does not arise from unconscious conflict between incompatible ideas; it is a straightforward biological injury, one that can be made to reappear, in ever more severe form, by subsequent stress. In order for (partial) recovery to take place, what the animal needs is a certain sort of restabilizing—remothering, a chance to model social skills, and a return to social integration.

If we turn to psychotherapy with humans, evidence from animal studies casts a favorable light on certain sorts of reparative work. For instance, throughout the middle decades of this century, the great hypnotist Milton Erickson practiced a psychotherapy in which he specifically avoided helping patients understand why they were neurotically stuck. Instead, he devised cunning strategies to catapult patients into age-appropriate successful social behavior. (When he encountered a vigorous young patient who claimed he was Jesus Christ, Erickson put him to work as a carpenter; the point was never to understand the delusion but, rather, to help the young person fit in socially.) This therapy-without-insight can be seen as a series of techniques for reuniting a traumatized and socially self-defeating person with the peer group.

Cognitive therapy, lately much in vogue, helps patients reframe environmental stimuli—redefining what is to be perceived as rejection, expanding the definition of "home"—so that sensitive or anxious patients avert their characteristic "functionally autonomous" responses. The cognition that the therapy reshapes is not unconscious inner conflict, but the definition of the trigger for demoralization.

Within psychotherapy, the variants that best take into account animal models of attachment and separation are those that emphasize empathy, more than insight, as the crucial tool in treatment, in effect giving patients the kind of careful, attentive parenting they lacked in early life. Such therapies assume that patients will always remain dependent on social supports.

By contrast, in classical psychoanalysis the goal of treatment is independence, and the method of cure is understanding of the details of individual development. There is nothing in the animal models that speaks directly against the tenets of classical psychoanalysis. Indeed, Freudian analysis can be seen as a therapy obsessed with a particular memory of separation, namely the Oedipus conflict, in which the five-year-old boy buries his sexual desire for his mother out of fear of his punitive father. But infantile sexuality, so crucial to Freud's view of the Oedipal stage, is unimportant in the animal models. And even if one sees the Oedipus conflict as a struggle over separation—the son's realization that he can no longer cleave to the mother—fear of the father seems irrelevant. (For monkeys, separation from the mother is traumatic, but it occurs in the absence of any significant relationship between offspring and father.) The whole notion of inner conflict—in this case, of desire thwarted by fear— is alien to the animal models. Mere repeated separation, followed by social stress later in life, is sufficient to produce not only indecisiveness and compulsiveness (which *look* in the adult human like products of inner conflict) but also anxiety and depression. And the notion that interpretation of conflict is curative finds no equivalent in the animal literature.

Much of this reasoning is, of course, circular. If you look to monkeys as a model for human psychotherapy, you will necessarily end in attending to issues of social integration and reparenting while devaluing the role of insight. Monkeys do travel in troops, and they don't respond to dream interpretation. Here is a distant form of listening to drugs: the success of medication makes animal models more attractive, and then the animal models shape our view of human behavior in a way that makes our uniquely human functions, such as symbolic reasoning, seem less important.

Beyond psychotherapy, animal research throws into question the validity of specific diagnoses for minor mental disorder. Traits of depression, anxiety, compulsiveness, and social inhibition are thoroughly mixed in the repeatedly separated monkeys. These monkeys are vulnerable to depression, but they are also abnormally anxious in the face of certain challenges. They engage in stereotyped behavior, such as insistent self-grooming, reminiscent of compulsive human behavior, like hand-washing. And, in other studies, they prove themselves, more than their untraumatized peers, prone to repeated alcohol consumption in response to stress. Like neurotics, these monkeys have "not specialized" in terms of their psychic vulnerability; depending on circumstance, they are liable to symptoms associated with a variety of illnesses that the current diagnostic system considers discrete. And the neural-transmitter pathways that are out of kilter in each of these symptom complexes appear to be similar, whether the illness is depression or compulsivity or addiction, and whether the animal under study is rat, rhesus, or man.

This welter of animal observations has colored the way I see certain patients who respond to Prozac. The animal models imply that a number of environmental factors, including stress, and perhaps especially the stress of social separation, can give rise to changes in the brain that then predispose the animal to ever more poorly modulated responses to subsequent stress. These changes can take place in animals, and presumably people, whose mood and behavior seem normal under ordinary circumstances. Such near-normal conditions may constitute the early stage of a progressive deteriorating condition; and the subtle collection of abnormalities may persist in a stable way over substantial periods of time, even in the absence of renewed gross trauma. Further deterioration may be lessened by certain forms of social contact. The animal models do not tell us whether medication can reverse injury, but they imply it can confer a protective effect against the consequences of further trauma. The animal models give "functional autonomy" a good name and make medication for "neurosis," and even for quite normal forms of chronic unhappiness, seem a reasonable option, perhaps a highly compassionate one.

•   •   •

It would be interesting to know how low-level, chronic disturbances of mood relate to abnormalities in serotonin. The animal studies give no consistent answer. Scientific understanding of the connection between affect and the biogenic amines—norepinephrine and serotonin—is in particular disarray just now, because Prozac has scuttled a very appealing theory that promised to connect events at the level of cell-to-cell communication to the chronic mood states of stressed mammals.

The biogenic-amine theory—the hypothesis that depression results from a deficiency of norepinephrine and serotonin—has had a series of differing incarnations. In the mid-1960s, it was thought that low norepinephrine levels cause depression. By the mid-1970s, the prevailing theory held that there are two kinds of depression: one related to abnormalities in norepinephrine, the other to abnormalities in serotonin.

But inadequacies in these theories—for instance, the observation that depressions that look as though they relate to serotonin sometimes respond to medicines, like desipramine, that work via norepinephrine—caused researchers in the 1980s to take a new slant on the amine hypothesis. They began to focus less on cells that *transmit* signals—the neurons thought to be depleted of serotonin or norepinephrine—and more on the downstream cells that *receive* signals. These cells are called postsynaptic neurons, because they sit on the far side of the synapse, or gap between cells, into which the transmitting cell releases neurotransmitter. According to the new theory, the common abnormality in depressions is an alteration in the sensitivity of the postsynaptic (receiving) neuron. In depressed patients and stressed animals, the theory held, these postsynaptic neurons have sprouted too many norepinephrine receptors. (The receptor is a molecular-level structure on the cell membrane to which the norepinephrine temporarily attaches, thus producing its effect on the cell.) The hypersensitive postsynaptic neuron overreacts to normal levels of neurotransmitter. This is a chronic abnormality; the receiving cell remains hypersensitive whether the animal is depressed or not.

The postsynaptic-hypersensitivity model meshes well with the animal studies we have discussed. The animal models say that stress affects the anatomy of the brain—and the new amine theory points to structural changes in the receiving cell. The receiving cells' chronic hypersensitivity to norepinephrine corresponds nicely to traumatized animals' chronic sensitivity to stress, even between episodes of depression.

The theory also explained patients' sometimes confusing responses to the "wrong" antidepressant. Pharmacologic studies demonstrate that tricyclic antidepressants—whether they block the reuptake of serotonin or of norepinephrine—"downregulate" the postsynaptic neuron in terms of response to norepinephrine.

The postsynaptic-hypersensitivity model is dynamic: mood is set by the relationship between the amount of neurotransmitter present in the transmitting cell and the number of receptors available on the receiving cell. In simplified terms, the working model goes like this: Acute stress causes such an outpouring of neurotransmitters that in time the transmitting cell is depleted. The receiving cell then becomes starved of transmitter, so it sprouts excessive numbers of norepinephrine receptors (in order to soak up every last bit of the scarce neurotransmitter). The animal or person now has too many norepinephrine receptors. Transmitter levels may rise and fall depending on stress, but the receiving cells remain chronically overexcitable. In the resting state, the level of transmitter is low, because the brain compensates for the hypersensitive receiving cells by diminishing amine production; but because of the postsynaptic hypersensitivity, the compensation may be imperfect to the point where the animal or person is always a little depressed or anxious, as well as vulnerable to catastrophic inner responses to stress.

The postsynaptic-hypersensitivity model explained the action of tricyclic antidepressants. Antidepressants make more amine available in the synapse, and they do so in a sustained way. At first, the patient receiving the antidepressant may feel a bit jumpy, as if on amphetamine—because the receptor-rich receiving cells have been revved up by newly increased levels of stimulus. But as the increased neurotransmitter level in the synapse persists (under the constant drive of the medication), the receiving cell is bombarded into submission. The chronic, constant, reliable presence of high levels of neurotransmitter causes the cell to "downregulate"—reducing the number of receptors, by drawing them back into the cell membrane, where they become inactive, or by otherwise uncoupling them from further events.

But, like the other versions of the amine theory before it, the postsynaptic-hypersensitivity model proved to be wrong. Many flaws have been found with the theory; the strongest in political terms is that Prozac does not downregulate norepinephrine receptors. It is hard to hold to a model of depression that does not fit one of the most widespread contemporary forms of treatment. If there is a final common pathway to depression, it is almost certainly downstream from the receptor—perhaps inside the receiving cell, in the sites where the biological concomitants of learning take place.

But the postsynaptic-hypersensitivity model remains influential in one way: it has focused attention on the chronic changes in state that persist in patients who have been traumatized or who have suffered discrete depressions. Henceforth, any interesting account of depression will need to say something about how the brains of injured people look between acute episodes, when they appear to be functioning well but remain exceedingly vulnerable to stress.

No single theory is able to encompass the vast and complicated body of experiments regarding the cellular basis of depression. As one of the pharmacologists who developed Prozac said to me, given the limits of our current stage of scientific knowledge, "If the human brain were simple enough for us to understand, we would be too simple to understand it."

● ● ●

At the cellular level, there is a kind of standoff. We have a number of inadequate models, most centered on norepinephrine, and we have a highly successful medication, Prozac, that works via the serotonin system. Not long ago, I attended a state-of-the-art conference on chemical correlates of animal models of depression. At the end of the first day of meetings, there was a cocktail party to honor the participants, and I had a chance to speak informally with a man who has worked for decades in this area. I asked him if he has an image of serotonin that guides his research.

The meeting was held in a medical school that sits uneasily within a tough urban area. The researcher waved his drink at me and said something like this:

"Maybe serotonin is the police. The police aren't in one place—they're not in the police station. They are a presence everywhere. They are cruising the city—they are right here. Their potential presence makes you feel secure. It allows you to do many things that also make you feel secure. If you don't have enough police, all sorts of things can happen. You may have riots. The absence of police does not cause riots. But if you do have a riot, and you don't have police, there is nothing to stop the riot from spreading."

Although it fails to explain much of what is known about the biochemistry of mood, I like the model of serotonin-as-police. Yes, serotonin is known to affect sleep, appetite, and the like. But, most dramatically, raising the level of serotonin seems to enhance security, courage, assertiveness, self-worth, calm, flexibility, resilience. Serotonin sets tone. As the researcher at the cocktail party implied, serotonin may not have much to do with depression at all, even though in its absence depression is more likely, and in its presence depression can disappear. Serotonin-as-police goes a way toward explaining why Prozac should be so effective in minor depression, and relatively less effective in major depression. In minor depression, a feeling of security goes a long way; in major depression, a more specific cure is called for. Serotonin-as-police also addresses Prozac's effectiveness in so many different disorders. Panic anxiety, for instance, may be caused by dysregulation of nerves that work via norepinephrine—but a sense of security, induced by adequate serotonin levels, may prevent panic anxiety from ever emerging. More generally, many things will go right when an animal, including a human animal, feels safe.

●　　●　　●

However promising the research, it is hard to leave a conference on the neurobiology of depression with a feeling of optimism. It seems that the neural pathways are like the joints in the musculoskeletal system. They are worn down over the years by inevitable trauma. If you injure your knee when young, you can perhaps compensate— stabilize the joint—by increasing the strength of the thigh muscles. But repeated injury, and even ordinary wear and tear, or age alone, may weaken the quadriceps to the point where compensation for the old injury is no longer possible.

Age alone seems a trauma in the cortisol model; the system deteriorates over time. The implication seems to be that if we live long enough we will all become depressed, just as we lose resilience in our skin, muscle, and bones. Perhaps we all wage a lifelong struggle against depression, even though those who are blessed with happy childhoods, peppy serotonin systems, and stable adult lives may never feel the effects of the growing dysfunction in their neural connections. There may be mechanisms of repair in these neural systems, ways to learn or relearn resilience. Then again, there is no good biochemical model of repair, only of injury prevention and of compensation. A good many of us may live in compensated states of depression, like the recovered patients on Prozac or MAOI who have become depressed within hours of having their serotonin depleted, perhaps not because their depression is "serotonergic" but because without the police the interrupted riot resumes.

Certainly the rate of suicide increases with age. Compulsiveness, worry, emotional rigidity, a tendency toward catastrophic reactions to stress—these are popularly understood to increase as well. But there is one disputed clinical phenomenon that seems to me to mesh especially well with the view that depression can be a condition of insidious chronic deterioration. I have in mind "late-onset depression," the distinctive mood disorder of those who first experience depression after age sixty.

People who have been healthy all their lives, if they fall prey to depression in old age, tend to be more anxious, hypochondriacal, apathetic, self-reproachful, and suicidal than elderly patients whose first episode of depression occurred early. Like other elderly people who become depressed, late-onset depressives are likely to be more severely depressed, and more often psychotic, than younger adults with depression. But, unlike other elderly depressives, those with late-onset depression stand out in terms of the normality of their background and even their current functioning. Compared with early-onset elderly depressives, late-onset patients are more likely to have normal personality traits, healthy interpersonal relationships, psychologically healthy relatives, and lower levels of recent loss or trauma. The picture of late-onset depression is of a person with no distinctive previous signs of mental illness who suddenly and inexplicably experiences severe depression in which worrisome features, such as the urge to commit suicide, are prominent.

Though the idea of late-onset depression is compatible with the theory that mood-stabilizing systems deteriorate over time, it seems to conflict with the notion of kindling. We might imagine that first episodes of depression, whenever in life they occur, should on average be mild. Yet here is a previously healthy group of people under an ordinary amount of stress who in their first episode of mental disorder suffer the most terrible sort of melancholy. Serotonin-as-police appeals to me as a way of understanding the severity of late-onset depression. Perhaps what we are seeing is a person whose depression-related neural systems (involving, maybe, cortisol or norepinephrine) have deteriorated over time, but whose resilience-related systems (involving, say, serotonin) have been so effective that quite extensive damage has been effectively masked. When the ordinary losses of old age arrive, a final straw—perhaps a very minor stressor, perhaps further age-related erosion of one or another neural network—causes the protective effects of the resilience system to falter, and extensive silent damage is revealed in a sudden and frightening alteration of mood and behavior.

I want to introduce a patient whose first depression occurred late in life, to show how animal and cellular models of mental illness can color the way we see the person in front of us—and the way we see the long near-normal period that precedes overt deterioration.

Daniel is a distinguished scholar who, in his middle sixties, retired from his university post in order to pursue research in fields beyond the narrow boundaries of his academic discipline. His wife, also a scholar, retired in the same year, and at first they both were happy in what seemed an ideal life, spending more time at their vacation house, attending national and international conferences in their professions, and moving ahead on long-postponed writing projects. Daniel, however, suffered from a debilitating flutter of the heart that proved so difficult to treat that he intermittently required brief hospitalizations. Only after much experimentation with combinations of cardiac drugs was the abnormal rhythm contained. Then, suddenly, he became depressed. Anxiety overcame him frequently and left in its wake a sense of depletion of spirit. His mind was filled with foreboding, he felt pangs of guilt that attached themselves to a variety of past events, and he wished for death, spending hours wondering how he could make it come about and not hurt his wife.

This depression did not abate, and in time Daniel was referred to me. He spoke with me for some time before mentioning the events of his adolescence. Born to a German Jewish father and a French Catholic mother, he had spent months early in World War II in a concentration camp—his family was able to buy him out—and later in hiding, and finally in a Swiss internment center. He had many terrible memories. But he had been young and resourceful. In the postwar period, he met an American relief worker, whom he adored, and moved to this country with her. She was assertive and dominant. He had always been rather shy. Despite his successful career, he spent the marriage in his wife's shadow. He had no history of depression —nor had anyone in his family—but he had sometimes felt vulnerable in a hard-to-define way, and he had restricted or circumscribed his life in response. He had chosen to have no children, partly out of a sense that children bring unmanageable disorder, but also because of his wartime experiences and his and his wife's careers. These inhibited aspects of the self were, he felt, minor. He had formed many friendships, was well liked by students, and was seen as an approachable and nurturant teacher, a productive and original scholar.

Daniel was crushed by the onset of palpitations. They seemed to him a constant reminder of death, and he had too many horrifying memories of deaths. In the face of the threat of death, he felt infinitely vulnerable, even though other illnesses earlier in life had not elicited this reaction. The recent hospitalizations, too, were traumatic, carrying overtones, as they did, of previous confinements. In this sense, Daniel's deterioration was understandable, and one could imagine other fruitful lines of inquiry as well. How had retirement affected him? Had extra hours with his still-dominant wife aroused resentment that conflicted with his belief that he owed her a debt of gratitude? And so forth.

Sitting with Daniel, I was struck most by the sense of depletion.

He seemed hollow, a man utterly without resources. His accomplishments, his family, his friends meant nothing. He had been emptied out, and what was left was exquisitely fragile. I had no sense of a struggle within, only of terror and exhaustion.

My first thoughts concerned medicine: perhaps a change in the cardiac regimen would reveal that one of the heart drugs had caused or contributed to the depression. But the balance here was so delicate that the cardiologist was reluctant to consider any change, nor was Daniel willing to risk the least chance that the arrhythmia might return. As an alternative, I suggested antidepressant medication, but this choice also was unacceptable. Daniel was unwilling to take any medication that would affect his mind, and, despite a cautious green light from the cardiologist, Daniel developed an almost delusional fear that antidepressants would make his heartbeat impossible to control. The antidepressant pills became an object for phobic and obsessional concern; he would carry a small number in his pocket and spend hours debating whether to take them, and then he would blame himself for his cowardice. Alternatives in these circumstances are electroconvulsive shock—it presents little risk to the heart, and sometimes it obviates the need for antidepressant medication—or hospitalization. I was reluctant even to raise these possibilities with my patient, and when at last I did, I discovered why. Daniel almost did not return to my office; the mere mention of these procedures made him see me as a sadist and a jailer.

One might imagine that this stalemate would resolve itself, but it did not. Daniel remained on the verge of suicide, unwilling to change his cardiac regimen, unwilling to risk a biological approach to his depression. And so we talked. I tried to create a setting in which this gentle, perceptive scholar could feel safe, in which he could discuss memories, fears, anger, grief. (The emphasis on safety before insight, in my therapy with Daniel, may already reveal my acceptance of a psychobiological model of damage and cure.) This approach was of some use. The relentless depression lifted and was replaced by a waxing and waning condition in which Daniel had days and sometimes weeks in which he felt normal. These good periods never lasted long, nor did Daniel seem to me entirely free of depression even at his best. He had a warm, lively, impish quality that now and then, pentimento-style, showed through the dense depression— a glimpse of how he would appear if well. Nothing we did restored him entirely, though in time he was able, as before, to write and publish, attend meetings, and travel.

Having seen other instances of late-onset depression (for I believe the category represents a useful distinction and that Daniel was suffering a representative case), I was not surprised by this chain of events. My image of the patient's inner state had disappointingly little to do with cognition and memory. I saw these terrible late years in an exemplary life as a consequence of the long-acting poison of trauma. That is to say, my sense of the patient was dominated by the animal and cellular models of depression. Here was a man whose hormone and neurotransmitter systems were battered by terrible inescapable stress early in life. Various compensatory mechanisms—and now I am alluding to biological compensation as well as defenses like repression, sublimation, reaction formation, and intellectualization —allowed him to lead a rather normal life throughout middle adulthood. But the covert progressive deterioration continued.

Although I am talking in highly speculative terms, my version of events corresponds to the consensus view of deterioration and overt disease held by scientists who work on the stress and kindling models in animals. Differing sources of damage can cause deleterious changes that may remain hidden, or only intermittently apparent, as long as they can be compensated for in a variety of ways. But there comes a day when compensation fails, and catastrophic changes in mood and behavior suddenly appear. (Indeed, we might guess that the stronger the individual is—and the more adept, biologically and psychologically, at compensation—the greater will be the extent of previously masked injury when the break finally occurs.) There are many examples in medicine of biological systems that can suffer major damage that remains inapparent. We survive easily with one kidney or the smallest fraction of working liver. But finally the balance is tipped, and the overwhelming damage is revealed all at once.

Certainly for Daniel the palpitations represented a new stressor, as did the brief hospitalizations. The immediate experience was traumatic, and it revived painful memories. We are symbol-centered creatures, and some of our worst stresses are symbolic. But to my mind these final causes were like the pebbles that finally turn a tenuously balanced collection of rocks into an avalanche. I had only a weak faith that repositioning the pebbles would cause the boulders to roll back up the mountain.

Daniel's own preference was to discuss his memories, a choice I would ordinarily welcome: what better way to treat depression than to explore its sources in repressed images of terror and suffering? But I found myself, in terms of my loyalty to the precepts of psychotherapy, something of an agnostic priest. Now that I had been exposed to the concept of progressive damage to transmitter systems, it no longer seemed as likely to me that re-examination of the events of half a century ago would reverse Daniel's catastrophic depression. I did try treating Daniel with psychotherapy. But as I sat with him, I was mostly struck by a sense that the biological underpinnings for mood had been badly weakened, and that what we were dealing with went so far beyond cognition that the patient's preference for psychological cures—for courage, for fortitude, perhaps for the very qualities that had permitted him to survive in earlier years—was now serving him ill.

I present this case as an example of the way in which the availability of medication, and the medication-supported predominance of biological models, influences the way we are likely to frame a human predicament. How extraordinary it is to see the depression of a concentration-camp survivor as finally a physiological event. It is conventional to call such an approach "reductionist," as if seeing mood and behavior in psychobiological terms diminished the person's humanity, and seeing them in purely psychological terms aggrandized or at least properly acknowledged that humanity. But I wonder if this dichotomy is always apt.

I am thinking of the late-life suicide of another concentration-camp survivor, the peerless writer Primo Levi. After his incarceration in Auschwitz, Levi, a paint chemist, returned to his native Italy and began writing essays, short stories, and novels of the Holocaust and its moral conundrums, all in an unerringly humane voice. Though he recognized the randomness of survival, he stood, through his person as well as his writerly persona, for hope, perseverance, and survival. It therefore came as a shock—even a personal injury—to his friends and his readers when, in 1987, he killed himself at the age of sixty-seven. So unwilling was a distant friend of Levi's—a British cardiologist who had met and corresponded with him—to acknowledge the suicide that he wrote an article propounding a theory by which the death could be seen as accidental. Levi's family declined to comment on his death, but certain facts are widely accepted. Levi was being treated for depression; his antidepressant regimen had recently been changed; his mother, to whom he remained close, had become ill; and he had recovered from minor surgery not long before his death.

Levi's suicide is hard to accept because it seems a failure of will. It disappoints us to think that human beings, especially those who have become icons, are not infinitely resilient—that they should change their minds and turn pessimistic and hopeless. To me, there is a sense in which the animal models, and the concept of late-onset depression, make Levi's suicide less shocking, less unexpected, more human; they may even enhance our appreciation of Levi's hardiness, in the face of the physiological forces tending to pull him toward dysfunction. The concentration camp attacks not just the soul but the animal part of man—attacks the soul largely through the animal. In this case, and in many others, we might want to say that biological models are not reductionistic but humanizing, in the sense that they restore scale and perspective and take into account the vast part of us that is not intellect.

The kindling model has the power to influence the way we see a range of mood states rooted in trauma, from Levi's suicidal depression to Lucy's sensitivity and Tess's seriousness. But how are we to understand the quite similar emotional difficulties of people—Sam, Gail, Julia—whose lives are devoid of dramatic losses and whose personality traits can be traced back to their earliest years? Here, too, medication response—especially that most puzzling phenomenon, the reshaping of personality traits by medication—may lead us to attend to a series of experiments and hypotheses it might otherwise have been easy to ignore.

6

Risk

Two of my patients entered into marriages while taking Prozac. The first, a constitutionally sunny woman who found herself increasingly withdrawn in the years following her divorce from an erratic husband, rediscovered on medication the vigor and confidence she needed to rejoin the life of her community. This result, though gratifying, was perhaps unremarkable. But the second patient was a woman who had since early childhood stood at the periphery of the social universe. For her, marriage was an extraordinary achievement, a sign of victory over a crippling aspect of the self.

Sally had been temperamentally shy for as long as she could remember. As a young child, she never left her mother's side. She needed to be coaxed to talk even to family members, and she was always uncomfortable in conversation. Except for walking to school, she spent little time with girlfriends, and she avoided boys entirely. Throughout grade school, she was afraid of her teachers and would vomit breakfast every morning. At night, she was prone to fears of darkness, witches, and death.

Sally's parents, who were themselves quiet and inward-looking —prone to depression and a variety of physical ailments—did not find her behavior remarkable. They were easily overwhelmed and intolerant of upset or intrusions. They expected Sally, from an early age, to care for her youngest sister, to behave while listening to adult conversation, and to socialize only at church and family functions.

This limited social circle did not protect Sally from trauma. Entering puberty, she was for a number of months sexually violated by an uncle who had heretofore treated her as a favorite niece. When Sally was twelve, her family suffered financial reverses. They moved into cramped quarters, where Sally was exposed to her parents' sexual behavior, an experience that left her troubled about her mother's submissiveness. Sally worried that the family would have another baby for her to tend.

By junior high school, Sally had come to feel that other children were more sophisticated than she, although she now was able to participate in group activities with girls. Sally's social inhibition did not prevent certain boys from telephoning her in high school, but the family discouraged dating and forbade makeup. Though she loved dancing, in all of high school Sally was allowed to attend only two dances, on chaperoned double dates.

After high school, Sally took an entry-level job at a large bank. At first she received promotions, but she remained afraid of entering a management position and soon was taken for granted and passed over by her superiors. She never had conflicts with her co-workers, but they kept their distance, because Sally seemed not to know how to act, have fun, or judge social limits. She stayed at the same job in the same department for eighteen years and began to worry more about losing her job than about progressing. She counted as friends a few women she had known since childhood; her contacts with men were infrequent and disappointing. Her home life remained remarkably unchanged—when her sisters moved out, Sally began caring for her parents—except that Sally's resentment broke through to the surface and she became openly desperate.

Before she came to the office, Sally wrote me a note. It began, "I am forty-one years old. I feel angry and hurt most of the time. I feel like my spirit has been shattered and fragmented with each piece having been trampled on and bruised. I am very, very anxious. I am afraid of everything, even centipedes and roaches. I keep thinking something very, very bad is going to happen to me, some great misfortune, or that I'll become handicapped and have to depend on people to take care of me. I don't know who I am, because that person stopped growing at the age of four, and it makes me very sad."

That Sally could formulate such a statement was a tribute to the psychotherapy she had engaged in over the course of many years with two talented social workers. The most recent therapy, however, had only made her more aware of her limitations and frustrations. At our first meeting, Sally had symptoms of depression: exhaustion, tearfulness, and poor concentration.

This story resembles others we have heard with one significant difference, the important role of inhibited temperament. Sally's shyness seems to have "been there from the start." Her mother, her mother's mother, her father, and her sisters all, to a greater or lesser degree, shared this trait. Because of Sally's entrenched timidity and social discomfort, there is a sameness to her life, a terrible monotony. In childhood, Sally's story has some of the lows but none of the highs we expect in a life history; in adult life, there are altogether too few ups and downs. Though before midlife Sally had never thought of herself as depressed, her social isolation and lack of confidence, combined with difficult circumstances, resulted in a life of intolerable bleakness.

Social introversion, when well established in adult life, is a difficult trait to change. I prescribed Prozac for Sally with an eye mainly toward her depressive symptoms but also with some hope of making a more profound difference.

Sally had been anxious in my presence at our first meeting, but she showed a touch of stubbornness, too—she was going to see treatment through, despite her fears. And though she looked younger than forty, there was nothing cloying or falsely naïve about Sally; she was going to work with whatever I could give her. After two months, she felt less depressed and much more angry. Indeed, Sally's anger was cause for concern, because irritability can be an early sign of mania, and mania is an infrequent bad outcome of antidepressant treatment. I lowered Sally's Prozac dose to half a capsule per day (ten milligrams), but I did not discontinue the medicine. Part of me was pleased to see Sally get angry: if we had been using only psychotherapy and not medication, I would have expected Sally's progress to include a period of anger—at her parents, at her superiors, at everyone who took advantage of her timidity.

In the third month, Sally remained angry and a bit too wired and bubbly. But after four months on Prozac, she looked brighter, calmer, self-assured, in firm control of herself. The most important effect of the medication, Sally felt, was that it cleared her head— made her more awake and aware, more confident of her perceptions. She said, "The medicine helps me to clarify problems. It takes me less time to find positive solutions. I don't panic. I don't feel my 'brain hurts' under stress, and I do not obsess."

After ten months on medication—her highest dose was one (twenty-milligram) capsule six days per week—Sally was decidedly more assertive at work. She negotiated a small promotion and pay raise at a time when the bank was cutting back staff, and she trained others to do some of the routine parts of her job.

More remarkable was the change in her private life. She started going to dances, making up for lost time. She even asked men to dance, and she dated a number of them. One she dropped because he drank; another because he bored her. After a year, she was dating two men steadily, without worrying how things would turn out and without letting either one pressure her into a premature choice. She was able to forgive men's faults: "They may be a little rough around the edges, but they can be fun." She was not afraid of men, or self-conscious around them.

I felt concern that Sally may have "overshot," that this new personality was too different from her old one. She demurred. She said the Prozac had let her personality emerge at last—she had not been alive before taking an antidepressant. Sally insisted I not stop the medication, but I tapered the dose slightly.

After a year and a half on a low dose of Prozac, Sally came in to tell me she was engaged. She was confident the man was the right one. He was divorced, with grown children, a successful businessman whose cultural background was similar to her own. She had been very strong in her dealings with him, negotiating her role in relation to finances, the children's visits, and other issues that arise in marriages later in life. "I never understood what people meant when they said things felt right. This is a big step, but I feel good about it. I am moving along fast, but not too fast. I love him, and he loves me. Before, I only felt closed in; now I feel happy."

•   •   •

Though Sally was abused in adolescence, her story—especially the persistence from early childhood of her shyness and timidity—raises questions about inborn predisposition to social behavior. We are talking, of course, about temperament, and, since inexactness is easy in this area, before going further I should say something about the words used to describe aspects of individual identity.

"Temperament" usually refers to an inborn, genetically determined and chemically mediated, predisposition to a cluster of responses and behaviors. Psychiatrists use the term sometimes to refer only to very basic functions, such as rhythmicity (is a person or an animal regular in its sleep-wake cycle, feeding and hunger schedule, etc.?), and sometimes to denote a cluster of functions, such as the optimism, heartiness, and energy of the sanguine temperament.

"Temperament" is generally contrasted to "character," which refers to stable, repeated behavior patterns arising from life experience. "Character" is also used to refer to a person's idiosyncratic traits or, more particularly, to a person's moral fiber; alternatively, it can refer to the defenses developed in response to different fears—a person's "character armor." "Character" describes acquired traits; it is environmental where temperament is inborn, psychological where temperament is biological.

"Personality" refers to the whole picture of habitual or characteristic social behavior and response to challenge, an amalgam of temperament and character. So permeated is our language by ancient scientific and philosophical theories that we can hardly discuss personality without falling back on words—"habitual," "characteristic," "typical"—that take sides in a centuries-old controversy.

Today, the dividing line between temperament and character is difficult to maintain. If trauma alters our biology, it changes our—what? Though the new traits are "acquired," and therefore constitute character, they arise from rewired neural circuitry, so we might want to say that what has changed is our temperament. And what about the effects of medication? The changed propensities that result, though surely they are acquired and not inborn, are due to altered brain chemistry. Therefore, we might want to say medication acts on temperament, except that, when it makes Tess less self-sacrificing, we want to say it has altered her (moral) character. For the sake of clarity, in this chapter I will use "temperament" to refer to the biological underpinnings of personality, even if the biology has been shaped or altered by circumstance or chemicals. In this sense, an adult's medicated temperament will differ from his or her "inborn temperament." It must—the neural chemistry with which we arrive in the world is inevitably modified by development, environment, life events, and now by discrete medicine. What we now know about the interaction of biology and experience tells us that the distinction between temperament and character will always be arbitrary and artificial.

• • •

For years, temperament in humans was the tar pit of psychological research. Whole careers disappeared into it. Every study that correlated childhood temperament with adult personality style was immediately followed by two or three refuting the same hypothesis. Worse, studies of temperament were sociologically suspect. The field was rooted in Carl Jung's concept of "attitudes"—introversion and extraversion—and was felt on a historical and also what might be called an aesthetic basis to be connected to Nazism, racism, and a denial of human equality and free will. In recent years, as much because of a change in zeitgeist as because of any dramatic shift in the evidence, temperament is once again fair ground for exploration. Indeed, when we try in today's climate to make sense of Sally's life, it is difficult to avoid consideration of a heritable predisposition to timidity—so difficult that we can perhaps scarcely imagine what a comparable discussion, omitting any such consideration, would have been like ten years ago.

The new research into inborn temperament has been both pioneered and popularized by the Harvard child psychologist Jerome Kagan. There are many components to temperament and personality. Kagan's genius lies in having focused on just one, inhibition. His work has been enormously influential.

Kagan began with three hundred twenty-one-month-old infants, a group from which he selected the 10 percent who were at each extreme—those who were most consistently shy, quiet, and timid, and those who were most consistently sociable, talkative, and emotionally spontaneous. The twenty-one-month-olds were tested by having their mothers bring them to an unfamiliar playroom with unfamiliar women and toys. In videotapes, the infants were rated for clinging to the mother, diminution of vocalization, and reluctance to approach objects or strangers. Later, thirty-one-month-olds (all of those tested ten months earlier and some others) were rated according to the time elapsed before they would interact, speak, or play with an unfamiliar child. Although the shy, timid children, for the most part, had experienced no serious trauma, their social responses paralleled those of the temperamentally normal but environmentally stressed young monkeys in Suomi's research—the ones who, after mild forms of separation from their mothers, showed inhibited behaviors, ranging from withdrawal in the face of strange objects to a diminished tendency to explore or affiliate.

The children in Kagan's study were retested in age-appropriate ways at two, three and a half, five and a half, and seven and a half years. For instance, by age seven and a half, a single unfamiliar child is not sufficiently stressful; the test condition involves introduction into a group of seven to ten children.

Kagan found that social inhibition tended to persist over time. In descriptive terms, he wrote of the seven-and-a-half-year-olds: "A frequent scene during the play sessions was a cluster of three or four children playing close to each other, often talking, and one or two children standing or playing alone one to several meters from the center of social activity. These isolated, quiet children were typically those who had been classified as inhibited 5 or 6 years earlier."

Children did not always remain "true to type." Supportive and assertive parents could sometimes move children out of the inhibited group, and there was a great deal of variability in the uninhibited group. Indeed, it looked as if *lack* of inhibition was not a special category—it existed on a spectrum with normal, and there were fluid changes in and out of the category. Nor did more minor degrees of inhibition make children special. But extreme inhibition appeared to be a distinct and relatively stable phenomenon.

These findings alone were not dramatic. Kagan believes that 15 percent of children are born inhibited. (In his study, however, Kagan did not identify nearly this many inhibited twenty-one-month-olds; he had an especially difficult time identifying inhibited boys.) Although as a group the severely inhibited children remain distinctive, a third to perhaps half of them are normally uninhibited by age seven. Kagan has estimated that, "for every ten children who are extremely shy in the second year of life, only five will be very shy in kindergarten and first grade; by adolescence, only three. By their twenties, only one or two will still be very shy. . . ." In other words, only 10 or

20 percent of the original cohort of 15 percent will remain shy. This amounts to 1.5 to 3 percent of adults. But not all shy adults will have been inhibited infants; some people—perhaps one in a hundred?—become inhibited on the basis of environmental trauma. The Kagan experiment, seen objectively, involves observing a group of, say, one hundred healthy toddlers and saying, "I will choose fifteen of the toddlers and predict that in this group are one or two who, in adulthood, will be among the two or three shyest of the original one hundred." This is not a very astounding achievement— and we do not yet know whether Kagan has pulled the trick off.

What has made the Kagan study more interesting is the extension of the inquiry into the realm of physiology. Kagan and his colleagues looked mainly at correlates of norepinephrine and the stress hormones. For instance, at age five and a half, children's urine was tested for breakdown products of norepinephrine, and their saliva for a form of cortisol. The neurotransmitter ratings correlated modestly with the children's current level of inhibition, and the hormone ratings correlated modestly with the children's original behavioral ratings as infants. In other words, both acutely and chronically, the inhibited children seemed to have the physiology of an animal under stress.

The strongest and most consistent findings, however, had to do with heart rate. Kagan looked at two measures: how fast the heart was beating and how much variability there was in the interval between heartbeats. Ordinarily, our heart rate rises and falls slightly as we breathe, and of course heart rate speeds when we are stressed. The two measures are related: the faster the heart rate, the less the beat-to-beat variability. From infancy, the inhibited children—who were selected according to behavior, not heart function—showed a high and invariant heart rate. They showed this pattern even when asleep. The children with the highest heart rates in infancy were those most likely to remain inhibited through age seven and a half. Children with intense fears at age five and a half or seven and a half (for instance, fear of kidnappers, of going to bed alone, of violence on television) were in the group with high heart rates; the group with low heart rates contained no fearful children. These and other measures (such as tightness of the vocal cords, as measured by analysis of quavering in tapes of children's speech) seemed to indicate that severely inhibited children are biologically different: they are in a state of constant arousal from infancy, and many of them remain in that state throughout childhood.

Having conducted these initial studies, Kagan speculated that "most of the children we call inhibited belong to a qualitatively distinct category of infants who were born with a lower threshold for limbic-hypothalamic [that is, norepinephrine- and stress-hormone-mediated] arousal to unexpected changes in the environment or novel events that cannot be assimilated easily." He made this statement, however, before having studied the physiology of inhibited newborns. Kagan had demonstrated that children who are socially inhibited around age two tend to have high and invariant heart rates. These children account for a high percentage of those who are socially inhibited as five- to eight-year-olds; and by that age inhibited children show the rapid turnover of norepinephrine and the high levels of cortisol typical of chronic physiological arousal.

Kagan also speculated that the translation of inhibited temperament into inhibited behavior requires environmental trauma—in other words, he propounded what is called a stress/risk model of inhibition, one in which the condition arises in children at risk only if they are also stressed. He predicted that inhibition as a behavioral trait would emerge primarily in children who had been stressed by such events as "prolonged hospitalization, death of a parent, marital quarreling, or mental illness in a family member," but the inhibited children in his sample had, in fact, experienced few such events. Kagan then looked elsewhere for stressors. Two-thirds of Kagan's uninhibited children were firstborn, as against only one-third of the inhibited. Kagan speculates, "An older sibling who unexpectedly seizes a toy, teases, or yells at an infant who has a low threshold for limbic arousal might provide the chronic stress necessary to transform the temperamental quality into the profile we call behavioral inhibition."

Kagan's more fundamental conclusion, that inhibition is largely grounded in inborn temperament, was modestly supported by his early experiments. The evidence was not overwhelming. Inhibition was a stable trait, but only to a degree: most inhibited infants blended with the average population in time, and a substantial number even came to overlap on test results with the children selected for lack of inhibition. Tests were not conducted over a long enough period to demonstrate a correlation with adult personality. There was no proof that the inhibition shown by the twenty-one- and thirty-one-month-old infants was inborn temperament rather than a result of yet earlier trauma. Nonetheless, the appearance, in *Science* magazine in 1988, of Kagan's overview of his research had a dramatic effect in legitimizing the discussion of inborn temperament, the part of personality that is innate.

Some of the impact had to do with who Kagan is and what he stands for. In the 1960s, Kagan was a leader in opposing the contention that intelligence is largely heritable. The debate over IQ—whether it measures intelligence, whether it measures the same thing in blacks and whites, and whether it is heritable—was especially heated. Those who concluded that IQ is heritable were branded as racists and sometimes banned from or shouted down at campus lecture halls. The assertion in the eighties that personality is partly heritable had greater effect coming from a thoughtful, eloquent Harvard professor who had in the sixties opposed an arguably more limited proposition of behavioral genetics.

Kagan's work on shyness was careful and comprehensive, and, relative to other sets of studies of inborn temperament, its results were strong. Kagan and others were also able, in the few years after the influential monograph in *Science,* to bolster the hypothesis that observed differences were due to nature rather than nurture.

For instance, Kagan's group had found inhibited children to differ in a genetic trait. Among white children, more inhibited children and their parents, brothers, and sisters had blue eyes, whereas more uninhibited children and their first degree relatives had brown eyes. There also turned out to be an excess of allergies among relatives of inhibited infants, so that the constellation of blue eyes, hay fever, and temperamental shyness may be a distinct syndrome.

These findings were followed up by further laboratory studies. A group at Brown University gave a novel stimulus to newborns by suddenly changing the content of what they were sucking from water to sugar water. All newborns increase their rate of sucking in response to the sugar water. But some infants change their rate of sucking dramatically; they are said to be more "avid." Avidity is thought to be a measure of arousal, vigilance, and awareness of novelty—traits that relate to later inhibition. And, indeed, those infants who are most avid on the first or second day of life were found to be most inhibited at a year and a half.

Kagan's group tested four-month-olds and found that those who had more motor movements (such as flexing and extending arms or legs, arching the back, and sticking out the tongue) and more fretful crying in response to unusual toys and sounds were more often inhibited at later ages. Kagan's work-in-progress, aimed at examining possible antenatal precursors of inhibition, is extending this inquiry into the womb, correlating high and invariant heart rates in fetuses with childhood temperament.

Researchers are also extending inhibited-temperament research in the other direction. Not enough time has elapsed for researchers to follow inhibited infants into adulthood, but adult relatives of inhibited infants seem unusually prone to conditions such as panic anxiety; and there is suggestive evidence that among these relatives is a greater-than-average number of inhibited adults. The result of inhibition may not be limited to anxiety; one study has found that among mildly depressed adults a disproportionate number had experienced extreme shyness in childhood compared to the general population.

This field of study, inhibited temperament, consists of a large body of modest, tentative experimental results. But the scope of the field is remarkable—from the fetus to the adult—and by and large the quality of the studies is excellent. As a result, something like a consensus has arisen in psychology and psychiatry that certain children are born different—different in terms of the reactivity of their stress-hormone systems, and therefore different in their response to novelty—and that this difference can lead to later social inhibition and probably to various disturbances of mood. People don't have to be made vulnerable by trauma: they can be born vulnerable.

•　　•　　•

We have seen that in rhesus monkeys early separation can produce a sensitivity to subsequent separations. The animals tested in those studies are either unselected or bred for genetic uniformity. That is, they are normal animals, and the chronic disturbances they suffer, including inhibition in the face of novel stimuli, can presumably be produced in any member of the species. But it looks as if monkeys can also be born sensitive, and work with those monkeys has lent strong support to Kagan's research on innate temperament.

In his observation of a breeding colony of rhesus monkeys, Stephen Suomi was able to identify individuals—20 percent of rhesus young—who appeared anxious and shy. Suomi called these monkeys "uptight" and contrasted them to the other 80 percent, who responded more flexibly to challenge, the "laid-back" macaques. Even more than in humans, Suomi found that in monkeys "differences in response to novelty and challenge show up very early in life and are stable over the life span." Differences are observable from the time infants first "stray from their mother and explore the environment."

Using four-month-old monkeys, Suomi replicated Kagan's research, starting with the sorts of challenges to which Kagan exposed
twenty-one-month-old children. As with the human infants, the uptight monkeys were slower to explore a playroom, and they tended
to have high and invariant heart rates and elevated levels of stress
hormones. On subsequent exposures to the playroom, this contrast
faded; differences in quickness to explore showed themselves only in
response to novelty.

Kagan's and Suomi's models were influenced by earlier monkey studies
looking at heart rate and behavior. Fifteen years ago, it was observed
that reactive monkey infants—those who at age one month have a
pronounced change in heart rate in anticipation of irritating noise—
develop, by age two and one half years, a heightened behavioral
disturbance in response to handling by humans. The study was remarkable for its findings regarding the origins of this variability. The
monkey infants were "nursery-reared" together, so all had received
the same environmental "mothering." Some of the monkeys were
also similar genetically: though they had different biological mothers,
groups of two to three shared a biological father and were thus half-
siblings. In terms of heart rate—and, later, sensitivity to handling
—monkeys grouped very closely according to their paternity. The
two monkeys with the greatest agitation when handled had the same
biological father. Three of the four monkeys with the least agitation
in response to handling had the same biological father. For a behavioral trait to sort out cleanly among *half*-siblings so far into the middle
of childhood implies the presence of a genetic factor with a very
robust influence.

A simple recent test using the Kagan/Suomi paradigm again demonstrates the strong impact of genetics on reactivity. Researchers
looked at monkey pairs who on first mating produced an uptight
infant. These parents were mated again, and the second offspring
were immediately given to adoptive mothers. These adoptive mothers

had been selected to be either uptight or laid-back. Whatever the adoptive mothers' degree of reactivity, these infants biologically at risk for inhibition emerged uptight.

In another study, monkey infants tested to be either uptight or laid-back were given to adoptive mothers who were more complexly selected. As in the last study, the adoptive mothers were chosen because they were either uptight or laid-back. In addition, they were selected according to whether they had been highly nurturant and protective or more punitive and rejecting in their maternal style with earlier offspring. Whether reared by laid-back or uptight new mothers—and whether reared by nurturant or demanding mothers —the infants tended to remain true to heritable type. The reactivity or nurturance of the adoptive monkey mother had no effect on the way her adopted infant reacted to novel challenges. Suomi concluded, "Clearly, for these infants the only significant predictor of scores on the neonatal measures was the infants' pedigree."

High reactivity or "uptightness" in rhesus monkeys looks a good deal like the minor disturbances of mood we have seen in human patients. Uptight monkeys behave normally when well supported. When separated from mother or peer group, initially they look more anxious than do their laid-back age-mates; upon longer separation, the uptight monkeys become withdrawn or depressed. The constant pattern throughout life is anxiety in the face of acute challenge and depression in the face of chronic stress. In adolescence, the monkeys who were uptight in infancy tend when stressed to fiddle in front of their cages or engage in other repetitive, stereotypic behavior. These tendencies—to anxiety, depression, and compulsiveness—increase with age and repeated challenge, as do parallel abnormalities in neurotransmitters.

Like traumatized monkeys, monkeys who are "born reactive" are nonspecifically "neurotic." Throughout life, they are especially prone to both anxious responses to novelty and depressive reactions to separation. When allowed to self-administer alcohol, they drink more when under stress than do low-reactive monkeys. Like "inhibited" humans, reactive monkeys are more likely to show allergic reactions starting in infancy.

What researchers have hypothesized about innate temperament in humans has been conclusively demonstrated by Suomi in rhesus monkeys. Monkeys do not need to be subjected to traumatic stress to become sensitive: they can be born uptight.

•   •   •

Seeing the monkey and human observations juxtaposed, the reality of inborn temperament may seem irrefutable. Some people are just born with a liability to grow up shy, quiet, timid, and vulnerable to stress or challenge, whereas others are likely to become, in Kagan's words, "consistently sociable, affectively spontaneous, and minimally fearful in the same unfamiliar situations." But it is worthwhile, I think, to remind ourselves that only a few years ago this same evidence might have been viewed differently—that for decades rather similar evidence was routinely dismissed. Studies showing high and invariant heart rates in inhibited dogs, for example, go back to the 1940s, as do reports regarding similarities in the degree of shyness in identical twins. And studies of reactivity among half-sibling monkeys were already quite advanced fifteen years ago.

Even before the era of formal studies of temperament, Carl Jung described "those reserved, inscrutable, rather shy people who form the strongest possible contrast to the open, sociable, jovial or at least friendly and approachable characters. . . ." Jung argued that these differences could not be accounted for by Freud's theory of sexual dynamism. Jung wrote, "The fact that children exhibit a typical attitude quite unmistakably even in their earliest years forces us to assume it cannot be a struggle for existence in the ordinary sense that determines a particular attitude." Citing the common occurrence of different personality "types" among children of the same mother, he concluded that, unless the mother's attitude is extreme, "Ultimately, it must be the individual disposition which decides whether the child will belong to this or that type despite the constancy of external conditions." Jung speculated that the cause of both extraversion and introversion is biological and based on evolutionary adaptation for the benefit of the species. "The one [extraversion] consists in a high rate of fertility, with low powers of defence and short duration of life for the single individual; the other consists in equipping the individual with numerous means of self-preservation plus a low fertility rate."

The extent of Jung's application of his beliefs regarding human "types" to contemporary racist dogma, and of his cooperation with the Nazis, is the subject of heated historical controversy. Certainly, late in World War II and afterward, Jung was horrified by the Nazis. But before the war, in 1934, Jung had accepted the editorship of the newly Nazified and Jew-free *Zentralblatt für Psychotherapie;* and he had opened the journal with an attack on Freudianism in which he argued, "The Aryan unconscious has a higher potential than the Jewish. . . . In my opinion it has been a great mistake of all previous medical psychology to apply Jewish categories which are not binding even to Jews, indiscriminately to Christians, Germans, or Slavs." It is fair to say that his views could be and were used to bolster the (already prevalent) concept of breeds within the human species, and to develop the Nazi depiction of Jews as the culturally destructive "antitype."

Because of the relationship of Jung's "types" to Nazi racism, and also because of the use of twisted biological determinism to bolster racism in the United States, the concept of temperament was culturally taboo throughout the forties and later, during the civil-rights struggles in the fifties, sixties, and seventies. Instead, the prevailing attitude was that enunciated by Margaret Mead in her studies in the 1930s of "primitive societies" in which women displayed personality traits associated in Western culture with maleness—namely, that "human nature is almost unbelievably malleable, responding accurately and contrastingly to contrasting cultural conditions." The concept of near-total malleability is especially appealing in an egalitarian society, and the idea of genetic determinism is especially alien. Carl N. Degler, a sociologist who has written an exhaustive study of the rise (and current descent) of cultural determinism in America, makes it clear that the role of scientific findings in the decline of biological determinism was limited: "The main impetus came from the wish to establish a social order in which innate and immutable forces of biology played no role in accounting for the behavior of social groups. . . . To the proponents of culture the goal was the elimination of nativity, race, and sex, and any other biologically based characteristic that might serve as an obstacle to an individual's self-realization."

Kagan has speculated that America was receptive to Freud precisely because of Freud's belief that experience determines personality. In introducing one of his recent studies, Kagan refers to "The return of the idea of temperament to discussions of personality after half a century of exile. . . ."

Forceful arguments are still made against the use of animal models in the study of human behavior. In a recent polemic against biological determinism, the evolutionary geneticist Richard C. Lewontin and colleagues repeatedly refer to the dissimilarity of human and animal brains. And, because human social behavior has never been linked successfully to particular genes, Lewontin contends that "all statements about the genetic basis of human social traits are necessarily purely speculative, no matter how positive they seem to be." But Lewontin's assertion sounds merely tendentious in today's scientific and cultural environment.

Without the related animal studies, we might conclude that Kagan's evidence for inhibited temperament is not overwhelming. Part of what makes Kagan's results convincing is that they confirm "what every parent knows"—namely, that infants are different, and that often parents do not so much influence personality as watch it develop. My sense is that, throughout our culture, the current assumption is that humans differ temperamentally, not just as regards inhibition, but in almost every aspect of personality.

• • •

Certainly hearing Sally's story makes it hard not to think about social inhibition, both as a matter of inborn predisposition and as an outcome of early stressors. Social inhibition, rather than depression or any distinct anxiety disorder, is the single quality most responsible for Sally's social and professional stagnation and for her unhappiness. Some psychiatrists and psychologists, however, would have difficulty with this point of view—not least because, if we attribute Sally's woes to personality rather than illness, when she recovers we must conclude that personality is what medication has altered. These clinicians have a different understanding of temperament: they believe it is less related to social qualities, such as shyness, than to chronic mood states.

In Sally's case, this alternative view would suggest that she becomes socially successful on Prozac because she is revved up. Patients prone to mania, the extreme and often psychotic state in which the brain is racing, sometimes enjoy a less extreme state of euphoria and energy, called "hypomania." "The goal is controlled hypomania," a pharmacologist once said to me. The relevant factor, according to this theory, is not what Kagan calls "inhibition" (and what Suomi calls "reactivity") but some broad measure of depression—whether Sally is sufficiently energetic, quick-thinking, sexually driven, optimistic, and sparkling.

The notion that people differ in affective, as opposed to social, temperament goes back to the beginnings of medicine, to the theory of the humors. The belief that both health and characteristic mood are governed by substances that flow through the body predates the earliest Greek medical texts available to us, from the fifth century B.C., and prevails in the medical literature almost to the present day. The classic humors are phlegm, blood, yellow bile (choler), and black bile, giving rise to the phlegmatic, sanguine, choleric, and melancholic temperaments. "Melan-cholia" is simply Greek for "black bile."

Hippocrates' *Nature of Man* is a treatise on the humors. Aristotle assumed that affective tone was set by the humors; like modern researchers who have found an association between mood disorder and creativity, Aristotle asked, "Why is it that all those who have become eminent in philosophy or politics or poetry or the arts are clearly of an atrabilious [that is, melancholic] temperament, and some of them to such an extent as to be affected by diseases caused by black bile?" The Greek concept of melancholic temperament is repeated in medical texts in astonishingly unaltered form throughout Western history— during the Middle Ages and the Renaissance and well into the eighteenth and even nineteenth centuries. Of Jung's "introversion" and "extraversion" we have already spoken; Freud's contemporary Kraepelin also recognized a depressive disposition. It is really only in the heyday of hidebound, theory-burdened post-Freudian psychoanalysis that the melancholic temperament drops from view and personality is assumed to be rooted mostly in experience. Today, in the era of the "neurohumors" (norepinephrine, serotonin), affective temperament has made a comeback, most notably in the work of Hagop Akiskal, a psychiatrist now at the National Institute of Mental Health who conducted most of his research at the University of Tennessee. Akiskal has devoted his career to the understanding and classification of minor affective disorders.

Akiskal believes that a good deal of what looks like personality, or personality disorder, is a *forme fruste,* or incompletely expressed version, of overt mental illness. Akiskal worked with a large number of patients in a private outpatient clinic in Memphis; he also collaborated with researchers who replicated his work in Europe. In these patient populations, he identified a variety of common personality types, including the depressive personality.

Before the advent of Prozac, Akiskal distinguished two forms of depressive personality. In both groups, patients reported having always felt depressed—since early childhood or adolescence. One group had a history of stress or loss; they tended to have had either a parent who was alcoholic or one who died while they were young. Akiskal assumed these patients' problems lay in the realm of character. Another group of patients with depressive personality reported a family history of overt depressive illness, especially manic depression. Even though they themselves were for the most part not acutely depressed, these patients tended not only to respond to antidepressants but also frequently to "overshoot" and become manic. Akiskal considered these people to have an "attenuated or 'subaffective dysthymic' disorder"—that is, to suffer a low-level chronic depression on a temperamental basis. Akiskal's subaffective dysthymia—a modern version of the melancholic humor—sounds like an alternative understanding not only of Sally, with her marked social inhibition, but also of certain other patients, such as Gail or Tess:

> These individuals, who are introverted, obsessional, self-sacrificing, brooding, guilt-ridden, gloomy, self-denigrating, anhedonic, lethargic, and who tend to oversleep, appear to be suffering from an attenuated but lifelong form of melancholia. . . . These dysthymic individuals were characterized by inability to enjoy leisure and overdedication to work that requires selfless devotion and much attention to detail. However, this stable adjustment in the vocational sphere was not paralleled in social adjustment. The somber personalities and intense attachment needs of these individuals may drive others away. Such interpersonal losses then cause them to sink into the lower depths of black humor.

Among the most enduring traits of depressive personality are introversion and social maladroitness, features reminiscent of inhibition in children.

Akiskal relies on a variety of evidence to argue that subaffective dysthymia is biological—that is, a result of temperament. In addition to family history and medication response, he has studied the sleep patterns of subaffective dysthymics. Depressed patients tend very early in the sleep cycle to enter the sort of dream sleep characterized by inactivity of the body except for rapid eye movements (REM). So characteristic is this pattern that "short REM latency" is considered a biological marker of depression. Even though they are not depressed, subaffective dysthymics have short REM latency.

For Akiskal, subaffective dysthymia sits on a spectrum of affective personalities. Elsewhere on the spectrum is the hyperthymic personality, understood to be an outgrowth of hyperthymic temperament. Many successful businesspeople and politicians are hyperthymics. These people are described by Akiskal with a series of adjectives, not all of which apply to any one person but the listing of which creates the image of a recognizable "type": hyperthymics are habitually "irritable," "cheerful," "overoptimistic," "exuberant," "overconfident," "self-assured," "boastful," "bombastic," "grandiose," "full of plans," "improvident," "impulsive," "overtalkative," "warm," "people-seeking," "extraverted," "overinvolved," "meddlesome," "uninhibited," "stimulus-seeking," and/or "promiscuous." They are habitual short sleepers, even on weekends. The traits are evident from early in life.

On first consideration, dysthymics and hyperthymics seem to stand at the extremes in terms of temperament. But there are similarities on a variety of levels. For instance, dysthymics are also driven in their careers. Throughout history, it has been known that melancholics, though they have little energy, use their energy well; they tend to work hard in a focused area, do great things, and derive little pleasure from their accomplishments. Much of the insight and creative achievement of the human race is due to the discontent, guilt, and critical eye of dysthymics.

Like hyperthymics, dysthymics can become extraverted and driven for brief periods of time. In symmetrical fashion, hyperthymics are liable to brief depressions. Both dysthymics and hyperthymics are prone to becoming revved up on medication. Like dysthymics, hyperthymics come from families with an excess of mood disorder and have a sleep cycle characterized by short REM latency. Both dysthymics and hyperthymics are at increased risk over time to suffer overt episodes of recurrent major depression. Thus, according to Akiskal's model, both depressive introverts and euphoric extraverts may owe their personality styles to a related biological instability in modulation of affect. Akiskal's writings suggest that both temperaments relate to manic-depressive illness rather than to depression alone—that there is a spectrum that runs from subaffective dysthymia (or melancholic temperament) through hyperthymia (or sanguine temperament) all the way out to rapid cycling.

Akiskal is a representative of the most ancient tradition in psychiatry, the humoral theory that links illness and personality. His signal contribution is the introduction into modern psychiatry of a new category of mental disorder, dysthymia (ill spirit—essentially, disordered humor), lying at the periphery of depression. The boundaries of dysthymia are hard to specify, but the term refers to a chronic condition in which a person has periodic intervals of depressed mood that are briefer or less severe, or involve fewer deranged functions, than episodes of major depression. Dysthymia sits in the penumbra of depression, and subaffective dysthymia sits in the penumbra of the penumbra.

Akiskal has reminded clinicians of what was understood from Greek times until the nineteenth century—namely, that dysthymia is not a matter of episodes alone. Dysthymics tend to have a gloomy and inhibited style between episodes, and there are those who have the style without the episodes but probably have the same underlying disorder. This view of the realm of disordered or variant personality raises a series of interesting issues regarding the patients we have encountered and their response to medication.

●　　●　　●

So far, it has appeared that changes in neurotransmission may have the ability to affect *social* temperament directly, turning a shy and conservative member of a human troop into an gregarious risk-taker. The concept of *affective* temperament raises another possibility. When Sally took Prozac, she at first became angry, wired, and bubbly. Perhaps medication "merely" transformed dysthymic into hyperthymic temperament.

Psychiatrists who are skeptical about the transformative powers of Prozac believe that what makes the drug popular is its ability to rev people up, to induce mild hypomania. The implication is that Prozac makes people silly, impairs their judgment, substitutes false euphoria for mild depression. Even if the skeptics are right, to turn dysthymia into hyperthymia is no minor achievement. A medication that can cause such a change in a stable, lasting way will alter personality. Specifically, it will take a person with a temperament that has led to loneliness and give him or her the equivalent of a temperament that, in moderation, often leads to social satisfaction.

My belief is different: I see hypomania as an infrequent but noteworthy side effect of Prozac, separate from its more common main effects. When Sally manages to date men, what the medicine helps her to overcome is decades of social inhibition. But is her interval of excessive energy mere coincidence? In the abstract, Akiskal's concept of temperament—at base, a chronic mood state—differs from Kagan's formulation, in which social inhibition is primary. But in particular patients, the distinction fades: Sally is both depressed and inhibited, and it is hard to say which is primary.

One of the most interesting understandings of the relationship between inhibited temperament and dysthymia comes from a novel perspective, that of sociobiology. The prime mover in this work is Michael T. McGuire, a California psychiatrist with a background in animal ethology. He is known for his work with monkeys, but he has done one fascinating study with humans. McGuire wanted to know what function dysthymia has played in the evolution of human behavior: Is it an illness, or a personality style? Did it confer evolutionary advantages? How has it persisted as a pattern of interrelating with the world?

To answer questions of this sort, McGuire and his colleagues created a center at which they could study dysthymic women not for a brief interview but for an average of 250 hours over an average of eighteen months each—an unheard-of degree of contact with experimental subjects, particularly outpatients. The testing and observations took place at a drop-in center. The atmosphere was such that the women got to know one another and the investigators; they began to function like a small society.

McGuire is still analyzing his data, but he gave a preview at a psychiatric meeting a few years ago. McGuire studied forty-six dysthymic women, ages twenty to forty, and forty-one age-matched controls who had no psychiatric diagnosis. Despite the use of very extensive test batteries, the researchers could not differentiate the groups in terms of cognitive function, such as intelligence or memory. But when they observed the women in social settings, the researchers found the dysthymics had a distinctive pattern of behavior. In contrast to the control subjects, the dysthymic women more often avoided social intercourse and were less likely to initiate social contact; they displayed more atypical social behaviors (such as decreased eye contact and atypical gesturing); they were more likely to express fear of negative evaluation by others; and they had "significantly limited capacities to develop novel behavior and interpretive strategies" and "significantly limited behavior capacities, including reduced capacities for: social maintenance, understanding social rules, self-maintenance, and communication efficacy." Interviews with both subjects and their relatives revealed that these tendencies were lifelong and had preceded the emergence of depressed mood. In other words, the dysthymic women had been *socially inhibited* but not depressed from an early age.

Accompanying the social inhibition were indications of chronic physiologic arousal. For example, the dysthymic women showed heightened responses to certain stimuli, such as anticipating a balloon burst. Behaviorally, these women—who were selected because of chronic minor depression, and not on the basis of social inhibition or anxiety—showed many of the traits we associate with Kagan's shy children or Suomi's uptight monkeys.

For these women, inhibition had social consequences. The dysthymic women differed from the control women in terms of access to life's bounty: "Experimental subjects had significantly fewer friends, social contacts, and living offspring. They had significantly smaller incomes, and significantly less living space per household." It seems dysthymic women's chronic temperamental characteristics —their social discomfort and their lack of flexibility—result in a restricted life with few social rewards.

McGuire was moved by his findings to apply to dysthymic women the sort of evolutionary theory that is more frequently, and perhaps more comfortably, applied to lower animals. The assumption of this theory is that animals, including humans, are "predisposed to achieve certain biological goals, such as acquiring resources, acquiring mates, developing social support networks, having offspring, remaining healthy, communicating efficiently, living in an optimally dense environment, and so on." Failures in these tasks, according to the theory, are the mediating circumstances that lead to chronic and recurrent depression. Inability to achieve goals or find access to resources—space, friends, mates—has direct adverse psychological and physiological consequences. The negative feelings may at first have adaptive value. For instance, anxiety may serve as a feedback signal—a warning—to the individual that goal achievement is suboptimal. The outward signs of depression may at first serve to elicit care-giving from companions. Later, the mechanisms for discontinuing anxiety and depression may be lost, and the conditions can become syndromic and almost wholly dysfunctional.

According to this evolutionary view, dysthymic women do not at base have an illness, depression. What they have is a characteristic strategy or mode of behavior that is not rewarded in contemporary society. People whom society does not reward—who do not find appreciation, love, career success, or a sense of competency—tend to become depressed; presumably this is a universal human vulnerability. But the fundamental problem is a mismatch between the women's coping style and the requisites for finding reward in this culture.

For example, McGuire's dysthymic subjects typically persevered at tasks beyond the point to which perseverance is rewarded in today's complexly demanding world. McGuire's staff made this observation after hearing the women, if they were scheduled at the center for morning and afternoon sessions, repeatedly complain that they had gotten little done during the lunch hour. Curious about what was going on, McGuire's staff followed the women as they took their lunch break.

A subject would leave at midday with a variety of goals—withdraw money from the bank, buy dinner supplies at the grocer's, pick up laundry at the dry cleaner's, and so forth. But, typically, if she arrived at the bank and found a long line, the woman would stand at the end rather than choosing to move on to the next task. She might make a commitment to the bank task, stand behind twenty people, advance, say, to the fourth spot from the front, and then abandon the line when she notices that it's almost time for her afternoon testing session. She would then return to the center without having accomplished any of what she had set out to do. So often did this phenomenon repeat itself that the researchers hypothesized half-seriously that the odds are that the last three people in any long line are chronically depressed.

This tendency to persist inflexibly at hopeless tasks was observed whether or not the women were acutely depressed: it seemed a "trait" as opposed to a "state" characteristic. Even at their best, the dysthymic women lacked the necessary quality—adaptability, optimism, aggression, sense of self-worth—to move on from a present, visible task that is likely to fail to other, imagined, unseen tasks that might possibly succeed. In terms of the virtues of an earlier generation, these women were single-minded, steadfast, loyal, and capable of remarkable perseverance. (This observation may lead us to wonder whether certain women's tendency to remain stuck in abusive relationships relates not, as much contemporary belief has it, to masochism or self-defeating tendencies, but, rather, to a specific quality of temperament having to do with persistence.)

McGuire's observations resonate suggestively with Kagan's and, more particularly, Suomi's work on social inhibition. The sequence seems to be that uptightness leads to social isolation, which leads to failure to achieve goals or acquire resources and then to depression. McGuire sees dysthymia as a secondary consequence of a "trait distribution phenomenon"—a normal human temperament that happens not to be rewarded in the modern world. McGuire's view combines sequentially the risk (inherited vulnerability, as in "children at risk") and stress (trauma) approaches to mood disorder: inhibited temperament (risk) leads to social deprivation (stress) which then produces dysthymia. The anthropological model resembles Jung's understanding of the sociobiological function of introversion: like introverts, the dysthymic women are evolutionarily adapted to take few chances and settle for few social contacts. But the social environment has changed, so that what was once a successful reproductive "strategy" is now the variant human trait underlying chronic and recurrent depression.

McGuire's hypothesis meshes with a larger body of work concerning conservative, as opposed to adventurous, social choices. Evolutionary biologists have developed computer models testing different behavioral strategies against different environmental conditions. For example, a simple mathematical strategy, using game playing or betting as the behavior, might be to make whatever choice you made the last time until you fail twice in a row; then make a different choice and continue with that one until it fails twice. It turns out that there are many computer "environments" in which conservative strategies lead to long-range survival for the individual. Moreover, inhibited temperament contributes to social stability. Again, consider the phenomenon of inhibited men and women who remain in abusive marriages; though painful to behold, relationships between domineering and dysthymic spouses are often remarkable for their longevity. More broadly, we can see how the survival of the tribe, or gene pool, might be enhanced by the presence of some dogged, methodical members.

This evolutionary reasoning implies that inhibited temperament may have been biologically adaptive throughout the hunter-gatherer stage of man's existence. It may even have been more adaptive in the Middle Ages or during the Industrial Revolution than it is now. The problem is that our modern technological society demands the ability to face outward, expend high degrees of energy, take risks, and respond rapidly to multiple competing stimuli. In our society, tribal and familial means of assigning mates and sharing resources have been superseded by demands for individual assertiveness. The environment no longer rewards the full range of temperaments that were necessary for human survival in prior settings.

Writing about Julia's fastidiousness, I said that certain personality styles are no longer socially favored or fashionable. If McGuire's formulation is right, the problem is not simply that extreme caution is no longer admired but that, in the ordinary course of modern life, it does not garner social rewards. It is not only that contemporary social convention demands that women be more assertive (here meaning aggressive, outgoing, and flexible—not firm in defense of the right to be passive and perseverative), but that social circumstances tend to frustrate women who use too cautious a strategy. If Julia is to be happy in a two-career marriage, she will need to tolerate disorder. For Sally to avert depression, it is required that she ask men to dance—that she have a more extraverted temperament. A degree of introversion that might have been rewarded in a different social climate here leads only to deprivation, disappointment, and depression.

• • •

Not long ago, I treated a patient whose story illustrates the social injuries that can arise from even a mildly inhibited temperament. Jerry was a surgeon who came to see me as he finished his residency training and set out to enter practice. He was quiet, reserved, and self-effacing, and had been so since early childhood. He had always wanted to be a surgeon, and he had achieved his goal, but not without difficulty. A solid student, Jerry had excelled in high school, but was then rejected by the college he most hoped to enter. He went instead to a less prestigious school, and again did well. However, to his surprise and disappointment, he was rejected by all the medical schools to which he applied.

Jerry went on with his life. He married his childhood sweetheart, took jobs in research laboratories, and continued to apply to medical schools. For three years running, he was refused entry. When at last he confronted the college office in charge of organizing his application, Jerry discovered that the summary letter of recommendation in his folder implied he was plodding—a word that did not relate to his achievements, which were substantial, but to his self-presentation. His conduct during interviews, where he tended to be retiring and tentative, had probably amplified this misimpression. The omission of certain offending phrases improved the application, and on his fourth try Jerry was admitted to a top-flight program.

There he excelled at first, but as the pressures mounted he became prone to such anxiety that he could barely function. Although he spent day and night in the library, self-doubt prevented him from translating his learning into academic success. A therapist at school identified the problem as overfastidiousness—the need to exercise more control than was possible in a complex program—and encouraged Jerry to study less. Jerry followed this advice and thrived.

When Jerry came to me, he was once again anxious, with an element of depression now added in. He was suddenly irritable, lashing out at nurses and colleagues in the operating room. He did not know whether he would be able to function in the "real world" outside residency. Just before coming to see me, he had put himself on Prozac.

What ensued was one of the simplest therapies I have ever conducted. I encouraged Jerry to review his history with me. It emerged that at every transition in his education his inhibition had been interpreted as incompetence—so he had been penalized for a particular personality style. This style had its productive side. It made him persistent in pursuit of his goals, allowed him to enter into a successful marriage without fuss, and made him a steady student and a clear-thinking, unimpulsive physician. Jerry's sense of self-worth and competency had been injured by the numerous rejections he suffered, rejections that had little to do with his ability and everything to do with various institutions' prejudice in favor of extraversion and "assertiveness." Toward the end of the therapy, one additional factor emerged. It seemed that in recent months Jerry had been seeing his son penalized—teased or excluded by peers—for the same quiet, retiring traits. Merely identifying this connection was empowering.

And it seemed that the Prozac did its job, too. Jerry found himself less frazzled by the complexity of the operating and recovery rooms, firmer in the outward expression of his opinions and decisions, at once more even-tempered and more commanding. I suspect the Prozac also helped quiet his reaction to "novelty"—that is, to the stress of leaving residency and entering practice.

The combination of therapy and medication in this brief treatment seemed to me especially effective. As Jerry reviewed his own history, he saw how he had been unfairly judged, and he changed the way he valued himself. This cognitive change was amplified by the Prozac directly, through visceral feelings of self-worth, and indirectly, through the good response of Jerry's colleagues to his new, more assertive behavior.

Jerry was not especially shy or affectively vulnerable; he might not have met Kagan's criteria for social inhibition, and he definitely would not have been studied by Akiskal or McGuire. But even in this mild case of social inhibition, Jerry's temperament interacted with an unfavorable environment to produce symptoms, and the sociobiological view of temperament and mood disorder was of use to Jerry in reshaping his sense of self.

●   ●   ●

Studies from a variety of perspectives—child development, animal ethology, descriptive psychiatry, and sociobiology—point to temperament as a crucial factor influencing personality and overall psychological well-being in a large and recognizable slice of humanity: the inhibited, the vulnerable, the highly reactive, the mildly depressed. What the different models have in common is an understanding that not only depression but also temperament rests on and is sustained by levels of neurotransmitters and stress hormones. One conclusion we might draw from this understanding is that medications that alter levels of, or transmission by, these substances *ought* to affect temperament. Indeed, we should be surprised if a medicine that resets the norepinephrine and serotonin systems does *not* directly alter temperament.

Psychiatrists have long recognized indirect effects of medication on temperament. If you give a child with attention deficits a stimulant, and if that child then succeeds academically and socially, you will—through the feedback from the external environment—produce a more confident child. The direct effect of medication on temperament is different. If you can alter serotonin and norepinephrine, you should be able, merely by virtue of that change in the biological interior milieu, to produce a more socially comfortable individual.

The medicines I have talked most about—imipramine, desipramine, the MAOIs, the SSRIs—are conventionally called antidepressants. But this label was applied as a matter of circumstance, because these medications were, historically, first found to ameliorate or end depressive episodes. The same medications are effective against panic anxiety, and they could as appropriately have been called anxiolytics. The term "antidepressant" encourages us to attend arbitrarily to one use to which these drugs can be put. Perhaps preferable is the old word "thymoleptic." A thymoleptic is a substance that acts on the "thymus"—Greek for the soul or spirit or seat of the emotions. ("Neuroleptic," a word in more common usage by psychiatrists, refers to antipsychotics, like Thorazine.) "Thymoleptic" comes close to expressing our understanding that medications act on the neurohumors, and that the medications' effects on anxiety, depression, and personality are particular manifestations of that deeper alteration.

Thymoleptic action is apparent in Sally's transformation in response to Prozac. On a chemical level, she is enhancing the activity of her serotonergic neurons; perhaps on a psychophysiological level she is altering her reactivity to challenge. But on the level we most readily observe, what is new about Sally is her reduced degree of social inhibition—a change in one of the most salient aspects of her personality. This change is more striking even than any decrease in depressed mood. There is, perhaps, no need to weigh these two consequences against each other: since both mood disorder and "reactivity" appear to be regulated by the same neurotransmitters and stress hormones, whenever a patient takes an antidepressant we will be uncertain whether what changes is illness or temperament.

Sally looks like one of the small percentage of people who remain shy into adulthood. Kagan believes 15 percent of young children are inhibited. Suomi sees similar tendencies in 20 percent of rhesus monkeys. The rhesus monkeys remain different—more "reactive"—into adulthood. If only 2 or 3 percent of adult humans remain inhibited, what has happened to the temperament of the other 12 or 13 percent of inhibited infants?

One possibility is that people "grow out of" childhood inhibition, so that their neurobiology becomes indistinguishable from that of their age-mates. This seems not to occur in monkeys, but monkeys may be less plastic than we are; monkey parents may expend a less focused effort on social education, may be more willing to write off a few unhappy offspring. If we are not very different from monkeys, however, a substantial percentage of human adults, though not outright shy, are walking around with highly reactive temperaments. Behaviorally, they may do fine under favorable circumstances; but they will become anxious and then depressed when confronted by novelty or social disruption. Indeed, we may wonder whether some of the patients we have met who enjoyed apparently tranquil childhoods came to their rejection-sensitivity by inheriting some element of the inhibited temperament.

Beyond Kagan's initial 15 percent, additional people may achieve a neural substrate similar to that of inborn inhibition through exposure to psychological or even physical trauma. If inhibited temperament and its inevitable variants are widespread, then a medication that affects the biological substrate of inhibition will be capable of altering personality in a substantial proportion of the adult population.

The vast majority of these people, including those who are outright inhibited socially, will be "normal" in psychological terms. Most of them will be highly functional in their careers and private lives. No one has ever called people with inhibited personalities mentally ill. The brief conclusion to this line of reasoning is that in patients like Sally, and in many others with less dramatic stories and perhaps with no history of depression at all, what we are changing with medication is the infrastructure of personality. That is, Sally is able to marry on Prozac because she has achieved chemically the interior milieu of someone born with a different genome and exposed to a more benign world in childhood.

I have talked often about the way medication colors our view of human nature, but there is also influence in the other direction. Once we believe that the state of biogenic amines determines aspects of temperament, we will expect amine-altering medications to influence personality. Indeed, we may wonder why antidepressants do not alter personality more often, or, if they do, why this effect was not noted in the past.

If altered serotonin levels change personality, this effect should have been seen in patients taking imipramine, as many as thirty years ago. There were, in fact, occasional mentions of the influence of imipramine on personality in the early literature. And after the reification of dysthymia as a diagnosis, even before the general use of Prozac, a few research reports appeared in the professional literature noting personality changes in depressed patients given conventional antidepressants. But for the most part, personality was the arena of psychotherapy. Indeed, what was called a "character disorder"—later "personality disorder"—was for many years a contraindication for treatment with medication.

Hagop Akiskal took this distinction into account when discussing depressive personality. Akiskal reserved the category of affective temperament ("subaffective dysthymia") for people with persistent biological markers of depression, a tendency to overshoot on medication, and a family history of manic depression. He distinguished these patients from people (the "characterologically depressed") who had come to their depressive personalities through trauma, such as growing up with alcoholic or absent parents. Akiskal for many years believed that characterologic depression did not respond to antidepressants—and, indeed, many of his patients did not improve on tricyclics.

According to Akiskal's early model, how you came to your personality mattered. Those who were born with a depressive temperament were considered likely to respond to medication, whereas those who were made depressive were not. This distinction corresponds well to the psychoanalytic view that problems of character require nonpharmacologic treatment, but it is curious. It corresponds poorly to the common observation that acute, major depression responds to medication whether or not an environmental cause is apparent. The idea that "characterologic" or environment-based depression does not respond to medication also flies in the face of animal research demonstrating that antidepressants can make genetically normal but behaviorally traumatized animals less vulnerable to stress.

Staking out a position more "biological" than Akiskal's, Donald Klein, the researcher known for his work on hysteroid dysphoria and phobic anxiety, weighed in on the side of medication treatment for characterologic depression. Klein holds that much chronic maladaptive behavior of all stripes arises from underlying physiological vulnerability.

The patients whom doctors most often diagnosed as characterologically depressed were those who had difficulty in social functioning—relations with others, job tenure, and the like. There was a derogatory cast to this distinction, as if to say that people with strong characters work whether they are depressed or not, and that characterologic depressives were complainers or "losers." Researchers never made such statements outright, but at worst character pathology carried the sort of stigma we have already seen attached to hysteria, and at best there was a sense that these patients were hard to help, not fully cooperative, perhaps two steps shy of malingering.

To test the relationship between medication responsiveness and character pathology, Klein's group looked at about two hundred chronically depressed adults almost all of whom scored as impaired on a scale rating social functioning, a measure of success in work and intimate relationships. After six weeks of treatment with imipramine or an MAOI, patients who responded in terms of mood (sadness, sleep, appetite, ruminations, etc.) also showed improvements in social functioning. Indeed, over 28 percent of those who responded to medication after six weeks showed social-adjustment scores as high as or higher than a general community sample—a remarkable phenomenon for a brief trial of medication. The greater improvement was in patients who had been given, and had responded to, the MAOI.

In strict terms, Klein had proved nothing. His study shows only that chronically depressed people who respond to antidepressants also show a rapid improvement in social functioning. But the ease with which "characterologic" handicaps disappeared on medication threw the utility of the concept "characterologic depression" into doubt.

Prozac settled this dispute. Once Prozac was available, Akiskal found that virtually all of his dysthymics and patients with depressive personality, whatever the origin of their pathology, responded to medication. Not all responded to Prozac, though responses to Prozac when they occurred were especially complete or dramatic. Some patients responded to imipramine or related antidepressants, some to lithium, some to a combination of lithium and antidepressant, some to anticonvulsants, but, one way or another, it was possible to get nearly every dysthymic patient to improve. In his research, Akiskal no longer divides patients with chronic low-level depression into the categories "subaffective dysthymia" and "characterologic depression." The distinction is of no clinical utility. There are no more "characterologic depressives," only dysthymics for whom the right biological treatment has not yet been discovered.

So strong is the influence of medication on the way we think about personality that a number of the psychiatrists charged with updating the standard diagnostic manual have suggested doing away altogether with the distinction between mental illness and personality disorder. Their assumption is that personality disorder and discrete mental illness are thoroughly intermixed—that much of what has been called personality disorder is the final, behavioral expression of a variant state of the biogenic amines. In the case of depression, this view holds that discrete bouts of depression are part of a recurrent illness which, between episodes, expresses itself as depressive personality. This illness has its more and less severe forms, and manifests itself differently in different people, just as atherosclerotic heart disease admits of different degrees, stages, and symptoms; but the distinction between recurrent depression, depressive personality, and dysthymia becomes superfluous. My own sense is that it is premature to lump all derangements of personality with acute illness. But I do think it is reasonable to use the word "dysthymia" to refer to depressive personality or chronic minor depression, whether the presumed cause is nature or (traumatic) nurture.

The conceptual leap Akiskal and others have made in recent years—all depressive personality is responsive to biological influence—raises the possibility that there is something special about Prozac. Perhaps "characterologic depression" did not in the past respond to medication because the medication available was ill-suited to the task.

Prozac is distinctive in a variety of ways. It may selectively treat atypical depression, thus filling a gap missed by tricyclic antidepressants like imipramine. It may be especially effective in minor depression. It can reduce compulsiveness. And it has a favorable side-effect profile, so it is acceptable to a wider range of people—certainly much more acceptable than MAOIs, which also seem to work through enhancement of serotonin. As for serotonin, it may have a broader effect on the stabilization of affect ("serotonin-as-police") than do the neurotransmitters altered by other medications; in particular, a serotonergic antidepressant might be more multipurpose than a medicine that acts on norepinephrine.

Certain researchers have speculated privately that Prozac may be especially effective in the full range of dysthymia because of quirks in the Prozac molecule. Prozac is particularly narrow in its locus of action. Most antidepressants influence multiple sites on the same neuron; they may, for example, increase serotonin production at one end of the neuron, but also diminish norepinephrine or serotonin production through ordinarily less marked effects at receptors elsewhere on the same cell. Perhaps Prozac's extreme specificity is overwhelming to the neuron; the cell responds at one site, in one direction, and cannot, through mechanisms that otherwise allow neurons to "compensate" for changes in state, return to a prior level of functioning.

Also, Prozac is especially long-acting. Its extended half-life in the body can be a pharmacologic disadvantage; if a patient experiences a side effect of Prozac, such as nausea or headache, the medication will not wash out for many days, and the side effect may persist for the whole of that time, even though the patient has stopped taking medicine. But long action may also have positive consequences. With short-acting drugs, the level of the chemical in the brain rises as the drug is absorbed and falls as the drug is excreted or digested. In contrast, the brain levels of Prozac are extremely steady. This lack of fluctuation may have peculiar neurochemical efficacy, or the invariance of the brain's chemical status may have psychological ramifications. In terms of sensitivity to disappointment, a very steady cushion against decompensation may translate into a new continuous sense of self—that is, the change may be experienced as altered temperament rather than temporarily altered circumstance. These speculations are untested—they are scientific table talk—but they suggest a willingness in the research community to consider the idea that our ability to influence temperament in pharmacologic terms is new and growing.

Or perhaps our ability to influence temperament with antidepressants is old and overlooked. In an era when personality was understood to be the summation of psychological defenses, and the defenses were understood as responses to trauma during development, it was threatening to see personality as responding to medication. It may be that Prozac is special in its effect on temperament, or that Prozac arrived at a propitious moment and as a result—because the time was ripe and also because the drug had few side effects and was given to many people—Prozac has allowed us to see an effect of medications that we should have attended to long ago.

• • •

The effect of medication on personality makes research on biological temperament look more interesting, and that research in turn makes plausible the idea that "antidepressants" are really "thymoleptics." In the midst of this reverberation between changed views of personality and of medication, it is impossible that our view of mental illness should remain constant. After all, what does it mean that the same medications can treat depression and anxiety? Antidepressants, or thymoleptics, are used in the management of eating disorders, especially anorexia. They can ameliorate attention-deficit disorder, compulsive behaviors, and a host of other syndromes and individual symptoms. Inevitably, this plethora of indications has made doctors wonder what it is they are treating when they prescribe these drugs.

A viewpoint that is gaining currency in psychiatry, under the rubric "the functional theory of psychopathology," is that mental states are best understood first through the consideration of particular mental *functions,* such as mood, cognition, and perception—and that multifaceted entities such as mental illness or personality should be considered secondary. An assumption of the theory is that variation in functions will turn out to arise from a particular state of one or another neurotransmitter.

The thrust of the theory is most easily understood through example. Herman van Praag, the psychiatrist most associated with this method of analysis, suggests that serotonin may regulate such functions as anxiety and aggression, whereas norepinephrine relates to pleasure or, more specifically, "reward coupling"—the ability to anticipate future pleasure in activities that have been pleasurable in the past. This theory accounts for the success of the antidepressant desipramine, which changes norepinephrine-based transmission, in treating both depression and anorexia, since a central element of both disorders is reward uncoupling (loss of the ability to experience pleasure in the case of depression, loss of appetite in the case of anorexia). Likewise, panic anxiety, chronic depression, and social inhibition, all responsive to serotonergic medications, can be seen as turning on issues of proper levels of assertiveness and inner comfort. Van Praag is quick to state that such formulations are premature.

The details are less significant than the perspective. Van Praag is asking us to look past complex diagnoses (such as depression and anorexia, each of which has many symptoms) to behavioral building blocks of illness and personality (such as aggression or "reward coupling") which are presumably influenced by particular neurotransmitter states.

A virtue of the functional theory of illness and cure is that it explains an apparent paradox of Prozac, a medication that is at once specific in its biochemical action and useful in a wide variety of disorders. The functional theory predicts precisely this relationship: "The greater the biochemical specificity of a drug, the greater is the chance it will be nosologically [that is, diagnostically] nonspecific . . ." Since the same functions are deranged in a variety of illnesses, a medicine that affects only one neurotransmitter, and therefore only a few functions, will have broad applicability.

The availability of increasingly specific medicines should open the possibility of increasingly specific modifications to temperament. There are at least five, and very likely more, subtypes of the molecule that binds serotonin at the cell membrane. Researchers have begun to identify drugs that are specific for particular serotonin-receptor subtypes. Perhaps the future will bring drugs that can influence narrower functions than "anxiety and aggression." These drugs might be applicable to a very wide range of problems (mental illnesses, personality traits, individual symptoms), but the function they address within those problems might be quite specific. You might get the confidence Prozac instills without getting the quickness of thought.

The research that yields these results will not be targeted at changing personality. But once we believe that temperament is ruled by the neurohumors, there is no separating progress in treating mental illness from progress in altering temperament. Necessarily, research on the treatment of major illness will also be research into cosmetic psychopharmacology. The better we are at changing specific transmission patterns in the brain, the better we will be at recasting the foundations of normal variants in personality. New drugs should be able both to modify inborn predisposition and to repair traumatic damage to personality that has become functionally autonomous on a physiological basis.

•   •   •

My speculations, though based on research into social reactivity and the affective temperament, are far ahead of the evidence. They are not, however, ahead of the field. An increasing number of psychiatrists believe the genetic set of the neurohumors governs personality in ways that go far beyond anything we have discussed.

One who has spoken out boldly is C. Robert Cloninger, a member of the department of genetics and head of the department of psychiatry at Washington University in St. Louis, the nation's most biologically oriented psychiatry program. In the mid-1980s, Cloninger published two widely read, and widely criticized, scientific papers outlining a "unified biosocial theory of personality." In Cloninger's monographs, theory has outstripped experimental results. Still, there is pleasure to be had in observing a fertile imagination at work, and Cloninger gives us a sense of where biological psychiatry wishes it were now and where it hopes soon to be.

Fully elaborated, Cloninger's theory is immensely complex. But at its heart is a straightforward set of tenets we can understand in light of concepts we have already discussed. Cloninger believes there are three biologically determined axes of temperament, corresponding to the three neurohumors: norepinephrine, serotonin, and dopamine.

The axis governed by norepinephrine Cloninger calls "reward dependence." A person who is "severely high" on this axis will be, in Cloninger's words, "Highly dependent on emotional supports and intimacy with others; highly sensitive to social cues and responsive to social pressures; highly sentimental, crying very easily; [an] industrious, ambitious overachiever who pushes [him- or her-] self to exhaustion; extremely sensitive to rejection from even minor slights, leading to reward-seeking behaviors such as overeating; [and] highly persistent in craving for gratification even when frustrated in attempts to obtain expected recognition or benefits." This constellation is none other than rejection-sensitivity. At the severely low end of the axis are people who are insensitive to rejection. In Cloninger's words, people with low "reward dependence" are "Socially detached, never sharing intimate feelings with others, content to be alone . . . insensitive to social cues and pressures." Such a person might be an alienated nonconformist, unmotivated by ambition to please.

There are less extreme positions on this spectrum. A mildly high "reward-dependent" individual prefers intimacy to privacy, usually conforms to social pressures, is usually helpful and industrious, and is sensitive to major rejections. Someone mildly low for this trait will have social contacts but few intimate ones, will for the most part resist social pressure, and will experience only a transient upset in response to rejection or frustration. In other words, the whole range of possible positions on this axis of temperament is seen as being governed by norepinephrine. We are no longer talking, as Kagan was, about 15 percent of infants or 3 percent of adults who are extreme in a particular personality trait. Every person's level of reward dependence (or social reactivity) is influenced by and encoded in the state of his or her norepinephrine-related neurons.

In the same way, the other neurohumors determine the whole spectrum of hues in their respective affective and temperamental colorations. To serotonin, Cloninger ascribes a trait he calls "harm avoidance." Harm avoidance resembles the uptightness and separation-induced fearfulness we have seen in rhesus monkeys. "Severely high" harm avoidance entails: inhibition in the face of unfamiliar people or situations, fear and anticipation of harm even in the presence of reassurance and support, pessimism, and easy fatigability. Those with very low harm avoidance are laid-back—confident, carefree, optimistic, energetic, quick to recuperate, and calm in the face of unfamiliar or threatening circumstances.

Dopamine, another biogenic amine that acts as a neurotransmitter, is the chemical that is thought to be too high in schizophrenia and too low in Parkinson's disease. Thorazine, the first modern psychotherapeutic drug, *blocks* dopamine in the brain, the presumed mechanism by which the medicine ameliorates the symptoms of schizophrenia. L-dopa, the drug around which the book and movie *Awakenings* revolve, effectively *increases* brain dopamine and is useful in ameliorating the symptoms of Parkinsonism. In the past fifteen years, many biological psychiatrists have speculated about dopamine's role in the temperament of normal people.

In Cloninger's model, dopamine levels set the degree of a trait he calls "novelty seeking." In similar theories, such as those of Monte Buchsbaum at the University of California, Irvine, the same trait is called "stimulus seeking" or "impulsivity." At one extreme is the person who "Consistently seeks thrilling adventures and exploration [and is] intolerant of structure and monotony." Such people make decisions intuitively, act and spend impulsively, and engage in a rapidly shifting series of interests and social relationships. They often take self-destructive risks. At the other extreme are people with low levels of dopamine transmission. Orderly, organized people wedded to routine and enamored of structure, they are controlled, analytical, frugal, loyal, stoical, and slow to change interests or attachments.

To relate Cloninger's axes to concepts we have already discussed: high reward dependence (posited to be a function of the norepinephrine system) corresponds loosely to sensitivity; high harm avoidance (serotonin), to inhibition; and low novelty seeking (dopamine), to fastidiousness or inflexibility.

These three axes—reward dependence, harm avoidance, and novelty seeking—allow Cloninger to cover a vast territory. Looking only at reward dependence and harm avoidance, we can imagine a person who is highly reward-dependent (signified by the capital letter R) and highly harm-avoidant (H). Such a person would crave reward but be afraid to seek it openly. Cloninger describes the RH personality with these adjectives: "passive avoidance; submissive/deferential; indirectly manipulative; dependently demanding." Given more courage (low harm avoidance, or h) we have the person (Rh) who is "heroic, persuasive/pushy, perseverant, and gullible."

Extremes on three dimensions correspond to personality structures that begin to look like psychiatric deviance. Nhr is psychopathy or antisocial personality, the profile of a man or woman who always needs a stimulus "high," ignores risk, and has little need for the rewards of social intimacy or acceptance; criminals and cool, manipulative salespeople may be Nhr; nHr is the obsessional, nhr the imperturbable, socially isolative schizoid. Some of the Prozac-responders we have met might be classed as nHR (avoidant of novelty, cautious, and sensitive), though none is at the extreme of the three axes.

Cloninger's is a true spectrum theory of personality. We are all brothers under the skin, the sociopath, the hero, and the working drone. What distinguishes us is the state of our neurohumors. Where normal personality ends and personality disorder begins is only a matter of convention—of how far along each axis we set the cutoff points. Every human being has a biological temperament parsimoniously described by three numbers—the values for reward dependence, harm avoidance, and novelty seeking.

For all that this spectrum aspect of Cloninger's work has humane implications—the sociopath is not of a different species, he is like many of us but more so—the model, taken as a whole, embodies a humanist's nightmare. Many people, even some who know a good deal about psychiatry, enter the consulting room with the fear, which is also a sort of hope, that the doctor will be able to classify them with great scientific specificity—"Oh, he's a 231010-XW." This fantasy is a complicated one. At its heart, I think, is the wish to be cared for, but not on account of one's idiosyncratic self. Implicit is the sense that one's intimate self is not lovable, and that the patient will do better to count on professional objectivity to ensure appropriate care. Implicit also is a degree of passivity or even masochism, a willingness to put oneself at the mercy of a medical Svengali. The certainty that they are known scientifically makes many patients feel safe, although that safety hides seeds of rage that may sprout rapidly when a patient discovers, to his or her disappointment and relief, the limitations of the care-giver. Cloninger's system indicates that this hope or fear of objective omniscience is a fantasy shared by the profession as well.

Speaking of disappointment and relief, we may feel both in the face of this oversimple model. No theory so mechanistic could possibly capture our essence: we have escaped again! No one, I suspect not even Cloninger, imagines this schematic formulation is "right." In the study of personality, even more than in the study of major depression, there is too much contradictory information to allow us to embrace simple answers. Cloninger's effort—and I have not done justice to the volume of supportive information he adduces, from genetics, neurochemistry, and drug trials—serves most importantly as a vision or an ideal, an example of the form biological psychiatrists might like our understanding of personality to take. His model does resonate with certain of our earlier discussions. For example, the multiaxial approach gives support to the notion of non-hysteroid rejection-sensitivity, the concept I attached to patients who are vulnerable to loss but who have not developed a style that caricatures femininity. Rejection-sensitivity will produce hysteroid traits only in the presence of high stimulus seeking and low harm avoidance (NhR). But rejection-sensitivity (high reward dependence, or R) in combination with other tendencies—for example, caution (H) and fear of novelty (n)—will produce very different pictures. The multiaxial model serves to remind us that the way any one attribute manifests itself will depend on the other attributes that accompany it.

The model serves also to underline the implications of the biological drift in our understanding of personality. It is not just "sensitivity" or "inhibition" but a wide variety of temperamental traits that we may come to see as reified, especially if advances in psychopharmacology continue to play a role. If someone develops a pill that makes people less gullible, we will see gullibility as a biological predisposition—shake our heads sadly behind the backs of parents of gullible children, express annoyance at gullible adults who fail to seek treatment, and wonder in a different way about ourselves if now and then in our social dealings we find ourselves taken in.

But when it comes to the specifics of Cloninger's model, even a modest background in the neurochemistry of personality induces doubts. Cloninger attributes harm avoidance to serotonin, but Suomi's monkey studies suggest that early in the traumatic process leading to inhibition it is norepinephrine levels that change; serotonin comes into play only after multiple traumas and challenges. Post's kindling model, with its evidence that first one neurotransmitter system and then another becomes disordered as a disease progresses, makes any one-transmitter/one-trait model suspect. If different degrees of depression involve complex changes in a variety of transmitters, it seems likely that different degrees of any one personality trait will as well.

Cloninger associates norepinephrine with reward dependence, but rejection-sensitive patients respond less often to medications like desipramine that affect norepinephrine, and frequently to medications like MAOIs and SSRIs that very likely work through raising serotonin levels. Moreover, in Prozac-responsive patients, it seems that this serotonergic medication has simultaneous effects on a variety of axes—decreasing inhibition and harm avoidance while increasing assertiveness and energy—casting doubt on the assertion that Cloninger's three axes are independent. In Cloninger's terms, Prozac decreases reward dependence, increases novelty seeking, and decreases harm avoidance. In summary, it takes a passive-dependent person (nHR) and makes her more of a sociopath (Nhr)—an observation that may make us wonder what it takes to get along in this society.

The truth is, scientists have a slender grasp of possible biological substrates for a few aspects of personality, prominent among them social inhibition and depressive personality. But we are a species of theory builders. Once we begin to believe that personality has biological underpinnings, we act as if the future were already at hand.

This speculation then drifts into the general culture, often in overstated form. I am thinking for instance, of the "Ideas" story in *Newsweek* that helped shape my awareness that we "listen to drugs." The article says genes "are estimated to account for . . . 30 percent of personality differences." A geneticist would deem this statement meaningless: the degree to which a trait is heritable varies according to the range of environments over which it is studied. Are we talking about a heterogeneous culture, or the culture within a single family? What is "personality," globally taken, and what measures it? The proportion of personality one finds to be heritable will depend to a great extent on how one defines and quantifies personality.

The *Newsweek* article is about why siblings differ. The writer says, "A child who is shy by nature will react very differently to having a social butterfly for a mother than does his outgoing sister." Hidden in the phrase "shy by nature" is a full acceptance, perhaps even an overvaluation, of the Kagan research. We have only modest evidence that even a small proportion of children are constitutionally shy; for the most part, the role of temperament remains a mystery.

The sentence about the social-butterfly mother and the shy-by-nature child made me think of *The Glass Menagerie*. I recently saw a performance in which the mother, played by Olympia Dukakis, seemed so sympathetic that the family conflict was drained of its tension. It is hard to remember how Tennessee Williams played a few years back, but part of the tragedy has always involved the mother's having destroyed her daughter. Today, I think we might just say it is difficult to raise a child who is shy by nature, and all the more difficult for a mother who is social by nature. Here is an example of how a reductionistic view of human nature at once takes something away, namely the force of the drama, and gives something back, by making the once-demonized mother a character with whose plight we can identify.

•   •   •

When Suomi studies monkeys separated from their mothers, he is investigating a stress or trauma model of mood regulation. Studies focused on inborn, heritable influences are called "risk" models; they concern subjects believed to be at risk on a genetic basis for various disorders or differences. Both trauma and risk seem capable of producing all the phenomena we have considered. Early separation leads to reactivity to novelty, but inborn temperament can have much the same effect. The prevailing developmental model of depressed or inhibited temperament combines these two factors into what is called a trauma/temperament or stress/risk model. According to this model, most manifestations of, say, dysthymia can be understood as resulting from different influences in combination—traumatic events in the life history of someone with a vulnerable temperamental predisposition.

The two factors can be interactive. To a "reactive" person, what might seem to others quite minor stress will be experienced as trauma. There may also be some clustering of stress and risk. For instance, when the California psychiatrist-sociobiologist Michael McGuire took careful histories of his dysthymic women, many of them reported having been (like Sally) abused as children; the dysthymic women were four times as likely to have been abused as the matched control subjects. For a variety of reasons, McGuire believes these women's social inhibition preceded the abuse. As girls, these women may have signaled their vulnerability in a way that made them more liable to be chosen as a target of abuse; this is a matter not of blaming the victim but of understanding the process of victimization. It is also possible that the relatives of dysthymic women are (biologically) predisposed to act dysfunctionally and thus to create harmful family environments; in the case of dysthymic mothers, through both their choice of mates and their behavior in the marriage. Even the penalties society attaches to depressive temperament—small living space, low income, social isolation—correlate with likelihood of abuse.

The work of all of the researchers we have discussed would lead us to believe that it is possible to come to dysthymia through stress, temperament, or both in combination. The type of stress may make a difference in humans, as it seems to in monkeys. For example, a recent genetic study of white twin girls and women showed that those who in childhood had lived through parental separation, generally through divorce, were more likely as adults to suffer major depression and generalized anxiety disorder—even though *death* of a parent did *not* have this effect. Death of a parent may well be a different stressor from parental divorce. The freedom to grieve death may be an important factor, as may be the sense that the parent did not choose to leave. And if a widow or widower remarries, a child may be freer to identify with the stepparent in cases of death than of divorce. As for separation, it is rarely a onetime event but, rather, a complex stressor over time, including perhaps family conflict before a divorce, social and economic disruption after, and prolonged pressures on the child from both parents.

Stress and risk commonly interact. A child born with depressive temperament may have a parent who suffered similarly. That parent, because of social handicaps or self-doubt, may have chosen a spouse poorly or may function poorly in marriage. The child at risk will therefore be a stressed child as well, and if the child is rejection-sensitive, whatever stressors he or she encounters will be psychologically and physiologically amplified. The child's growing dysfunction then affects the family, not least the temperamentally vulnerable parent.

The stresses the child suffers are encoded physiologically, as altered neurotransmitter systems. They are also encoded psychologically, as characteristic defenses, defenses that will be all the more necessary as the child's psychophysiologic vulnerability increases. The "highly defended" adult who emerges from these difficult circumstances will tell a story that makes sense in strict psychoanalytic terms—that is, a story of trauma, self-blame, loss, and so forth; but part of what maintains his or her dysfunctional status can also be understood as functionally autonomous, biologically maintained patterns of response to stress or novelty.

———

The stress/risk model admits of complexity. It attends to the mind, and to the broader social setting, as well as to the neurons. It illuminates the stories of patients we have met. And it corresponds to the commonsense belief that there should be biological as well as environmental components to personality and that they should interact in intricate ways.

But the psychological element in the stress/risk model is often overlooked. Implicit in the model is an openness to the sort of statement often made to psychiatrists at the initiation of treatment: "That's just who I am." As recently as ten or twenty years ago, the therapist would likely have responded that who a person habitually is, is largely a matter of defensiveness—that is, of characteristic ways of avoiding disorganizing thought and emotion. This point of view—in truth, not alien to the risk/stress model—demanded that patients take responsibility for broad areas of personality and try to reshape them through self-understanding and courage. Today a patient who protests, "But that's just who I am," is in line with the prevailing wisdom, and it may be harder to convince the patient to see the role that experience plays in the formation even of behaviors and traits that feel automatic, visceral, and unchangeable.

In light of the rapid efficacy of medication, psychiatrists and, increasingly, the public lean toward the belief that personality is "biological." In both Julia, the fastidious housewife and nurse, and Jerry, the self-effacing surgeon, it seems that inborn temperament played a major role in personality formation; Lucy, the student whose mother was murdered, seems shaped by trauma; Sally, both inhibited and abused, is most clearly a mixed case. But medication was transformative for all these patients, suggesting that, before treatment, temperament had a large role in shaping their personalities.

"Temperament," in the risk/stress model, is a biological substrate for adult personality that has inevitably been modified by life events such as profound trauma. But it is easy—seeing the effects of medicine, reading about differences between monkeys bred for laid-back or uptight temperament—to ignore the role of experience and focus only on the role of inborn "type." This point of view—a pure "risk" model—is one our society has resisted for decades, on grounds that it is antidemocratic or racist or sexist. Such a psychology raises questions about human malleability, about free will, about models of child-rearing and education, and about the degree of responsibility and level of effort we should expect of people vis-à-vis their personality traits. Even if we understand the complexity of temperament, to the extent that we believe personality is largely a matter of biology, we experience ourselves differently, and we may be less curious about psychological avenues of change.

Our view of psychotherapeutic drugs has changed already. Earlier, I said in passing that through medication Sally may have been given the interior milieu of someone born with a different genome and exposed to a more benign world in childhood. Is it not remarkable that such an assertion can now be made "by the way"? The capacity of modern medication to allow a person to experience, on a stable and continuous basis, the feelings of someone with a different temperament and history is among the most extraordinary accomplishments of modern science.

Part of what makes medicine seem so powerful is an ambiguity in the word "personality." On the one hand, it means what the researchers are able to measure—gross traits such as shyness, aggression, impulsivity, and the like. On the other hand, it refers to the many small and consequential features that make each person unique. When Sally took Prozac, she was able to change the most socially handicapping aspect of her personality. But after the transformation, she was still Sally. Most of what we would call her personality persisted in a recognizable way. Though no longer inhibited, she is the same woman, with the same determination, the same opinions, aspirations, bêtes noires, mannerisms, and memories—although each of these might be changed a bit, too, by medicine, and she would still be recognizably the same.

Tess's reaction to the return of her symptoms when she was off Prozac was: "I'm not myself." But many patients stress a continuity of self on and off drugs. "I am myself without the lead boots," "myself without swimming through Jell-O," "myself on a good day, although I never had days this good," "myself without fears"—these are words inhibited and dysthymic people use to describe the effect of thymoleptics. Their reactions acknowledge aspects of the personhood that medication does not alter.

Some months before her wedding, Sally said, "I am myself, but no longer shut out of everything. I am more comfortable in myself —not empty inside." She seems very much this way: liberated, filled out, at once grounded and lightened, but still very much Sally. Self and personality turn out to be greater than the sum of their parts. They are gestalts, hard to tease into factors, hard to pin down. Here is an additional effect of medication: When we see how essentially unchanged a shy person is without her shyness, we will want to say that personality extends far beyond the limited traits or axes researchers are able to study.

We may even ask: Is Sally's fiancé truly marrying the shy woman with the difficult history? The past self is not hidden from her fiancé, but neither is she fully present. However Sally experiences it, we may feel that her self contains a discontinuity. And if we sense this discontinuity, we are also saying something about the extent to which a person "just is" her stable, continuous biological inner self.

Still, we should be proud to dance at Sally's wedding because of the pleasure this sign of her liberation brings her. The wedding may stand also as an icon for another union in progress, that between biological and psychological views of personality, and therefore of self. Though it is not free of ominous portents—is it a match between equals, or will biology dominate?—after half a century in which physiologically based temperament had been banished from society, this marriage should be welcome.

Formes Frustes:
Low Self-Esteem

A reviewer of a recent book about antidepressants complains; she wishes that the author's "argument did not extend to such a huge and varied list of ailments." Recalling the syndromes we have seen Prozac treat, ranging from minor degrees of depression, anxiety, and compulsiveness to melancholic temperament and social inhibition, we may express a similar wish. It seems that any human frailty whatsoever is likely to be caught in our net. Worse, each of these conditions is itself composed of a list of symptoms, from alterations in bodily functions, such as sleep and appetite, to disturbances of mental functioning, such as memory and concentration, to distortions of self-assessment, including body image and global self-worth. But multifaceted syndromes can appear in incomplete forms—what Freud, in his discussion of anxiety neurosis, called "rudimentary" or "larval" presentations of the illness, or illness-equivalents, and what are now most often called *formes frustes*. The same underlying biological condition that in some people is expressed as the full picture of dysthymia will appear, in other people, as a single symptom.

Insomnia, for instance, may be the solitary symptom of what, in biological terms, is chronic minor depression. Sometimes a person with a long-standing sleep disorder and no depressed mood will find, on being given an antidepressant for an incidental indication (of which there are many—including prevention of migraine headaches), that the sleep problem disappears. This may occur even in response to a "stimulating" antidepressant whose side effects include arousal rather than sedation. Biologically, the insomnia was an isolated symptom of dysregulation of the biogenic amines. What is only mildly remarkable regarding sleep disturbance is more noteworthy in the case of such complex human functions as the assessment of self-worth or the ability to experience pleasure. These functions may be altered in depression, but they are also highly personal aspects of the self, linked closely to the individual's sense of who he is and how life events have shaped him.

●　●　●

Self-esteem is the most autobiographical of traits. A person's private assessment of his or her history, it contains, in integrated form, the victories and failures he or she has achieved and the cruelties and kindnesses with which he or she has met. Self-esteem is largely thought of as an intellectual function—the opposite, for example, of self-doubt, thinking ill of oneself, or undervaluing one's own capacities.

Self-esteem is hot as a defining and explanatory concept in today's culture. The goal of all modern parents is to give their children high self-esteem. Popular magazine articles debate what best fosters self-esteem in children: support or challenge, implicit trust or firm boundaries, room to grow or encouragement to excel. Every private organization that serves children, from preschools to summer camps, advertises itself as nurturing self-esteem, in the way that schools and camps of an earlier era stressed building character.

Alcoholics and adult children of alcoholics strive to reassess themselves in terms of past injuries to self-esteem. Low self-esteem is understood as a common impediment in women's social and professional struggles. Motivational tapes for businessmen purport to bolster self-worth. In myriad ways, American culture promotes self-esteem as the key to success and happiness, usually expressed as self-fulfillment, with the implication that self-esteem can be achieved through the experience of success or through the retraining of habitual patterns of thought.

This popular focus on the importance of self-esteem follows an evolution in the assumptions of psychotherapy. Self-esteem entered the psychiatric agenda through the rather odd theories of Alfred Adler. Though Freud later dismissed him as a dissident, Adler was part of Freud's inner circle in the first years of this century. Adler believed that many people suffer from defects, largely hereditary, in their bodily organs—he was especially interested in the bladder and kidneys. He maintained that people with "inferior" organs tend also to have defective nervous systems, and the already compromised nervous tracts become more strained as they try to compensate for the bodily defects. This "organic inferiority" is ultimately experienced by the person as a "feeling of inferiority" or insecurity. From insecurity comes neurosis—the result of a person's varied attempts to deny or compensate for the feeling of inferiority, perhaps through false bravado, perhaps through meekness and timidity. Though obscure and difficult to read, Adler's work had enormous popular influence in the 1920s, when the term "inferiority complex" became a near-synonym for neurosis.

Though Adler's ideas about the origins of low self-esteem were odd, his account of the effects of low self-esteem was prescient, presaging modern work on inhibition, reaction to novelty, and the role of self-image in family life. But to Freud, Adler's work was heretical: Adler grounded neurosis (albeit circuitously) in biological constitution; and Adler ignored unconscious inner conflict—the struggle of desire and guilt—in favor of the central role of the feeling of inferiority. Freud responded by arguing that low self-esteem was an incidental phenomenon, essentially a variant form of guilt. According to Freudian psychoanalysis, a person with low self-esteem typically had an overly strong conscience (in the language of psychoanalysis, the superego), which he attributed to an inner image of the exigent father. When psychoanalysis was employed to confront the sense of inferiority, its goal was to temper the power of the superego by making the (male) patient aware of his exaggerated sense of his father's power. (The less-developed theory regarding women centers on fear of loss of the mother's love.)

But Adler's concept of inferiority left its mark, and in time even faithful Freudians became interested in low self-esteem. In recent years, analysts have focused less on guilt as a source of low self-esteem and more on the role of childhood deprivation, or of misunderstandings between parent and child. Over the past twenty years, a consensus has formed that self-esteem arises, intact or damaged, from a person's experience of being recognized and appreciated at critical junctures in childhood.

The new guiding metaphor for the source of self-esteem is the gleam in the mother's eye. (Research on nurturance as a factor in the development of self-esteem shows attachment to the mother as of primary importance, with the father's role, in most cases, as surprisingly inconsequential, though that may change as fathers take on more of a nurturing role.) "What a lovely drawing!" the empathic mother says. In this, she is authentic; she does not praise what she does not see. She takes genuine pleasure in the child's stage-appropriate accomplishment, and she communicates her pleasure in a way that is neither overwhelming nor secretly demanding. She is aware of the child's needs more than of her own. And if she manages to gleam most of the time, she will be a "good-enough mother," providing sufficient security so that her occasional failures in empathy do not damage her child's sense of self. What a "good-enough mother" induces in her child is "appropriate grandiosity," the ability to imagine great things, without the need to scurry compulsively after superficial indicators of success. The values instilled by the rule-giving parent, traditionally the father, are still believed to influence self-worth, though, again, they are accorded relatively less importance.

Self-worth is a product of family experience and the family culture as they are absorbed by the growing child. Most developmental theories also recognize the role of later environmental influences outside the family. Children encounter success and failure in friendships, studies, sports, and their private play and exploration; adults succeed or fail at love and work. Self-esteem can grow, in response to achievements and the experience of competency, and it can be damaged by disappointments, humiliations, and losses.

But the effect of experience on self-worth in adult life is limited by the self-esteem with which a person enters adulthood. People with low self-esteem seemingly "do not know their own worth" and habitually discount successes. Typically, they are most aware of failures that confirm their negative self-image.

All the different maladaptive personality types that make life difficult and unhappy, ranging from the overscrupulous to the sociopathic, from the socially avoidant to the exhibitionistic, can be seen as outcomes of early failures in parental empathy interacting with painful life experiences. From this point of view, the diverse personality types represent responses to differing needs to shield the self from awareness of its own vulnerability, and then to conceal the imperfect, fragile, devalued self from the world. Psychotherapy allows change by helping a person reassess threats to integrity of the self, and by providing a person with a reparative relationship in which he or she is understood empathically, or empathically enough.

What is missing from this account is any appreciation of the factor Adler began with—the effect of biology on mood and temperament. To be sure, psychotherapists have begun to think about the issue of mismatched temperaments—the "swan raised by ducks" or a "bad fit" between child and parents. (Again, consider mother and daughter in *The Glass Menagerie*.) Certain parents have more trouble understanding certain children. But even this perspective may not be "biological" enough. Theories of parent-child mismatches may not explain a person's level of self-esteem. Temperament—sanguine or melancholic, for example—interacts with the environment both in childhood and in adult life. Positive mood leads to behaviors that are rewarded in the world and to full appreciation of those rewards —thus further enhancing self-regard and reinforcing the sanguine temperament. In the complementary sequence, melancholic temperament leads to maladaptive behaviors, which lead to disappointments, and thus to ever lower self-worth and ever more melancholy. The dysthymic women studied by Michael McGuire—the ones always at the end of long lines—suffered this constant sequence of maladaptive behavior, injury, and demoralization.

Some biologically oriented psychiatrists believe that self-esteem is directly related to mood—in the extreme, that low self-worth can be little more than a *forme fruste* of chronic minor depression. A happy, expansive, optimistic, energetic temperament includes positive self-regard as one of its elements; a more passive and pessimistic temperament includes low self-esteem. There are patients whose sense of self-worth seems to rise and fall in immediate response to the state of the biogenic amines—without any change in the degree of empathy they receive from others.

Donald Klein has written about such a person, a successful lawyer in his forties who, despite "a reasonably happy marriage, well-adjusted and successful children, and a career of moderate accomplishments and continuing upward social mobility," suffered persistent low self-esteem. The lawyer, whom the authors call William M., came to know himself better through psychotherapy, but without diminution of his sense of inadequacy or intermittent depressions. After six months of increasing feelings of groundless free-floating anxiety, the lawyer was referred for medication treatment.

Expecting an awkward and socially inept patient, the consulting psychiatrist was surprised to find William M. "good-looking, urbane, witty, intelligent and psychologically sensitive"—far from dysthymic or socially inhibited. William M.'s only chronic problem was low self-esteem. The psychiatrist prescribed an antidepressant. First the acute anxiety and depression faded. Then:

The patient's low self-esteem, which had been present since his earliest childhood, began to disappear. He began to re-evaluate his aptitudes and assets in a thoroughly realistic manner. The insights gained in psychotherapy, which heretofore had had no emotional impact, were now accompanied by a different attitude toward himself. It was as if William M. had been subtly depressed throughout his life and as if his low self-esteem had been a superficial manifestation of the depression.

On medication, William M. experienced a sense of self-worth superior to any he had felt before. What is more remarkable is that each time the medication was tapered—in the hope that William M. would be able to do without the antidepressant—the low self-esteem returned. When medication was reinstituted, his self-esteem improved.

The case of William M. has a number of implications. For him, medication—an impersonal, ahistorical intervention, far from the realm of empathy or revised autobiography—affected self-esteem dramatically and decisively. The success of medication suggests that in some people levels of self-esteem may be largely a matter of neurobiology, related more to inborn temperament than to life experience.

Most important, beyond the question of how self-esteem arises, this case makes plausible a new understanding of what self-esteem is. For William M., psychotherapy was useful only when he was on medication; off antidepressants, he was unable to use insight. The beliefs that accompany low-self esteem—I am a failure, what I have achieved is of no importance—appeared and disappeared, or gained and lost potency, in conjunction with the changed feeling regarding the self. Neurologists use the term "proprioception" to refer to perceptions that monitor the self; proprioceptive pathways tell us where our hands and feet are, so we know where we are in the world. In the story of William M., low self-esteem seems a matter of altered emotional proprioception—a neurological distortion in self-awareness.

*   *   *

I have treated a number of patients like William M., people plagued by low self-esteem for whom medication works. The story of one such patient, Allison, reinforces this metaphor of proprioception—low self-esteem as an almost neurological inability to locate the self.

Allison wavered for over a year before coming to me. Her psychotherapy with a social worker had focused on issues of self-esteem; she had made slow, steady progress and then plateaued. The social worker had seen other such patients improve on Prozac but could not convince Allison to seek a consultation. Allison feared that an antidepressant might cause her to gain weight, and she believed she would be even more worthless and intolerable to others if she were not thin and unobtrusive. The more Allison obsessed about whether to make an appointment, the more the psychologist believed she was right in urging her on. At last, while trying in psychotherapy to face her feelings toward her mother, Allison hit a period of paralysis and found herself spending whole weekend days in bed, consumed with self-pity and vague fears. It was at this point that she wrote me an autobiographical letter in preparation for an appointment.

Allison began by describing her persistent feelings of sadness and fear. "It's like woe-is-me and doom-and-gloom are my partners," she wrote. "I want to be happy but can't give up the negatives, and can't get to that point of feeling self-worth."

Allison, an only child, saw her self-valuation as grounded in family life. Her father, she wrote, lacked the ability to assert himself. Instead, like Zelig, Woody Allen's chameleonlike film protagonist, he took on the personality of whomever he was with. To his daughter, the father was confusing, consistent only in his unhappiness, his focus on money issues, and his rejection of almost all members of the extended family. "He never knew me," Allison said, "and I never knew him."

Allison's mother was disappointed in her husband and lived through their daughter, dressing her like a doll but also comparing her with her cousins in ways that made Allison feel stupid. As a child, Allison was frail. She spent many hours alone—her favorite form of play was dressing paper dolls—but she had little sense of privacy, because her mother, who demanded that Allison confide in her, divulged Allison's secrets to cousins, aunts, and uncles. Allison's mother seemed content to have an ill daughter. The mother was gentle, but she used the excuse of Allison's infirmity to make all the decisions for her daughter and acted wounded if Allison tried to make any choice independently.

In adult life, Allison felt physically weak, intellectually second-rate, and socially awkward, although there were intervals when she was healthy and had friends. With the help of a supportive husband, she achieved many of her dreams. She raised three reasonably well-adjusted children and rose to a responsible position in her work as a fashion designer. But Allison never felt connected to her successes. She took no credit for the children's progress, doubted even that they had felt the effect of her love for them. And she behaved as if her design work had been done by someone else; she could not look at the clothes and see them as her own.

Her family complained that Allison repeated herself in conversation. She could not help it—she never believed that anyone ever listened to her. Even her body felt alien. She found herself occasionally staring at her own face or hands, or looking at photographs, to remember what she looked like. What she was searching for included and went beyond the physical self. She remembered in fifth grade having seen her image in the mirror and thinking, "There is a person there," but being unable to connect that person with Allison. The month before she to wrote me, Allison's husband bought her a sports car for a special birthday. She found she would adjust the side-view mirror so she could see the car, or adjust the interior mirror so she could see herself in the car, so difficult did she find it to accept the gift as real or connected to her.

When she showed up in the office, Allison's low self-esteem was written all over her. Though attractive and well dressed, she maintained a self-conscious posture for much of the interview and then apologized for her unease. Her conversation gave no indication of the slowed thoughts or impaired concentration typical of depression, but when I tried to check these functions by asking her to do simple mental tasks—recalling four phrases after five minutes, counting down by sevens from one hundred—self-doubt impeded her performance.

In the realm of pleasure, Allison's problem was her inability to believe that anything good would, or should, befall her. She lacked any certainty of her right to live and be. She said she was not outright depressed but, rather, "always on the verge of tears."

Because of her apprehensions and her acute sensitivity to any changes in her body, I started Allison on half the usual dose of Prozac. Even so, she felt side effects: excessive energy at first, and a sense of spaciness or difficulty concentrating. These diminished rapidly, and within a month Allison declared herself better.

The feeling of impending tearfulness had disappeared. With this change came a profound alteration in self-regard. "I am convinced my husband loves me," Allison said. She was able to experience the sports car as her own, able to appreciate and enjoy the fact that her husband had meant to give it to her in particular. And she found she no longer needed to repeat herself, no longer feared being overlooked.

A problem had arisen at work, and her first thought was "I can get over this hurdle," something she was not aware of ever having thought before. She threw herself into the fray. "I was always a watcher," she tried to explain. "I did not want to make waves. I was constantly afraid I would make people angry. Now I am more forward, and at the same time I feel I am a more gentle person, a more loving person. My staff has noticed it."

After three months on Prozac, Allison developed a rash, and we interrupted treatment. Off the drug, she again felt devastated, unworthy, and physically clumsy. The rash turned out to have had an unrelated cause, and when we restarted the Prozac, the sensation of confidence and connectedness returned. Allison's self-esteem, like William M.'s, was exquisitely medication-sensitive.

A few weeks after she resumed taking Prozac, Allison related a telling story. She had just been to visit a cousin she adored. She had always wanted red hair and green eyes like this cousin; Allison had blond hair and blue eyes, but somehow the family had made her feel this coloring was second best. As a grade-schooler, Allison ate carrots and beets in the hopes that her hair would turn red. She made over her dolls in the cousin's image. Over the years, everything about this cousin had been better: her native intelligence, the college she went to, her field of study, the man she married, the part of the country she lived in. And, of course, the cousin was taller and thinner.

But this time when she visited the cousin, Allison no longer felt like the dumb one: "So she went to a better college. What does she do with it? She sits home and reads women's magazines. I would never trade my children for her children." The two went grocery shopping, and the cousin tried to convince Allison that sea scallops were better than bay scallops. "I almost believed her—any other time I would have believed anything she said. This time I said, 'Whatever do you mean?' What I meant was, 'I am not an ugly idiot.' And then I noticed I was taller than she was—and I had been for thirty years."

Two things struck me as remarkable about Allison. Before she responded to medicine, she impressed me with the variety of ways in which she described low self-esteem as a perceptual experience. It was hard not to listen to her accounts with the ear of a literary critic in search of a subtext, underlining the frequency with which she referred to an inability to find the self. She was virtually invisible to herself, except for her faults.

After the Prozac "kicked in," I was impressed with her instantaneous change in self-image. Though I suspect that the medicine would have been less effective without the prior and concomitant psychotherapy, when the change occurred, it seemed a matter of changed self-valuation leading to changed self-understanding, rather than the reverse: the medication allowed her to locate herself. Before seeing Prozac work in this way, I would have said that to alter your self-image you have either to understand yourself differently or to live through a relationship in which you experience being valued differently. Surely a pill cannot reshape the inner representations you carry of your disconnected father and narcissistic mother. But Allison's self-image had indeed changed, on Prozac. And prior to her change in proprioception, Allison's marriage and her psychotherapy, both of which offered new forms of self-understanding and appreciation, seemed powerless to improve her self-esteem.

Other patients we have met, Tess and Julia prominent among them, responded to medication with rapid changes in self-image. The story of Jerry, the self-effacing surgeon, could be retold making self-image the central theme. What distinguishes these stories is the immediacy of the metamorphosis. We think of self-image as something accreted over time, acquired through living, subject mostly to incremental change. But in my practice I have seen case after case in which self-image changes overnight.

Patients who do well on medication quickly take on positive beliefs about the self. The new valuation of self seems to come from nowhere. The visceral sense of self-worth, positive or negative, appears to have an enormous effect on self-image, social efficacy, and overall well-being. And, as in the cases of William M. and Allison, medication works like a switch. When the patient is taking medication, self-esteem is high; when medication is interrupted, self-esteem is absent. There is nothing incremental about this change. The switch flips, and the whole package of self-valuation changes: beliefs about the self, assessment of personal history, sense of place in the world. The response to medication is independent of self-understanding.

Psychotherapeutic drugs have the power to remap the mental landscape—lithium makes manic depression seem ubiquitous, Xanax does the same for panic anxiety. But pharmacotherapy is not the only technology that has this effect; psychotherapy is a technology as well, and it has shaped the modern vision just as surely. In the half-century before the development of antidepressants, the facilitation of self-understanding was the most reliable way to alter low self-worth. Reasoning by inverses, and starting from the observation that improved self-understanding results in improved self-esteem, we have come to believe that a disorder of self-understanding causes low self-esteem, or even that low self-esteem is simply a disorder of self-understanding.

This belief is reasonable on other grounds. People with low self-esteem often say or believe bad things about themselves. And, historically, we find that many people with low self-esteem were taught in childhood that they are inferior to others. In Allison's case, we could conclude that her mother undermined her by criticizing, while her father injured her sense of self-importance through his emotional unavailability. Allison came to see herself as unworthy among women and unlovable among men. This view appeals to our sense of man as a creature of reason even as regards his unreason.

The way that negative belief about the self tends to accompany feelings of low self-esteem, and the way that effective psychotherapy fosters self-esteem, encouraged the belief that self-valuation is primarily a matter of self-understanding—that is, of cognition. In retrospect, however, there have always been reasons to question this idea. For one thing, self-esteem often does not respond to changes in cognition. There have always been patients like Allison and William M. who progress intellectually in psychotherapy without benefiting in terms of self-worth. Indeed, the distinguishing feature of the damaged sense of self is its poor responsiveness to evidence, even to evidence that is cognitively appreciated.

If we had looked at drug abuse as carefully as we now look at the licit use of medications, we would long have been aware that self-worth can respond to biological interventions. One reason amphetamine is popular as a drug of abuse is that people feel good about themselves on it. Uppers enhance users' sense of their place in the world. They feel big, important, worthy of attention. The classic experience of college students writing papers while on amphetamines is to overvalue the composition while the drug is active—even to imagine they are great writers and have dashed off a masterpiece—and then, as the drug wears off and they "crash," to undervalue their work and themselves. The problem with amphetamine as a treatment for disorders in self-image is precisely that it exposes the user to dramatic ups and downs. But its ability temporarily to alter self-valuation might have told us something about the physiological nature of self-esteem.

Even without referring to drugs, we know that self-worth has a distinct visceral component. Think about being overcome by a sudden failure of nerve. Like an attack of shyness or an urgent desire to gain the attention or approval of an admired person, this sensation is gripping and poorly responsive to reason. Accompanying it are profound bodily sensations: butterflies, flushing, weakness, and dizziness. The physical aspect of self-esteem is encapsulated in the common statement "I just don't feel good about myself." Feeling bad about oneself is an affective, not a cognitive, state, although feeling bad about oneself and thinking poorly of oneself are clearly related.

If psychiatry has ignored the physical aspect of self-image, it is in part because the autobiographical model of self-image has been so predominant and in part because there have been no alternate models around which to organize discrepant evidence. This is changing. First, there has been a re-emergence of the James-Lange theory of emotion, known in America through the writings of the nineteenth-century philosopher and psychologist William James, brother of the novelist Henry James. William James argued that the bodily elements of emotion, the parts we usually think of as secondary phenomena, are its core: the rapid heartbeat *is* fear, and we come to think "I am afraid" only after we sense palpitations. James was largely forgotten in the psychoanalytic era. But Donald Klein's explanation of panic anxiety has made James's psychology more appealing. As we have seen, the new dominant theory holds that the bodily sensations of anxiety, including the sense of dread that is so characteristic of panic attacks, can arise spontaneously and then accrete around them a series of explanations that are the mind's way of integrating this over-whelming emotion into a coherent experience. In a similar way, the cognitive element of self-esteem, far from being primary, might be a response to negative feelings about the self. Just as, when parents divorce, a child will make the world coherent by taking on the belief that he or she is bad, a person with a visceral sense of low self-worth will take on negative beliefs about the self, in order to make sense of the bad feelings.

Once again, the animal world provides an analogy for the problem of high and low self-esteem. Human experiences of self-worth seem to bear a relationship to pecking orders in the animal kingdom.

Much mammalian social behavior revolves around what is formally called "dominance hierarchy." We think of hierarchy as a reproductive strategy. The strongest lion is able to impregnate a group of females and then defend enough territory to guarantee that his lionesses are well fed and rival males kept at a distance. But hierarchy is also a way of organizing social behavior, of introducing an element of order into the pride to prevent what otherwise would degenerate into a war of all against all.

Those who watch natural-history specials on television will be familiar with the dominant-submissive rituals of a variety of animals. How are these encoded? Consider the alpha-beta hierarchy of pack animals like wolves, in which certain males lead and others follow. How does a wolf know he is the alpha wolf? Yes, the experience of success in combat must have something to do with it, but surely we do not believe that the feeling of being the alpha wolf is maintained in the wolf's mind by cognition. To be the alpha wolf must be a pervasive experience, a feeling that informs every action, a state of the neurons that differs every minute of the day from that of the low-status "babysitter" wolf. And this visceral superiority probably exists in the absence of anything we would recognize as autobiographical memory. Rather than say a wolf learns to feel worthy of leadership, we might say that, on achieving alpha status, a wolf has become, neurochemically, a leader. This analogue of self-esteem pervades the wolf's physiology. He grows bold and voracious.

A research team—including Michael McGuire, the sociobiologist who studied dysthymic women—observed dominance hierarchy in multimale, mixed-sex troops of captive vervet monkeys. They noted that in each troop there was one male monkey in whose bloodstream there was a distinctly elevated level of serotonin, the mood-setting amine whose reuptake is blocked by Prozac. The level of serotonin in this male was about one and a half times that in other males, and in every instance the high-serotonin male was the dominant male in the troop.

The researchers first looked at groups that experienced a spontaneous change in leadership. Barring a change in status, blood-serotonin levels over time are remarkably stable in individual monkeys, as they are in man. But when a monkey changed status, his serotonin level changed dramatically. The serotonin level in newly dominant monkeys rose almost 40 percent, whereas the level in newly subordinate (formerly dominant) males fell almost 50 percent, to a level below that of the average subordinate male.

Dominance hierarchy can be manipulated in captive monkeys. Researchers remove the dominant male from the troop, and a new male takes on the dominant role. If the original leader is returned to the troop within ten weeks, he will resume the dominant role, and the interim dominant male will again become submissive. Here the changes are even more dramatic. Serotonin levels in the submissive monkey rise over 60 percent when he becomes the interim dominant male, and then fall to below their original level when the old leader returns. The old leader's blood serotonin falls to the levels of a subordinate monkey during the period of isolation, and returns to its usual elevated level on restoration to the troop and his former status. Subordinate males' blood serotonin is unaltered by social isolation. The factor that affects and sustains a high serotonin level is active dominance within the troop. Even removing a dominant male from a multimale group and housing him with three females causes his serotonin level to drop.

This research leads to the conclusion that, at least in vervet monkeys, serotonin levels are influenced by social status. In particular, receiving submissive behavior from other males elevates serotonin levels. Conversely, do serotonin levels influence social status?

To investigate this issue, the same researchers influenced vervet monkeys with drugs (including Prozac) that raise serotonin levels, as well as with drugs that lower them. The researchers looked at twelve social groups, each consisting of three males, three females, and their offspring. There were two experimental conditions.

In the first, the dominant male was removed from the group and one of the two remaining males was given a drug that increases serotonin levels; the other male was given a drug that lowers serotonin levels. The monkeys were observed for eight or more weeks, and then the dominant male was returned to the group, and all medicines were withdrawn.

After the group was given eight weeks to restabilize, the dominant male was removed again. This time, the monkey that had been given the serotonin-elevating drug was given a serotonin-depleting drug, and the monkey who in the first trial had been given the serotonin-depleting drug was given a serotonin-elevating drug. This is called a crossover design.

The results were dramatic. In every instance, after three or four weeks, the male monkey given a serotonin-elevating drug achieved dominance over the monkey given the serotonin-depleting drug. Dominance was complete and stable—the dominant monkey always won over 85 percent, usually 95 to 100 percent, of aggressive encounters. Because of the crossover design, it is clear that the effect had nothing to do with inherent traits in the monkeys selected. Whichever monkey got Prozac, or a drug with similar effect, dominated.

When the originally dominant monkey returns to the group, he assumes dominance once again, even if a formerly subordinate male is kept on a serotonin-enhancing drug. Mostly this is a function of the extreme stability of dominance hierarchy in vervet monkeys; monkeys instinctively remain loyal to old leaders even after relatively protracted absences, a trait that must provide continuity to troop life. But perhaps it is also an indicator that serotonin status is not the whole story: dominant males have other features, beyond high serotonin levels, that make them leaders. When coexisting in a group with a naturally dominant male, a Prozac-treated male achieves intermediate rank. The researchers have concluded that "serotonergic mechanisms seem to promote dominance acquisition only when hierarchical relationships are in flux."

There is suggestive evidence that serotonin levels in both humans and monkeys are under genetic influence. In juvenile rhesus monkeys, a breakdown product of serotonin has been shown to correlate with their fathers' levels of the same metabolite, even though the fathers do not raise the children. The vervet monkey researchers hypothesize that, in nature, certain male monkeys are endowed with high levels of serotonin. This endowment causes them to engage in successful behaviors—affiliation with female monkeys seems particularly important—which in times of flux can lead to the assumption of the dominant role. This status then leads to yet higher levels of serotonin, as well as to stable behaviors that reinforce dominance status.

Comparable studies of serotonin levels in man have not been carried out; it is difficult to vary status hierarchy experimentally in humans. But the monkey studies suggest that self-esteem, or the tendency toward assertiveness, is maintained by the serotonin system, and that the setting of the serotonin system is important in predisposing to levels of both self-esteem and certain kinds of social success. The vervet-monkey studies also suggest that self-esteem is a function of social reward, whether or not mediated by complex cognition. Perhaps in some people low self-esteem may be less a result of biography than of genetics: a low serotonin setting in a sense *is* low self-esteem—a feeling of unworthiness or submissiveness—and leads to low self-esteem by engendering unassertive behavior and an acceptance of low social status. Perhaps there are even people with a serotonin system so unresponsive that they do not experience high self-esteem whatever their social good fortune. Other people may come to low self-esteem by experiencing social deprivation, but even their self-image may be encoded less in cognitive memory than in the condition of their neurons. However low self-worth is acquired, a medication that raises serotonin levels might move a person biochemically from the feelings of subordinate status toward the feelings and even the behaviors of dominant status.

Low self-esteem is so closely related to other concepts we have considered—depressed mood, social inhibition, reactivity to novelty—that it can be conceptualized in terms of a now familiar model. Though it is a far stretch from dominance hierarchy in lower primates to self-esteem in humans, it is possible to imagine that for us low self-worth is either "biological" on a primary basis (that is, inborn, perhaps through serotonin levels) or else biological on a basis that is mediated by social status and in which self-understanding is a secondary, compensatory process.

Still, no one is likely to abandon the idea that self-esteem can be autobiographical. Constantly critical parents do often destroy the confidence of their children. Much research attests to the role of parenting in the formation of self-esteem. For instance, an often cited study of children in Connecticut concludes that self-esteem in ten-to-twelve-year-olds correlates with measures of "parental warmth, acceptance, respect, and clearly defined limit setting."

But after acknowledging the role of autobiographical memory in self-esteem, we will likely end by saying that much of the autobiography is stored in transmission patterns of mood-setting neurons. I can imagine a "kindling" model of low self-esteem parallel to that for depression: Over the years it may take less and less humiliation to set off—neurochemically—the same feeling of low status. As such feelings become endemic, low self-worth may become relatively insulated from the reparative powers of success. I can also imagine a sort of "failure-sensitivity," an analogue to rejection-sensitivity, in which minor humiliations strongly reinforce feelings of worthlessness. As in the case of kindled depression, such models would presumably entail progressive change in a number of neurotransmitters, not just serotonin. The concept of kindled low self-esteem implies that idiosyncratic, autobiographical experience does shape a person's sense of self-worth, but in the context of biological constraints. Those constraints may be inborn or may arise from trauma, or persistent low social status—perhaps enforced by insensitive, domineering parents.

We understand Allison's biography differently once she has responded to medication. We see her father's role as partly biological; perhaps his chameleonlike social behavior was a response to his own (neurochemically determined) inability to locate the self, a handicap he has passed on genetically to his daughter. The father's low self-worth has led him to attract and marry a woman who is dominant enough to lead but sufficiently inhibited to confine her expression of power to family matters. A child with a temperamental vulnerability to low self-esteem experiences the father's absence and the mother's stifling presence as neglect and abuse. With the extended family defined as the troop, Allison finds herself at the bottom of the pecking order. Her sense of self diminishes progressively to the point where she disappears from view, an absence that is encoded as a hard-to-influence, functionally autonomous trait, perhaps one maintained by anatomical changes in serotonin-responsive neurons. Later in life, not even marked social success can reverse the process. Medication restores to Allison the neurochemical substrate that appropriately corresponds to her adult social status, and she reappears to herself at last.

•   •   •

I perceived a complex interaction of medication and self-understanding in another patient with low self-esteem. Paul consulted me for what he called "problems arising from a crummy childhood." He had not thought about his own childhood until his struggle to be a proper father to his own son exacerbated feelings of inadequacy he had experienced for years.

Paul was a sensitive youngest child born into a family of noisy, volatile, and controlling go-getters. His parents were constantly annoyed at him. "They tried to break me," Paul said, as he recalled the parents' draconian methods of curing him of thumb-sucking and other minor bad habits. Throughout Paul's childhood, his father, who prided himself on his rugged masculinity, called Paul a sissy and tormented him over his lack of interest or ability in sports, an area where the older boys excelled. Paul's mother seemed overwhelmed by the number of sons her husband had, as she saw it, foisted on her. She was constantly yelling, something the other children seemed to tolerate. Paul recalled going to bed every night in tears. To Paul, childhood was a series of overwhelming family fights punctuated by teasing directed especially at him. He emerged into adulthood feeling inferior, unmanly, misunderstood, and cheated of love.

Paul dealt with his discomfort by burying himself in his studies. With the encouragement of teachers, he pursued an academic career and went on to teach and write about Renaissance history at the university level, a calling his family considered inferior to the practical professions favored by his brothers. Paul managed to hook up with an equally sensitive and accomplished young woman, and in time they had their first child, a son.

As the boy grew, Paul became aware of keen feelings of inadequacy as a father. One day, a college student came to Paul's office, seeking not so much help with his studies as moral support. Feeling he had nothing to offer, Paul broke into tears in front of the student. From that moment, a sense of inadequacy became foremost in his consciousness, and after some weeks he decided to consult me.

Once Paul had poured forth stories about his childhood, he saw how his identity as a father related to his feelings of inferiority. He had become paralyzed with his son, whom Paul saw as sensitive and unathletic, the way he had been as a child. Paul was afraid to get angry with the son, for fear of replicating his own father's behavior, and equally afraid of hugging and kissing him, for fear of turning the boy into a sissy. After Paul had verbalized these concerns, they seemed foolish. He understood that, even if he expressed anger, it would not be in the relentless, destructive way his father had. And he knew that a boy would not become a sissy because a parent was too affectionate; on a conscious level, Paul believed the opposite was the case, that sensitive children do best if they feel secure and loved.

This new self-understanding gave Paul substantial relief, and after five sessions he pronounced himself cured. I wondered whether this early end to therapy arose from Paul's need not to be weak: psychotherapy was an activity his father would have derided. But I was happy to see him take charge and move on with his life.

Eight months later, Paul returned. The hiatus had been an occasion for intense self-examination. He had puzzled over his relationship to his father, whom he now considered openly abusive, and he had immersed himself in reading about family relations. Paul believed that he had come a long way toward handling the consequences of his father's rage; but now he was troubled by insistent, highly emotional memories of rejection by his mother. He feared that these feelings were damaging his marriage. He saw himself as a constant disappointment to his wife, and he felt wounded by any hint of disapproval from her. Just as his father had needed him to be strongly masculine, his mother, surrounded by men, had badly wanted her last child to be a girl. Paul saw how he had been caught between his parents' contradictory wishes and subjected to anger rooted in their ambivalence and discord. Talking to me, he focused on his struggle to distinguish his wife's reasonable demands from his mother's impossible ones. Again, after a few sessions Paul disappeared.

Paul did not return until a year later, after the birth of his second son. Again he felt overwhelmed and worthless. This return of the sensation of low self-esteem was accompanied by signs of depression. We discussed parenting, but I did not feel my words or even his own reached him. I suggested Prozac, saying it might help with the depression, expecting it to do more as well.

Three weeks after he began the medication, Paul felt back in control. And, as I had hoped, the drug worked on the chronic issue of self-worth. Paul reported he no longer felt globally inadequate and inferior. He realized he had long been somewhat afraid of his wife, for no discernible reason; now he felt her equal. He was even able to stand up to his father, who until then had continued to dominate any one-on-one interactions.

Paul tried to describe his new state: "I just feel strong. I feel resilient. I feel confident. I can get bombarded and still feel in one piece. I no longer lack resolve when it comes to the children. This is who I am." He felt masculine enough to be a father of boys, and still sensitive and gentle enough to avoid becoming the type of father his own father had been. This feeling was a necessary complement to the insights that had reassured him about his capacities as a father.

Paul noted another remarkable difference. In the past, he said, he had been able to recall certain painful experiences and to *imagine* how he must have felt as a child. Now, when he remembered such incidents, he *felt* what he had felt as a child. He could not tell whether this striking change in the affective quality of his memory—just the connection between thought and deep feeling that psychotherapists hope to inspire—was due to a direct action of medication or, as he believed more likely, an increase in his tolerance for strong, disturbing emotions. The medicine, he said, gave him the will and the means to continue to face himself, and he soon left psychotherapeutic treatment again, to continue his private exploration, returning to see me only for brief, infrequent meetings to discuss medication management. This statement of independence, Paul felt, differed from the others. In the past, he had wanted therapy but denied himself; now he just felt beyond the need for psychotherapy. He did consider Prozac a "crutch" but said, "What the hell. Some people need a crutch to walk."

I find this case telling, because it speaks to an interaction between insight and medication in reversing a focused problem regarding self-worth. Psychotherapists talk about insight's not having impact until it is connected to the relevant affect: reattaching "split-off" memories to the feelings that accompanied them is a central task, for example, of psychoanalysis. For Paul, medication provided that link. In addition, the medicine seemed to give Paul a feeling of dominance that was helpful in dealing with his father and his sons, as well as his mother and his wife.

Paul's sense of low worth had been relatively circumscribed: he managed fairly well except around the birth of his sons. Medication gave him a sense of strength, with regard both to the people he faced and to his memories. Paul's feelings of low self-esteem could hardly be called meaningless; they related to his childhood experiences. Yet they seemed to have a physiological component—the neurochemistry of membership in a family that valued only leadership—that was dealt with most parsimoniously through drug treatment.

The question of medication as a crutch is interesting here. Ordinarily, we understand confidence to be a response to accomplishment, to overcoming obstacles through sustained effort; we might therefore imagine that taking medication would lower self-esteem. Here, and in most cases I have seen, the reverse was true: medication allowed Paul to experience what had heretofore meant little to him —namely, the truth that he had already perdured many difficult trials. Medication allowed him to reinterpret history—although this phrasing perhaps understates the role of the antidepressant. It might be more honest to say, "Medication rewrites history." Medication is like a revolution overthrowing a totalitarian editor and allowing the news to emerge in perspective.

As medication helped Allison locate her self, it helped Paul give his history flesh and blood. One of the functions of a psychotherapist addressing the abused is to say, "Yes, it was as bad as you imagine it must have been." Medication played that role for Paul: it made his injuries more real, his response to them more comprehensible. Paul's is a case in which, rather than say self-understanding promoted self-esteem, we might argue that chemically restored self-esteem catalyzed self-understanding. This new self-understanding then reshaped self-valuation. The medicine also worked directly, combating both a biological predisposition and the effects of family life that had assigned Paul the lowest position in the dominance hierarchy.

Alfred Adler identified low self-esteem as an organic handicap. Traditional psychoanalysis emphasized fear of the domineering father in fostering inferiority. More recently, psychoanalysts have deemed low self-esteem to result from failures in parental empathy. The ability of Prozac—in both humans and low-status monkeys—to alter self-valuation now adds a new dimension to the understanding of self-esteem.

From the viewpoint of biological psychiatry, it is possible to conceptualize low self-esteem as one of many possible expressions of low serotonergic transmission. Like the melancholic temperament, a predisposition to low self-esteem can be inborn, or can be induced or exacerbated by trauma. Perhaps there are particular sorts of trauma that lead more often to low self-esteem than, say, to compulsiveness or inhibition to novelty. Certainly humiliation by domineering parents, or by competitive siblings or classmates, might be as much a factor in low self-esteem as empathic failures by otherwise nurturant parents.

Low self-esteem may be grounded in unconscious conflict or cognitive self-doubt, but the efficacy of medication is evidence that low self-esteem exists as a state of the neurons and neurotransmitters. If insecure humans are like low-status monkeys, to have low self-esteem is a particular neurochemical state, one responsive both to the experience of social dominance and to the effects of serotonergic drugs. Self-esteem is not primarily a set of thoughts about the self; it is an aid or an impediment to locating the self, and a lens through which the self's history is viewed.

The various models of self-esteem remain to be integrated. But with the belief that self-esteem is as much physiological as psychological, we have moved a long distance toward ending the hegemony of mind over brain in our concept of the self. The change in paradigm to a perspective that is highly aware of the bodily aspect of mental functioning is sometimes called psychiatry's "loss of mind." And it is true, if we were to deny the obvious—namely, that ordinary life experience influences self-esteem—we would have lost our minds. But it can equally be said that by recognizing the visceral or perceptual aspect of the self we will save the concept of mind by making it more complete. As regards such issues as self-esteem, the contemporary mind is like a stroke victim who had lost both recognition of the physical self and memory of its own past but is now, with the help of medication, regaining both proprioception and an awareness of its history.

Formes Frustes:
Inhibition of Pleasure,
Sluggishness of Thought

*A*nnie Hall, Woody Allen's film about a man who on neurotic grounds can enjoy the pleasures of neither intimacy nor Los Angeles, was made with the working title *Anhedonia*. Anhedonia, the illness, is a quaint Victorian variant of neurasthenia in which a person cannot experience pleasure. Freud redefined the inhibition of pleasure as psychological. A girl who is forced, through fear of loss of her mother's love, to forsake her desire for her father may in adulthood suffer a global muting of desire, a numbing of the hedonic senses; she is then "repressed," which is to say she has repressed her capacity to enjoy. The ability to experience pleasure is a trait that has now for many years been understood in purely psychological, as opposed to neurological, terms. Repressed people are "too hard on themselves" or, more deeply, afraid of pleasure. Anhedonia has disappeared as an illness; it persists in the language as a social or political metaphor, a sign of discord with contemporary culture, like "anomie," "ennui," and "alienation."

But anhedonia exists. It is another element of depression that can stand by itself, so that a patient may come to the consulting room complaining that there is nothing particular wrong with her except that the salt has lost its savor. I don't believe I have ever seen a case of pure anhedonia—in the absence of other signs of depression—but I worked for almost two years with a patient whose most persistent complaint was that she did not experience pleasure.

Hillary had tried a number of cures for her ailment. She had been in psychotherapy on and off throughout adolescence. Her last therapist became so intrigued or frustrated that, after many months of a failed traditional psychotherapy, he took to massaging her, according to the precepts of a fringe therapy called Rolfing. By the time she came to me, early in adult life, Hillary's problem had been labeled depression. But the gist of it was that she had no passion, no enthusiasm, no drive, no initiative, just a sort of lazy passivity grounded in her indifference to the pleasures of life. This take-it-or-leave-it attitude was so pronounced that, although she was funny and attractive and had the ability to consider situations with great originality, Hillary had few close friends and no boyfriends; men invariably developed the impression that she was bored with them. An admittedly overly sensual image of Hillary might be Marlene Dietrich in Alfred Hitchcock's film *Stage Fright,* where she sings the Cole Porter song "The Laziest Gal in Town." I have a pronounced memory of Hillary smiling languorously in a way that makes a therapist imagine his insights are less than compelling.

Hillary complained that she was bored, lonely, and underscheduled. She never had the willpower to bring order to her life. Nothing touched her or meant much to her, which was strange, because she came from a family of achievers, and on an intellectual level she shared their values. She loved her parents and wanted to please them, and she wanted to please herself, but without enthusiasm it was hard to sustain projects. She had limped through college and professional school, doing adequate work; she had been offered an interview with a respected firm on graduation, but she had not bothered to go to the interview, and now she was unemployed, paying her rent through odd jobs. She felt isolated because, as she put it, "The whole world seems to be in on something I just don't get."

Hillary had some of the traits of dysthymia or atypical depression:

sad mood, poor concentration, and constant sleepiness. (One doctor I consulted in her behalf suggested she suffered not from a mood disorder but from idiopathic central-nervous-system hypersomnia, a rare neurological condition in which patients sleep too much. Certainly Hillary yawned a lot.) Other than the sleepiness, most of Hillary's depressive symptoms seemed secondary or intermittent. The problem Hillary had early in life, and the one that persisted month after month, was an inability to understand what the fuss was all about.

Hillary combated her anhedonia in various ways. For instance, she learned how to hang-glide—and felt little thrill. (Her efforts made me think of the writer Graham Greene, who in his youth felt such ennui that he went to a dentist and feigned the symptoms that would lead the doctor to pull a tooth—to provide momentary respite from boredom.) She went to art galleries and concerts, but complained, "I don't see anything; I don't hear anything." Her isolation, low productivity, and lack of progress in a career all led to self-doubts.

Hillary's history with antidepressants was unusual. She responded to Prozac with a burst of activity that soon faded and did not return even with higher doses. Hillary would read her diary from the brief good period and ask, "Where did all the ideas come from? How did I manage to make so many plans?" She was angry at the medicine, because it had given her a taste of normal life, and now her emptiness was all the more poignant.

Though her last psychopharmacologist thought Hillary had suffered a major depression, he believed many of her problems were related to character and would respond best to extended psychotherapy. He wrote me: "She is a talented, creative individual who is stymied in her own mire of conflicts; I sincerely hope that she can allow herself to engage in the kind of treatment she would need in order to genuinely become unstuck." Hillary did enter psychotherapy with me for many months, but she found the process frustrating and considered me not a little foolish in my efforts to make connections between her affect and her life story. She herself could produce many plausible theories: "Being out of touch keeps me from being loved. Am I so afraid that I anesthetize myself?" But one hypothesis sounded as empty as another, and none of them helped her.

Because it had worked, if only briefly, I tried Hillary on Prozac again; with each increased dose, she got a slight effect which then faded. I added another drug (lithium) that sometimes acts synergistically with Prozac, but to no effect. At last, Hillary found a full-time job, one that demanded so many hours she could not find time to see me. Using the supply of Prozac she still had in the medicine cabinet, she resumed the medication in the hope that it would give her a little energy. On this third trial, the Prozac worked dramatically, and the effect was sustained.

"Now I understand what people were talking about," Hillary said. There were a hundred things to enjoy in life. She had no need to hang-glide: exhibits, concerts, films, and theater all spoke to her. She laughed about her relations with men. "They no longer intimidate me. I get a lot of attention from men these days, and frankly most of them are disappointing and unconvincing." She was able to enjoy dates even though she had her doubts about each man. She moved into and out of relationships with surprising ease. "I am in good control of my emotions," she said. "I don't get hurt. When I break up with a man, I have no bad feelings whatsoever, and I don't worry about whether I'm hurting him. Sometimes I wonder whether I haven't suffered a loss of moral sensibility." As for work, she was openly enthusiastic: "This is the perfect job for me." And it seemed her skills at work were enhanced; she loved what she was doing and could do it well.

I should emphasize that Hillary was not in the least manic, or even hyperthymic. Her social behavior seemed appropriate; her reasons for starting and ending liaisons sounded plausible, and if she was getting some of her own back with men, who could blame her?

I have no explanation for Hillary's initial failure and subsequent transformation on Prozac. Patients do occasionally improve on an antidepressant that previously did nothing for them. Sometimes I think the effect has to do with a synergy between the medicine and circumstances in the person's life that catalyze the cure—in this case, the job. I also wonder about the role of psychotherapy, as if some patients, through insight and a nurturant relationship, can be made psychobiologically "ready" to recover from a dysthymic syndrome. (If Prozac works best for lesser degrees of depression, perhaps in some patients it will only "kick in" when they are already psychologically and neurochemically on the mend.) It would be most honest to say that I do not know what factors allow medications to work where once they failed. But I have no doubt that what I saw in Hillary was a response to Prozac.

Here again, the medication seemed to flip a switch, to turn black and white into Technicolor. Prozac did things we have seen it do before—reduce rejection-sensitivity and increase liveliness—but it also seemed to provide access to a vital capacity that had heretofore been stunted or absent. Hillary's story made me appreciate how crippling the disregulation of "hedonic capacity" can be. The inability to experience pleasure as others do not only interferes with the motivation necessary to ambition or affiliation, it also leaves a person subtly uncomprehending of social behavior, and therefore utterly isolated.

Researchers have given a good deal of thought to the neurobiology of pleasure. Pleasure is essential to most social activity. In the form of reward, it influences attachment and learning, particularly social learning, and willingness to participate in groups and obey rules. It regulates appetite, for food and other substances. And it reaches broadly into every aspect of personality through enthusiasms, passion, aesthetic sensibility, and feelings of self-satisfaction. A host of disorders have been related to abnormalities of pleasure or reinforcement. Autism, schizophrenia, learning disabilities, delinquency and psychopathy, anorexia and bulimia, drug abuse, and depression have all been hypothesized to relate to dysfunction in the experiencing of pleasure in response to ordinary stimuli.

A variety of neurochemical systems and brain centers have been implicated in disorders of pleasure. Different neurotransmitters and different forms of injury are thought to be involved in, say, an autistic toddler's failure to respond to his parents' warmth and an anorexic adolescent's stubborn resistance to sustaining her body. Pleasure is so important to the establishment and maintenance of social and self-preservative behavior that its encoding in the brain is likely to be extensive and complex.

Though researchers have not elucidated the cellular biology of pleasure, theoreticians have given a good deal of thought to anhedonia. The modern reformulation of the concept began in the middle 1970s, when Paul Meehl, a psychologist at the University of Minnesota, published a critique of the prevailing psychoanalytic understanding of hedonic capacity. Meehl stepped back and looked from a distance at the Freudian view of psychological aberration. Freud assumed that all people strive for pleasure, and what distinguishes people are the forces that impede the striving. (To be fair, Freud also thought people differed in the strength of their drives, but that aspect of his thinking was never well elaborated.) The essence of psychoanalysis is the remove of defenses and resistances—various impediments to effective behavior and a full emotional life.

Meehl considered the impedance of drives to be only half a theory. Yes, people might come to mental illness through fear of various negative consequences; but why should they equally not come to it through the absence of positive reinforcers? His own observations led him to believe that, "just as there are some organisms impeded by fear, so there are other organisms whose fears are insufficiently softened, attenuated, or, I may even say, impeded by adequate pleasure."

In the normal population, there are, Meehl asserted, some children who are observably less capable of experiencing pleasure than others, just as there are adults who appear to have been "born three drinks behind." He suggested that, when a person reports he has just never gotten the same kick out of life that others do, therapists might consider, besides searching for impedances to pleasure, taking the patient's statement at face value. Just as McGuire saw the inflexibility in his dysthymic women as a an aspect of temperament that exists on a continuum, Meehl saw "cerebral 'joy-juice' " as a spectrum trait. Some people can take pleasure from almost any situation. Meehl wrote: "I conjecture that these people are the lucky ones at the high end of the hedonic capacity continuum, i.e., they were 'born three drinks' ahead." Both high and low levels of joy-juice are normal variants, not illness.

Anhedonia, however, can produce illness. Life at the low end of the continuum is difficult. People with little hedonic capacity must tolerate the same stresses as others, but without many of the rewards, and depression may result. Arming such patients with insight or even strategies for success is of little use. Their problem is precisely that success does not serve as a reward, because they do not experience the pleasure that ordinarily accompanies success. Meehl admitted that his formulation was speculative, but he conjectured that low hedonic capacity (hypohedonia), of the sort that leads to depression, can be a genetically heritable trait. Meehl might well say that a patient like Hillary is primarily hypohedonic; any depression she feels arises secondarily, from her inability to attain or appreciate life's bounty.

For the moment, Meehl wrote, the best treatment for (or prevention of) the depression that results from low hedonic capacity is a diminution of secondary guilt: the person who is socially limited because of hypohedonia ought not to blame himself for his social isolation; not everybody gets the same pleasure from affiliation. Meehl was not impressed, though, with strategies designed to encourage patients to "learn to live with a 'scarcity economy of pleasure' "; people just cannot maintain their mood or self-esteem without pleasure. Meehl believed that the best approach to hypohedonia would ultimately be psychopharmacologic.

———

Meehl's rejection of the "impedance" model of anhedonia was as challenging to the prevailing view of human nature as Klein's concept of rejection-sensitivity, and it suffered a similar fate. That is, in the absence of effective medication, it remained an interesting idea but one that was addressed by only a smattering of research. Much of that research is the work of a Chicago-based psychiatrist, Jan Fawcett, and his psychologist colleague, David Clark. In the early 1980s, Fawcett and Clark looked at hospitalized depressed patients and found that 12 percent complained of anhedonia. On a variety of psychological tests, the anhedonic group looked different from the other depressed patients. In particular, they showed fewer signs of neurotic conflict—that is, they seemed to have come to their ailment directly through a deficit in hedonic capacity, and not through guilt or anxiety. Anhedonic patients tended to recover faster than did other depressed patients, but even upon recovery they remained unable to experience pleasure. These results lend support to Meehl's conjectures. Fawcett and Clark's findings argue that hypohedonia is a chronic trait, that it is not especially associated with neurotic conflict, and that it results in a distinct subtype of depression.

Research regarding hypohedonia in normal populations has been more confusing. There are hints that low capacity for pleasure is a chronic trait, persistent throughout the life cycle, and that it correlates with difficulty in establishing or maintaining intimate relationships. These studies do not show that anhedonia results in depression, but the research has focused on very high-functioning populations—medical students, medical interns, and senior executives of Fortune 500 companies—in which anhedonic traits would likely have been compensated for in some way. And, of course, Meehl's assumption is precisely that, although low responsivity to reward can result in depression, for the most part it exists as a variant trait and is expressed differently depending on life circumstances and the additional temperamental traits that accompany it. One adaptation to low hedonic capacity is overachievement, in hopes of maximizing what little pleasure one can attain. Like Akiskal's dysthymics, the hypohedonic people Meehl describes can be driven in their careers.

When Meehl's monograph appeared, Donald Klein had just published an article that contained a different approach to anhedonia. Like Meehl, Klein was critiquing a basic tenet of psychoanalysis, but instead of impedance, Klein focused on Freud's claim—long since rejected even by most psychoanalysts—that there is only one sort of pleasure: excitation reduction. (According to Freud, pleasure is the replacement of irritating excitation, such as hunger, by satiation.) As usual, Klein's work rested on pharmacologic dissection.

Before studying imipramine, Klein had worked with drug addicts, and he noticed that addicts had distinct preferences. Those who favored morphine could generally be distinguished from those who favored cocaine or amphetamine. And though both types of drugs give a rush of pleasure, the eventual effects are different. Opiates satiate an addict, at least while they remain effective. Cocaine and amphetamine do not satiate but, rather, excite further desire; stimulant addicts will tend to "go on a run" and rapidly use all the drug at their disposal.

To Klein, these varieties of pharmacologic pleasure-seeking corresponded to varieties of ordinary enjoyment. Some pleasures, like eating a big meal or sexual orgasm, are satiating and do accord with Freud's concept of excitation reduction. But others, like "foraging, hunting, searching, and socializing," or sexual foreplay, are excitatory. Klein labeled these two sorts of pleasure "consummatory" and "appetitive."

Klein later looked to imipramine for clarification of this distinction. He pointed in particular to certain depressed patients who respond only partially to imipramine. These patients recover in terms of sleep and appetite, but they remain uninterested in work and other activities; adding amphetamine to the imipramine revives their interest and energy. Klein described such recovery as a two-step process.

Imipramine restores patients' responsiveness to the consummatory pleasures, but only on the second drug do they rediscover the pleasures of the hunt.

In his work with depression, Klein tried to distinguish those patients who were best treated with imipramine from those best treated with MAOIs (monoamine-oxidase inhibitors). Klein found that imipramine was most useful in the treatment of severe depressive episodes with a definite and rapid onset. Patients who looked less depressed, had arrived at depression more gradually, and complained mostly of boredom and apathy did not respond to imipramine but might respond to MAOIs. This second group could sometimes be interrupted by distractions or amusements; in the midst of a hospitalization for depression, they might be seen on the ward chatting happily. Yes, they were impaired. But the impairment extended only to appetitive pleasures. Though they had lost the capacity to forage, if pleasure landed on their plate, they consumed it.

Klein's theory holds that the pleasures of the hunt are neurobiologically distinct from the pleasures of the feast. The normal process of desire and satiation would go something like this: Encountering an appetitive stimulus (say, some mouth-watering prey), the organism experiences "hopeful expectancies and images." These lead in an excitatory fashion to heightened drive and heightened anticipatory pleasure. As the organism pursues the consumable object, it receives feedback from a "central comparator"—some part of the brain that mediates between desire and action—indicating it is doing well and encouraging further pursuit; in the case of impending failure, the comparator produces demoralization and energy conservation.

Atypical depression—the type in which patients eat and sleep too much—is nicely modeled by this theory; atypical depressives do not forage, but they do consume. They have appetitive, but not consummatory, anhedonia. Typical depression, in which appetite and sleep are lost, relates to consummatory anhedonia, which includes and supposes appetitive inaction: if you have no interest in eating, there is, *ipso facto*, no point in hunting.

Klein's account of anhedonia is often contrasted to Meehl's. But if we understand Meehl's "low hedonic capacity" to overlap with Klein's "appetitive anhedonia," Klein's work adds a nice refinement. Meehl's account is useful in underscoring the probability that responsiveness to pleasure is a spectrum phenomenon, and that unresponsiveness may be either a matter of defensiveness (impedance) or a deficit state (a low ability to experience pleasure) that exists as a normal variant. Klein's account helps explain a contradiction between what we see and what patients tell us. A patient may be perfectly charming in conversation and yet complain that she cannot function socially. The problem is that she can enjoy pleasures that happen to come her way, but she does not anticipate pleasure, and she is not moved to pursue it.

Hillary's case does not fit Klein's categories in any neat way. Like an appetitive anhedonic, she is lethargic and indifferent to anticipated pleasure; she also finds no (consummatory) thrill in art, music, or hang-gliding. But Klein's idea of an imperfectly inclusive anhedonic condition does go some way toward accounting for Hillary's ability to stumble through professional school as well as many of her pleasant traits, including her sense of humor. Both of these similar models help to make us comfortable with a biological approach to Hillary's frustration. If she is born with too little joy-juice, we should supply her with more; if her "central comparator" is misfunctioning, we should recalibrate it. And once Prozac works, it thoroughly undermines the Freudian hypothesis that "inhibition" of pleasure is merely a matter of defensiveness, guilt, and sexual shame.

The treatment of anhedonia with Prozac helps to clarify the distinction between drug use and drug abuse. Prozac does not provide pleasure; it restores the capacity for pleasure. It is neither excitatory like cocaine nor satiating like heroin. The drug taker does not crave Prozac and does not feel relief when it enters the system. The desired effect, a change in responsiveness to ordinary pleasures, occurs gradually and is unrelated to the daily act of consuming the drug.

But this is not to say that the use of medicine to alter the capacity for pleasure is without its accompanying questions, call them ethical or sociological, according to your taste. If we accept the proposition that hedonic capacity exists along a continuum, then in treating hypohedonia we are shifting a normal person from one part of that continuum to another. As long as we move from the extreme toward the middle—from atypical depression toward appetitive wellness—that exercise is unexceptionable. But should we aim for the precise center? Surely patients would prefer to be rendered a little hyperhedonic, to have an enhanced enjoyment of the ordinary. And then there is the question of people who are not patients—who begin with hedonic capacities close to the norm. If the drug is developed that will, with minimal side effects, make the ordinary taste richer—psychopharmacologic MSG—will we accept its use by people whose hedonic capacity is average and who have reasonable self-esteem and social skills? What is reasonable? Certainly Meehl sees the whole range of hedonic capacities as normal. Most decisions regarding continua are arbitrary: Who can say that this much hedonic capacity is standard and that much is above standard? Where does treatment end and—to use the word—hedonism begin?

These questions are not solely hypothetical. Often patients say they feel all right if they take one Prozac capsule four days a week, but they feel better still if they take the medicine more frequently. And there are patients who, once successfully weaned from Prozac, want to restart it, not because they are depressed, but because life seemed brighter when they were medicated. If we believe that hypohedonia is a chronic trait intermittently expressed as depression, we will expect exactly this difficulty. Forced to decide what level of hypohedonia bears treating, we may *tell* ourselves we are making the determination on quite different grounds, that we are weighing the possible risks of exposure to Prozac against the countervailing risks of recurrent depression. But in truth the deciding issue, which is largely aesthetic, or related to a modern tribal standard, is just how much zest a person ought to have.

To look again at drug abuse: An untested but widely accepted hypothesis regarding drug abuse is that it is in large measure a form
of self-regulation by people whose high rejection-sensitivity, low self-
esteem, and low hedonic capacity leave them vulnerable to painful
emotional states for which there is little counterbalancing pleasure.
According to the "self-medication hypothesis of addictive disorders,"
a formulation of the Harvard psychiatrist Edward Khantzian, addicts
use cocaine to treat affective states very similar to those I have discussed in relation to dysthymia; opiates, in contrast, may be used to
mute the disorganizing effects of rage. In other words, drug abuse,
particularly stimulant abuse, is not merely the pursuit of pleasure
or, as was once thought, an attempt at regression, but, rather, a
complex behavior aimed at coping with intolerable feelings in a person
who, without medication, may experience little enjoyment. Indeed,
the self-medication hypothesis has led to the treatment of certain
drug abusers with antidepressants in the hope that antidepressants
will at once increase addicts' hedonic capacity in their daily lives and
decrease their vulnerability to loss or rejection. These projects generally meet with mixed success—so much in the addict's culture
determines whether he gives up street drugs. But many addicts do
kick the street-drug habit once on antidepressants; and many report
that the prescribed medication makes them feel less empty and better
able to enjoy ordinary pleasures.

The difference between use and abuse rests on such issues as
legality, excitation, the characteristics of the drugs employed, and
the relationship of drug procurement and use to the rest of the person's
life—but not on the underlying purpose for which the medication
is taken. Both the anhedonic on Prozac and the drug abuser on cocaine
are trying to compensate for diminished hedonic capacities. In terms
of treatment, for both the neurotic and the drug abuser, the goal is
to adjust the capacity to experience pleasure in response to ordinary
events. Psychiatrists have always worked on this goal with the "repressed" neurotic, by questioning his or her unconscious need for

self-denial. For the addict, the hope is to enhance the ability to "postpone gratification," something antidepressants may do by increasing the ability to imagine future pleasure. In both cases, the problem may best be seen as anhedonia, and we may prefer to approach it pharmacologically, in the hope that, if the comparator is reset—if ordinary pleasure becomes appealing—self-understanding and self-control will follow.

●　　●　　●

Prozac alters an additional aspect of dysthymia that has been the subject of little research but that stands out prominently in case after case. Starting with the first patient we discussed, Sam, the architect who on Prozac found himself quicker of thought and more fluent in his presentations, we have met a series of people who, however else they responded to Prozac, also became more mentally adept. Tess, Julia, Gail, Jerry, and Hillary all responded to Prozac with a new fluency of thought. Most "good responders" to Prozac say that they think faster and function better at work when they are on the medication.

Perhaps this response should not surprise us. Impaired memory and concentration are characteristic symptoms of depression. And though dysthymics are generally normal in their mental functioning—McGuire's depressives were not distinctive on traditional tests of memory and concentration—"sluggishness of thought" has for centuries been recognized as a constituent of the melancholic temperament.

It follows, according to the principle we have been discussing—any single aspect of depression can stand for the whole—that there should be people who, despite the absence of other symptoms, can use antidepressants as a mental tonic. I do not imagine that otherwise contented people are flocking to psychiatrists to have their minds sharpened, nor do I know how psychiatrists would respond to such requests. But I recently worked with a patient who in her own way made this issue real.

Sonia is a talented graphic artist referred to me by a social worker for medication consultation concerning her minor depression. My first impression, on meeting Sonia, was of what might once have been called an ethereal young woman. She had that vague, hesitant habit of speech sometimes characteristic of artists and often affected by members of the British aristocracy. For Sonia, even mild depression carried some urgency, because other members of her family had suffered serious mood disorders. I started her on Prozac, and the depression lifted. But she changed in other ways that will now sound familiar: she became more energetic and more assertive socially than she had been even in the years before the onset of her depressive symptoms.

In Sonia's case, an additional change was especially striking. She became more fluent of speech, more articulate, and better focused. Depression can cause "paucity of speech" and "psychomotor retardation"—a tendency to produce few utterances, and those slowly. But Sonia said she had never enjoyed such clarity of thought. This was not about recovering from a depression; it was something new.

I was able in time to withdraw the medication. In the ensuing months, Sonia reported that she was not quite so sharp, so energized, as she had been on Prozac, but she considered herself cured—back to normal.

Case closed.

And then, after another few months, Sonia called for an appointment. She was not certain she needed to see me. But she was still in psychotherapy with the referring social worker, and the social worker thought Sonia was again becoming "disorganized." Sure enough, the stumbling speech pattern had returned. Though it had once seemed appropriate to Sonia—in accord with some ideal of the tongue-tied artist whose true expression occurs on the canvas—now it was disturbing, even painful, to hear. Having experienced this young woman as articulate, I now considered her halting speech a symptom.

But a symptom of what? Sonia and I reviewed the indicators of depression, and we found she had few of them. Some early-morning wakening, yes, but early rising had been a lifelong pattern. Social withdrawal? Only to the degree that had characterized her throughout her adult life, and she had, after all, a husband and numerous family friends. No tearfulness, no guilt, no ruminations beyond the ordinary. She was not even sad, unless a tinge of *Weltschmerz* constitutes sadness. And even to mention these patterns is to exaggerate.

Sonia was not depressed. She was herself. But her fumbling speech now sounded pathological, and it was accompanied by a certain lack of precision in her ideas. I doubt she or I would have remarked on this mental vagueness had we not the hope of altering it with medication. What we were considering treating was a lifelong manner of thought and expression about which a friend might lovingly remark, "Oh, that's Sonia all over!"

Sonia had just finished a major exhibit, and she would be able to relax for a while. Since she was in reasonable spirits, I was somewhat reluctant to restart the medication. Whether from pharmacologic prudence or prudery, I suggested we hold off, and Sonia readily concurred. At the same time, we agreed that, if we saw any further deterioration, any indication that her fumbling speech was the prodrome of depression, she would resume medication.

The grace period was two days. By then, both the social worker and Sonia had called back. They had decided Sonia's mental disorganization—difficulty planning, difficulty following through—was too pronounced to go untreated. Sonia was having difficulty showing up on time for scheduled events, she seemed to lack the interest or ability to manage her finances, her husband had remarked on her murkiness of thought. And, contrary to what I had believed, her upcoming calendar included a number of difficult transitions. I called in the prescription—Prozac to treat ethereal temperament.

Sonia responded again, and at a very modest dose. Her focus was clearer, her speech crisper. Her characteristic pattern of thought, one that had not been remarked on in her schooling, one that she just considered a part of her makeup, was now a fit target for medication. In her husband's mind, and perhaps mine and her own, Sonia's habitual way of approaching problems, and her vague speech, are no longer delightful eccentricities but, rather, a biological handicap.

The question is: Which biological handicap? What is it in Sonia's thought that changes on medication? The answer is of scientific and, I would argue, philosophical interest. In medicating Sonia, am I curing an ailment or merely moving her along a continuum, in this case from lesser to greater mental quickness? The former use of medication is unexceptionable; the latter, perhaps problematic. We are justly suspicious of tonics for the normal brain.

One answer to what ails Sonia—the wrong one, I think, but worthy of a brief digression—involves the ability to pay steady attention to tasks. Attention deficit is both a legitimate arena of inquiry and something of a cult subject within the profession. Some psychiatrists believe that attention deficits are among the most poorly recognized and widespread of mental conditions, and whenever I write an essay about a patient like Sonia I hear from these partisans. At first blush, the suggestion that Sonia—and with her possibly Tess, Julia, Gail, Jerry, Paul, Tom, and Hillary—suffers from an attention deficit is an odd one, as a description of the concept should make clear.

Attention-deficit disorder is a condition that first manifests itself in childhood, where it is noticed by parents and teachers. Children with attention deficits are poor listeners. They are easily distracted, and fail to complete tasks, whether at schoolwork or in play. They are impulsive, a trait that tends to get them in trouble in school, where they fidget, have difficulty organizing work, speak without being called on, and require frequent special supervision. Many of these traits disappear in the face of challenge or novelty and reappear when routine reasserts itself.

Attention deficits in children often occur in conjunction with hyperactivity, the condition in which children are always on the go, as if driven by a motor. So common is this pairing that the standard term for marked attentional problems in children now is "attention-deficit hyperactivity disorder," or ADHD. In their play with peers, children with hyperactivity can be aggressive and domineering. They often have trouble falling asleep, and wake frequently at night. They have normal memory and produce no distinctive pattern on neuro-psychological tests. In the laboratory, children with ADHD display the skills to organize tasks, but in daily life, they do not use those skills. Although most of the children have otherwise normal developmental histories, studies of ADHD often find increased rates of intrauterine or birth complications, and minor neurological abnormalities can often be detected when these children are examined in detail. It is also believed that ADHD can be produced by certain environmental toxins, such as lead.

ADHD typically begins before age seven and is most evident during the school years. But it sometimes continues into adult life, where it may manifest itself in impulsive conduct. One would imagine that, on the basis of failure to gain rewards, ADHD would be associated with depression. But, although children with ADHD may show anxiety and sadness and may develop low self-esteem, as adults they do not suffer an excess of major depression. Other problems, however, such as criminal behavior and drug abuse, arise disproportionately in adults with residual attention disorders.

The dysthymic patients we have met seem to stand at the opposite pole from ADHD. Typically well organized, driven, and somewhat compulsive, they are extremely obedient and may overachieve in school, even in the face of disrupted home lives. They are good at following through on tasks, tend to sleep too much rather than too little, are rarely impulsive or domineering, and, indeed, tend to be timid and risk-averse. They do better in the face of routine and worse in the face of novelty. And they are prone to depression.

Why, then, would anyone say these patients have attention deficits? One reason rests in the history of the profession. It has been difficult to get ADHD recognized in children—so many children have social and school difficulties for so many different reasons—and even more difficult to accustom psychiatrists to look for the syndrome in adults. As a result, aficionados of ADHD tend to have in their sack a sheaf of histories of patients in whom the diagnosis was missed and for whom, once the diagnosis was made, the relevant drugs (usually stimulants, like amphetamine or Ritalin) were all but miraculous. They believe that symptoms of demoralization paired with a subtle disorganization of thought often represent ADHD.

But objective problems in memory and concentration are typical of ordinary depression. There is even a condition called "pseudodementia." People with pseudodementia look for all the world as if they were suffering a dementing biological illness, like Alzheimer's disease; but they recover with biological treatments for depression—antidepressants or electric-shock therapy. Their problem was precisely a *forme fruste* of depression. Most psychiatrists tend now to say that pseudodementia is not pseudo- at all; rather, major depression should be recognized as a reversible dementing condition. By analogy, minor depression in *forme fruste* can have as its primary symptom a minor impairment of mental agility.

Is disorganized thought in "neurotic depression" more like ADHD or more like melancholia? You might imagine that this dispute could be settled through pharmacologic dissection. The problem is that the treatments for ADHD overlap with those for depression. The drugs of choice for attention deficit are stimulants: Ritalin and the amphetamines. But stimulants are sometimes effective in depression. And the stimulants act on two neurotransmitter systems: dopamine, thought to be aberrant in ADHD, and norepinephrine, the neurotransmitter that is sometimes deficient in depression. So stimulants might help people with either disorder, perhaps through quite different mechanisms. The second-line drugs for ADHD are the antidepressants, including those, like Prozac, that act primarily on serotonin.

My own belief is that Hillary, Sonia, and the other patients we have discussed do not have ADHD. Quite the contrary. These are people who tend toward compulsiveness, social inhibition, and steadfastness. The disorganization of thought they suffer may have to do with a general mental slowing to the point where connections are not made rapidly enough for the system to function efficiently. One gets a different impression with attention-impaired, impulsive patients. They may make connections too rapidly, but the problem is not speed alone; it is that they occasionally skip certain intermediate steps that allow for continuity of thought processes, consideration of alternatives, and the application of mature judgment.

What is it, then, that improves in patients like Hillary, Sonia, and the many others who think more clearly and speak more fluently on Prozac? What they experience, and what we see, may entail a number of changes. The loss of social inhibition and increase in confidence they feel on medication leaves them less tongue-tied. The restored or enhanced sense of pleasurable anticipation makes them more present in the world, and thus more alert and responsive. But my impression is that these people also experience an alteration in a spectrum trait having to do with rapidity and agility of thought. Just as some people are less social, more risk-averse, or less responsive to pleasure than others, certain people think more slowly and are less intensely alert, whereas others think fast and are habitually highly focused and neurologically aroused. The features that typify hypomania or hyperthymia are "press of speech" and "flood of ideas"; dysthymia is characterized by a relative paucity of thought and speech. Antidepressants can reposition people along this continuum.

I believe that when Sonia speaks and thinks with her charming hesitancy, she is displaying a *forme fruste* of dysthymia; I have raised the issue of ADHD not because I think the diagnosis is right but because the contrast between the two explanations highlights the complexity of the ethical issues embedded in the treatment of patients like Sonia. Someone with ADHD presumably has a subtle neurological deficit; someone who is similarly handicapped on an "affective" basis is not neurologically damaged but, rather, comes to her condition by virtue of sitting toward one end of a normal continuum of speech and thought patterns.

Imagine the following. Into the office comes a patient who says she would never have consulted a psychiatrist but for the remarkable change she has seen in her identical-twin sister, who has responded to psychotherapeutic medication with a marked increase in productivity at work and a new crispness of thought in ordinary conversation. The as yet untreated twin has always felt ponderous in her thought, thick of tongue, a bit unfocused on the task at hand. Might the doctor recommend a medicine for her as well?

If the twins had been subtly injured in the birth process—if they both suffer from what used to be called "minimal brain dysfunction"—and as a result display a derangement of attention, then we will feel justified in applying any medical technology that might correct or help compensate for this damage. If we believe the twins have an attention deficit due to lead poisoning, we will rush to treat the problem. We will step in even if the attention deficit never causes the twins' performance to dip below the (low) normal range for every function we test.

But if the twins have suffered no birth deficit and no lead poisoning, if they just display a temperamentally based sluggishness of thought—if their deliberateness is a normal trait that has persisted, evolutionarily, because of the selective advantage it confers on the tribe—ought we to intervene? Let us say we diagnose Twin A with depression and notice that her thought becomes more agile on antidepressant medication; will we then treat Twin B, who has never been depressed?

Here is a peculiar situation. If the first twin had ADHD, we would not hesitate to treat the second mentally sluggish twin. In contrast, if the first twin experienced her improvement incidentally in the course of pharmacotherapy for depression, then we might have scruples about treating the second twin. But the two imagined twin pairs—one where the index twin has ADHD, one where she has depression—may have the same levels of concentration and agility of thought. There are circumstances in which we sanction the treatment of normal variant traits with medication, but we are more comfortable with the use of medication to treat illness.

Had she not experienced acute depression, no one would have medicated Sonia for vagueness of thought or speech. Having responded to medication with a sharpening of her thought processes, she became her own "twin." We now consider her mental disorganization and vague speech to be a handicap, not an eccentricity, but the handicap is not one of illness. Or, rather, if we do now label her ill, we will have redrawn our diagnostic map and once more allowed medication to tell us who is normal. What began as a consultation of a psychiatrist regarding medication will have become the consultation of a medication regarding psychiatry.

Sam, the architect whose personality lost some of its edge in response to Prozac, resumed taking the drug long after his depression had disappeared (as I learned when I ran into him at a social function). He found he drafted, thought, and talked more fluently when on medicine, so he "chipped" Prozac, taking a small dose daily, despite the misgivings of his wife. He had assumed that I, too, might disapprove of this use of medication, so he had asked his internist to arrange for an open prescription. And Sam had read me right. I would have been uneasy about prescribing Prozac to make him more mentally agile, although I might finally have done it.

The issue of using medication to improve mental acuity is not new. Jean-Paul Sartre wrote his last books while on amphetamines, fully believing he was hastening his death but preferring his version of Achilles' choice: the short, productive life. In the United States, we do not grant the individual this option. We know that many people feel more alert and productive on amphetamines, certainly in the short run. But amphetamines are addictive and cause paranoia—they are drugs of abuse—and for these reasons we allow them to be prescribed only for very narrow medical indications, chiefly ADHD. An American doctor would have to say to Sartre, "The choice is not yours: the book goes, you stay; we are caretakers for a whole society, not potentiators of your work."

The example of Sartre makes clear the arbitrary or contingent nature of our boundary-setting. Surely the moral calculus might change if the facts were to change. What if we knew that for certain people we had a nonaddicting, relatively safe drug that increases alertness, quickness of thought, and verbal and mechanical fluency? Should each person be permitted to weigh the risks and benefits and choose to take the drug, even in the absence of illness?

Perhaps traditional antidepressants can decrease mental sluggishness in people whose deliberateness of thought is set by their affective temperament. Until the advent of Prozac and other potent and specific medications, the prevalence of dangerous or even just troublesome side effects spared us from the need to make certain decisions about the socially acceptable use of medication. Now we have to ask the question: ought medicine to be used for self-enhancement? We might be quite pleased to find a pill that has few side effects and that speeds thought processes. But this option also gives rise to nightmare scenarios.

In his syndicated column, the management consultant Tom Peters recently wrote an essay, titled "The Quick and the Dead," whose central thesis is that executives who make decisions well tend to make them quickly, whereas those who make slow decisions tend to make poor ones. There are settings in which quickness of thought may be all but mandatory. We may well wonder whether the availability of licit mind-quickening drugs would lead to pressures on managers to use those drugs to become as quick of thought as possible. Think of the self-effacing surgeon, Jerry. Were he a junior executive in a fast-paced corporate atmosphere, might not a concerned superior suggest he go for a psychopharmacology consultation?

This nightmare view of the use of medication to increase mental agility—not to repair brain damage but to alter a spectrum trait—helped form the basis for my coining the term "cosmetic psycho-pharmacology" and speculating about the use of antidepressants as "steroids for the business Olympics." In the face of this vision—the all-but-coercive setting in which normal people must use drugs to keep up—the term may sound superficial and glib. If we put science fiction aside and think about the patients we have met who have responded to Prozac, the phrase may seem unfair in quite a different way: though the drug is altering spectrum traits, the help it provides is far from trivial.

When I first used the expression "cosmetic psychopharmacology," Edward Khantzian, the psychiatrist who proposed that drug abuse is often a form of self-regulation, wrote to ask whether his model might apply to the "cosmetic" use of Prozac. He suggested that the drug helps because it modifies "atypical or sub-clinical states of distress or suffering that are admittedly more subtle or less apparent." That objection applies well to some of the conditions for which we have seen Prozac used: the medication is treating subtle distress that is subclinical in the sense that it does not rise to the level of illness but exists on a continuum with illness.

There are a number of perspectives from which to see the Prozac-responsive minor conditions whose manifestations are limited to a single symptom, or a few of them. From one point of view, they are mild or early forms of illness—on the continuum with depression and even rapid cycling; this is the viewpoint that justifies treating Sonia. From another vantage, they are aspects of temperament that sit on a different sort of spectrum and relate to illness only insofar as the environment disfavors the traits that arise from that temperament; in this sense, Sonia needs treatment only because the contemporary world is so demanding. From a third point of view, to medicate these conditions is just to tamper with normal minds.

Categories aside, these minor and partial disorders entail a wide range of suffering. Hillary, unable to experience pleasure, is clearly in constant pain; Sam, if we believe his claim that he was taking medication only for the mental adeptness it offered, comes close to using Prozac "cosmetically"; Sonia falls in the middle. She was once comfortable enough but now sees herself as defective. And yet the responsiveness of all three to Prozac may be on a quite similar basis—a low-normal setting of a serotonin system in the brain.

When depressed patients respond well to Prozac, they often report that their mental processes run faster and more smoothly than they did before the onset of the depression. If we think about Sam and Sonia, it is easy to imagine that many people who have never suffered an episode of depression—and who do not routinely experience other symptoms of dysthymia—would discover an increase in mental agility or acuity in response to an antidepressant. We can say these are people whose hesitancy of thought is minor depression in *forme fruste*. Alternatively, we can say that they are normal people, and that if they ask for Prozac they are requesting, according to our point of view, legitimate enhancement, legalized cocaine, or a neurochemical nose job. If I am right, we are entering an era in which medication can be used to enhance the functioning of the normal mind. The complexities of that era await us.

They await us, and they are with us already. I do not want to give the impression that the ethical and aesthetic dilemmas around medication of long-standing traits exist only in some science-fiction future. I recently treated a patient who without knowing it used words similar to those I had written about Prozac. She was a social worker who suffered not dysthymia but the real thing, full-blown major depression. I had treated her for the acute episode, and on medication she seemed to me to have the increased acuity of thought we have been discussing, as well as a new verbal fluency that was noticed by her colleagues. Off medication and free of depression, she was again more fragile and vague—I might once have said sensitive and psychologically attuned. When she was in the course of applying for a new job, a terribly stressful undertaking for her, I asked if she might not want to go back on medication, in the hopes that she would feel and appear more focused. She objected, "Wouldn't that be like taking steroids?"

Maybe I was acting toward this patient like an anxious or even pushy parent. It is painful to see someone fail where she can succeed; one wants to give all the help one can. I found it hard to contemplate the possibility that my patient would stagnate in her career because of a fuzzy style of thought that remained untreated. Having worked with so many people who responded well to Prozac, I was now "out ahead" of a patient, eager to give medicine in a circumstance that seemed to her to call for a different approach. The social worker did not take medication before her job interview, though she later resumed antidepressant use when it seemed her major depression was beginning to recur.

Social definitions change through the accumulation of particular instances. If other doctors are tempted to use medicines to treat vagueness of thought in patients with *formes frustes* of dysthymia, then in time as a society we will find ways to understand this practice as acceptable. Perhaps we will expand the definition of disease, so that patients like Sonia are considered ill, even in the absence of depression. Alternatively, we may expand the indications for which medicine is given, so that they encompass an increasing variety of characteristics that are acknowledged not to be illness but that exist as normal variants in healthy people. Either way, we are likely to see a variety of traits associated with dysthymia as indications for pharmacologic therapy.

We can now see that the possibilities of cosmetic psychopharmacology extend far beyond the brightening of mood. Each of the *formes frustes* of depressive temperament and personality should in principle be reachable through medication: a variety of individual traits will be treatable in people with otherwise unremarkable psychological histories. We may not be quite at this point: Prozac seems to me most often to be transformative in a grand way, not merely influential of single functions. But as we have access to yet more specific drugs, our accuracy in targeting individual traits will improve.

We have talked about medication as altering personality, taking a person with dysthymia and making her temperamentally hyperthymic, sunny, and social. This potential has disturbing overtones; it may lead us to imagine a future in which the culture at large considers the depressive personality to be illness and the hyperthymic type to be optimal health. But perhaps the treatment of *formes frustes* is more disturbing yet. It raises the possibility of taking a normal individual and reaching into his or her personality to alter a particular trait—in the instances we have discussed, to reset self-esteem, or hedonic capacity, or mental agility. Here medication allows for tinkering with personality and particular mental styles. This possibility has worrisome implications, not only as regards the arrogance of doctors but as regards the subtly coercive power of convention.

At the same time, we should be aware of the moral tension in failing to tinker with particular traits. Returning to the thought experiment involving pairs of twins, it hardly seems right that equally handicapped people should be treated differently based on the category (dysfunction or normal variant) into which the hypothesized origin of their handicap is placed. Illness or spectrum trait, the vagueness of speech or hesitancy of thought is the same; whether the as yet untreated twin should be allowed the benefit of, say, an antidepressant ought not, in human terms, to depend on whether the co-twin had ADHD or dysthymia. We may want to rethink our reticence to treat normal variant traits with medication. The availability of potent and specific drugs is dislocating in many arenas. Once these medicines have colored our view of how the self is constituted, our understanding of related ethical issues inevitably will be affected.

The Message in
the Capsule

In *The Thanatos Syndrome,* the last novel by the Southern writer
Walker Percy, a maverick doctor finds that plotters have introduced
an insidious chemical, Heavy Sodium, into the water supply. On
Heavy Sodium, shy and anxious women—the first example is "a
housebound Emily Dickinson"—become erotic, bold, competitive,
slim, un-self-conscious, and insensitive to the point of perfunctori-
ness. They shake off "old terrors, worries, rages, a shedding of guilt
like last year's snakeskin."

Percy was writing before Prozac was marketed, but Heavy Sodium
is like Prozac in so many respects that we must credit him with
creating the art that life imitates. To Percy, the drug's effects are all
to the bad. On Heavy Sodium, people are "not hurting, they are not
worrying the same old bone, but there is something missing, not
merely the old terrors but a sense in each of her—her what? her
self?" Heavy Sodium reduces a person to his or her ignoble, animal
being, a point Percy emphasizes by having the book's villains, over-
dosed on Heavy Sodium, take on the posture and behaviors of apes.
By reducing human self-consciousness, the drug robs individuals of
their souls. What links men and women to God is precisely their
guilt, anxiety, and loneliness.

Percy's novel of ideas, written from a Catholic viewpoint, presages much of the controversy that followed the medical community's discovery of Prozac. Like Percy, medical ethicists asked: Is it a good thing?

Shortly after I saw my first patients respond to Prozac, I raised that question in a series of essays for psychiatrists. While I was struggling in print to put my finger on what was troubling about Prozac, colleagues had been doing much the same thing in private or in local hospital rounds. Those discussions gave rise to an interesting consideration of the ethical dilemmas raised by drugs like Prozac.

•   •   •

The debate about Prozac was catalyzed by a young Harvard psychiatrist, Robert Aranow, who challenged his colleagues to consider the ethical implications of "mood brighteners," a phrase he coined after seeing Prozac exert a dramatic effect on certain of his less ill patients. Aranow defined mood brightener as a medicine that can "brighten the episodically down moods of those who are not clinically depressed, without causing euphoria or the side effects that have accompanied the mood elevators of abuse," such as cocaine or amphetamine. Aranow stressed the lack of side effects in order to sharpen the discussion: once we set aside the argument that drugs are bad because they harm people physically, we are forced to focus on whether we really want to be able to use drugs to improve normal people's mood.

Until the advent of Prozac, most ethical questions involving psychotherapeutic drugs turned on clinical tradeoffs: For which indications may highly addictive medications be prescribed? Ought coercion to be permitted in the administration (to gravely disturbed or dangerous patients) of drugs that alleviate psychosis but can cause neurological damage? What constitutes informed consent regarding risks and benefits of medications given to the mentally ill? And so on.

Prozac made Aranow wonder about the ethical implications of a drug that demands no tradeoff. He further highlighted this issue by formulating a second concept, "conservation of mood." Amphetamine, cocaine, heroin, opium, alcohol, and other street drugs used to elevate mood all ultimately result in a "crash." Under conservation of mood, there are, Aranow notes, no shortcuts to happiness: "In effect, there has been an unspoken assumption that . . . any substance that induces an elevation of mood above an individual's long-term baseline will eventually result in an opposite equivalent or greater decline." What goes up must come down. What interested Aranow was the consequences of mood-elevating drugs that violate the principle of conservation of mood.

Aranow's inspiration was a familiar-sounding case. The patient was a forty-four-year-old woman who two days each week tended to feel apathetic and unable to complete her usual tasks. She met criteria for none of the depressive disorders, though she did appear to have a "personality disorder" characterized by dependency and passive aggression. One gets the impression that the patient may have struck her doctors as a whining complainer. She requested Prozac to give her energy on her down days. Her doctors suggested that psychotherapy would be more effective, but at the patient's insistence Prozac was prescribed. Six weeks later, she reported that she had much more energy, optimism, and self-confidence: "This is the way I have always wanted to feel." Twice she was weaned off Prozac, and each time she returned to her normal, unsatisfactory level of functioning. Back on the medication, she found her energy and optimism returned. She never became manic and never suffered a collapse in mood.

This case led Aranow to challenge his colleagues to think about the implications of a harmless drug that could "reduce the common experiences of drudgery such as going to work Monday mornings for those who, at present, are not seen as suffering from a mood disorder. . . ."

The first to respond to Aranow's speculations was his co-worker at McLean, Richard Schwartz. Although Schwartz had not read my essays, his stance was akin to the one I took upon seeing Sam and Tess respond to Prozac: he was disturbed, but he had some difficulty saying why.

In a paper published in 1991, Schwartz suggests that mood brighteners interfere with a person's relationship to reality in a way that traditional antidepressants do not. If depression entails a distortion of perception—the sufferer sees life as more bleak than it is—then antidepressants make a depressed person once again responsive to reality: "Recovery from a depressive illness therefore involves an act of connection, an act of integration." But when normal people experience pain, they are merely in touch with reality and their own human vulnerability. To use a pill to improve their mood is, Schwartz asserts, "an act of disconnection. You bring about a break, however small, between the individual and either his external reality or his humanity, by which I mean his tendency to react 'humanly' to external circumstance."

Schwartz acknowledges problems with his own line of argument. For one thing, studies show that depressed people tend to be more accurate in predicting probabilities than "normal" people, who are too optimistic; it is the "normal" whose view of reality is distorted, however adaptively. Giving an antidepressant to a depressed patient thus disconnects him or her from (bleak) reality. But no one faults that intervention—so to use a medicine to make a person more optimistic than strict realism allows must not be inherently unethical.

Nor is medication unique in tempering harsh reality. Psychotherapy sometimes helps a person confront unpleasant truths, but many psychotherapies entail support rather than confrontation. For example, a patient may feel strengthened because he comes to identify with an idealized, and therefore unrealistic, image of the therapist. If we value such therapies—and Schwartz does—it is because the result, not the means, of the treatment is reality-enhancing. But the result of a supportive psychotherapy is likely to be similar to the result of a mood-brightening medication—namely, improved mood.

Conceding the inadequacy of the argument that mood brighteners disconnect people from reality, Schwartz turns to his central idea, "affect tolerance," the ability to "stand to feel what you feel." Affect tolerance has its own history in psychiatry; it is the contribution of one of the most beloved and influential American psychoanalysts, the late Elizabeth Zetzel. Zetzel considered the capacity for emotional growth to be grounded in the capacity to bear anxiety and depression. To Schwartz, a mood brightener fails to induce the capacity to bear depression (it actually obviates the need to bear depression), and therefore it stunts emotional growth.

Schwartz's concern is not just at the level of the individual. He fears that mood brighteners have the capacity to reinforce oppressive cultural expectations. The issue he uses to make his argument is bereavement. Psychiatrists have reported success in using antide-pressants in prolonged bereavement. But what is prolonged? Schwartz reports that American research psychiatrists prescribe antidepressants about one year after the death of the beloved. Schwartz contrasts this standard with that of rural Greece, where formal grieving, of a mother for a child or a wife for a deceased husband, lasts five years. Schwartz comments, "Here is a culture with impressive affect tolerance." When doctors pharmacologically mitigate the pain of bereavement after one year, they may be using medication to reinforce cultural norms and encourage conformity. The medication seems to justify the standard that is in place by labeling those who deviate from a cultural norm as ill and then "curing" them.

Schwartz's ethical arguments were immediately echoed from another quarter. Randolph Nesse, a University of Michigan psychiatrist who has collaborated with Michael McGuire, criticized mood brighteners from the viewpoint of evolutionary biology.

Nesse argues that bad feelings are useful. Pain, diarrhea, and nausea are distressing, but all carry information vital to the survival of the individual and the species. Unpleasant mood states are similarly adaptive. Anxiety reminds animals of circumstances in which they have encountered danger. In the modern world, anxiety protects humans from heedlessly attacking powerful leaders. More generally, anxiety and the internal threat of depression moderate primitive urges that would otherwise cause people to pursue ephemeral gain at the expense of stable social relationships. Sadness, Nesse says, helps allocate energy resources: mild depression causes an animal that is failing to near its goals to slow down and return home. And a depressed mood helps people who are low on the totem pole to adjust to their social position.

Nesse's argument seems to be careening toward quite ghastly conclusions, that the downtrodden should be glad of their depression and anxiety, and that people should tolerate every form of pain that is natural and was once adaptive, an argument that would ban analgesia and anesthesia as well as efforts to mitigate the feelings of low self-worth caused by low social status. Psychotherapy, which—beyond diminishing sadness and anxiety—aims directly, by analyzing Oedipal inhibitions, to allow people to be more assertive in the face of authority, would be as suspect as mood brighteners according to Nesse's line of thought.

But Nesse slams on the brakes and concludes mildly that psychiatrists should recognize that negative feelings may not be signs of family or developmental dysfunction but, rather, of adaptive mechanisms appropriate to a different environment, presumably mankind's hunter-gatherer phase. Nesse believes awareness of this point of view can be a relief to patients: "The new perspective allows them to quit blaming themselves and others and to concentrate instead on making their lives better." Nesse hopes the evolutionary perspective will convince sad-but-not-ill people to avoid mood brighteners and instead to welcome their own discomfort as useful.

As Schwartz and Nesse see it, mood brighteners stand indicted on a number of grounds: they (unhelpfully) free the taker from struggling with reality and thus achieving affect tolerance; they act to reinforce dehumanizing social expectations; they interfere with adaptive mechanisms developed over eons of evolution; and they encourage people to understand as illness aspects of the self that are normal.

Aranow, in an article co-authored with Schwartz and Mark Sullivan, a psychiatrist and philosopher at the University of Washington in Seattle, adds to these philosophical objections a list of concrete issues that would follow from the availability of a harmless mood elevator. The concerns include the influence of mood brighteners on the role of the clinician, professional standards regarding use of medication for enhancement as opposed to treatment, and insurance coverage and general availability of drugs for such use. What drives these issues is an altered relationship of risk and benefit. With the hypothetical mood brightener there are no adverse effects, so there is no risk. And since the drug is used for people who are not ill, benefit is ambiguous. Doctors are adrift, without a yardstick against which to measure particular choices.

In his role as philosopher, Sullivan suggests "autonomy" as an ethical yardstick to replace the lost standard of risk and benefit. In judging whether the use of a medicine is for good or ill, Sullivan proposes we ask whether it promotes or retards a person's capacity to run his or her own life. An addicting drug may make a well person happier, but, by virtue of the compulsion inherent in addiction, it compromises autonomy. Illness also compromises autonomy, so an addicting drug might be used in the treatment of illness and on balance meet the ethical guideline. This standard of autonomy makes us rethink what our objections might be to a mood brightener, a drug that is by definition not addicting. In the end, Aranow and his colleagues return to Schwartz's concerns, that, even in the absence of the sorts of effects that normally give mood elevators (like cocaine) a bad name, mood brighteners might decrease true autonomy by distancing man from an aspect of his humanity—his legitimate despair—and by reinforcing dehumanizing cultural expectations, such as the requirement always to be happy and productive, even in the face of a world that deserves a more complex emotional response.

●   ●   ●

My impression, on listening to the medical ethicists and reading their essays, was that they had captured important concerns regarding the potential corrosive effects of mood brighteners on individuals and on society. Their arguments expressed in formal terms certain quiet worries I had felt on first working with Prozac. At the same time, I found the mood-brightener discussion unsatisfying.

After struggling to put my finger on what was lacking, I concluded that the problem had to do with the vast discrepancy between what the ethicists were imagining and what I was seeing in my office. The potential drug users in their model—the people whose level of distress did not rise to the level of illness—did not resemble the struggling, handicapped, often socially isolated patients I had seen respond to Prozac. And, more important (since I could imagine even healthier people taking medication), the effects they ascribed to a mood brightener bore only a vague resemblance to those of Prozac, the drug that had inspired the discussion. Much of the problem, I concluded, was inherent in the abstract concept "mood brightener," which fails to take into account the characteristics—the personality —of any actual drug that might affect an actual human brain. The mood-brightener discussion showed how elusive a target Prozac is, how quicksilverish in its resistance to being grasped.

For example, the argument that a mood brightener interferes with a person's development of affect tolerance might apply comfortably to a short-acting pill that gives people an hour or two of happiness (or relief from sadness, in the way anesthesia gives relief from pain) in the face of loss or humiliation. Given access to such a medicine, someone who is afraid of life might take it intermittently to avert sad moods, while failing to act in the world or face her or his own fears and weaknesses. But Prozac does something quite different: it lends people courage and allows them to choose life's ordinarily risky undertakings.

Schwartz is afraid that mood brighteners will rob life of the edifying potential for tragedy; but when Prozac works well—as it did for Sally, who chose to marry, or Julia, who took on pediatric nursing, or Gail, who simultaneously applied for an administrative post and re-engaged her husband—it catalyzes the precondition for tragedy, namely participation. Prozac both elevates mood and increases emotional resilience, perhaps because these two qualities are biologically represented by the same neurotransmitters. The example of Prozac thus raises the possibility that mood-brightening drugs necessarily, because of the way the brain is wired, will increase affect tolerance.

Of course, the phrase "affect tolerance" is ambiguous. The expression comes from psychotherapy; but when psychotherapy enhances affect tolerance, what exactly is it doing? Psychotherapy might make people more capable of bearing deep, disorganizing depression and anxiety in response to small, predictable losses. Alternatively, it might make people less likely to experience disruptive emotion in the face of ordinary loss. No doubt it does both—allows for more profundity of feeling and for more resilience—but which of the two is affect tolerance?

Turning to Elizabeth Zetzel, whose work sets the stage for this discussion, I have the impression that she, like most modern therapists, used psychotherapy as a means to make easily disorganized patients less disturbed by loss. (Secondarily, as they became less vulnerable to hard knocks, they would need fewer defenses against experiencing deep feelings.) If so, what happens to people in psychotherapy is similar to what happens when they take Prozac. The result is not so much that they are better at tolerating the most excruciating emotions—no one would do well with the sense of inner disorganization that the rejection-sensitive feel—but that they are more experience-tolerant.

In some patients, Prozac quite directly increases the ability to bear troubling emotions. On Prozac, Paul, the Renaissance history teacher, no longer just imagined but, for the first time, felt his childhood memories of trauma. His emotional palette expanded quite directly because of medication. In many patients, Prozac lets feelings emerge in new settings. Allison, the fashion designer, was able on Prozac to display her gentle and concerned side in the office, because she felt less anxious. Certainly people who become less obsessional on the drug are thereby made more open to emotion. Not only does Prozac increase resilience, in some people it increases the profundity of emotion available to them as well. Yes, there are some patients —Tess, perhaps, depending on how we value the muting of her intense concern for others—whom Prozac makes less "serious." But any theory of mood brighteners must take into account the many other people for whom medication produces an increase in depth and range of emotion. If we are uncomfortable with the use of mood brighteners in such people, it can hardly be on the grounds that the drugs decrease affect tolerance. Indeed, Prozac raises the opposite issue: how comfortable are we with a pill that *increases* affect tolerance?

Richard Schwartz anticipates a question of this sort when he writes of psychotherapy: ". . . a person grows by taking something human from another person, a process that I find more appealing than taking a pill. . . ." Schwartz's argument has the flavor of what has been called pharmacological Calvinism, the sense that there is something bad *per se* about taking pills. Cure by pill is seen as dehumanizing when compared with psychotherapy, even the parts of psychotherapy that provide support rather than insight. The problem is not that the medicine fails to confer affect tolerance or fails to move people toward an adaptive interaction with reality but, rather, that it succeeds. In doing just what psychotherapy aims to do, Prozac performs chemically what has heretofore been an intimate interpersonal function.

Both Schwartz and Nesse worry about the capacity of medication to diminish a person's experience of sadness: Schwartz because sadness is morally and developmentally salutary; Nesse because it is evolutionarily adaptive. Again, these concerns seem to apply to a different drug, a psychic anesthetic that makes people preternaturally invulnerable to grief or dismissive of danger. Exposure to the effects of Prozac raises an alternative possibility, a mood brightener that moves people from one common human state to another.

Prozac shifts people from dysthymia to hyperthymia, to use a shorthand for relative vulnerability and invulnerability to psychic pain. Dysthymia and hyperthymia are normal human states. Both have survived centuries of evolution. To say that a Prozac-style mood brightener is maladaptive, Nesse would have to believe a normal variant condition like hyperthymia is maladaptive. Similarly, Schwartz can argue that Prozac diminishes people only if he simultaneously holds that hyperthymics are, by virtue of their temperament, immoral or inferior in their humanity. Melancholy is often engaging. And congenitally sunny people can be annoying; it is sometimes suggested that such people might be improved by the experience of suffering. Cynics might even favor the use of a pill to make bland and happy people more vulnerable. But I doubt that Schwartz and Nesse would support this intervention by arguing that it favors the aims of morality or evolution.

Nesse hopes that evolutionary theory will help us decide whether to continue to medicate a patient who requests a renewal of a prescription for Prozac. The patient Nesse describes in his essay is one of our classic good responders. She says, "I used to be uncomfortable with strangers at parties, but now I can go up to anyone and say anything I want to. . . . I don't feel nervous or worried about what people think of me. Also I am more decisive, and people say I am more attractive. . . ." This quote is intended to make us worry that the woman now lacks an evolutionarily adaptive defense, social anxiety.

If the drug has made her manic or silly—if in effect it has made her ill—she is at a disadvantage in terms of self-protection. But if, despite her reduced anxiety and vigilance, she is nonetheless as self-protective as certain other normal people, we cannot worry about her from an evolutionary perspective. It may be bad for the species to have too many risk-takers and too few worriers in the population. But for the individual, every position on the dysthymic-to-hyperthymic spectrum has been adaptive over time, and the hyperthymic position is well rewarded today.

Evolutionary theory cannot tell us whether to refill that prescription. Nor would I want to be the one to tell that patient that the sadness and anxiety she experienced before she was medicated were normal adaptive states and that therefore she should accept them.

As a clinician, I will worry about Nesse's patient if she too readily accepts the conclusion that her pain is a normal state, the result of her inborn temperament. Vulnerability to depressed and anxious feelings probably can be inborn, but it certainly can be caused by trauma. Adults who were abused in childhood are all too ready to hear that their pain is a random force of nature, and the therapist's challenge with these patients is precisely to give historical meaning to symptoms. An understanding of inborn temperament does not excuse the therapist from the obligation to approach each patient with an eye toward personal history.

It strikes me, in the end, that Nesse has his worries backward. If the woman has anxiety or depression based on hidden wounds, we might conceivably worry about medication as a form of collusion with her traumatic history: we would want to help her gain awareness of her past. But if her pain—perhaps even a "normal" level of pain that she, as an individual, finds excessive—is a mere atavism, an evolutionary adaptation to a bygone environment, medication may be a particularly humane intervention—indeed, a singular accomplishment by a science that aims to free man of certain of his animal constraints.

Nor am I certain, as I once was, that the availability of mood brighteners would disrupt medical practice. Aranow has concerns about the effects of a mood brightener on various parts of the medical system:

Will it redefine the doctor's role? Will it present challenges to the Food and Drug Administration? These questions echo worries I have raised about the proper use of a drug that can increase mental agility or hedonic capacity. But, having worked with Prozac for some time now, I have the sense that, if mood brighteners are like Prozac, the disruption to current arrangements will be subtle.

For one thing, enhancement of normal functioning, as opposed to treatment of illness, is an established part of medicine. In the field of pharmacotherapy, the drug Rogaine is used to treat a normal condition, male pattern baldness. The concrete issues regarding Rogaine have not been especially complex: the FDA does regulate it, insurance does not reimburse for it, the rich can have it and the poor cannot. Much of office-practice medical dermatology, such as treatment of uncomplicated adolescent acne, can be seen as treatment of normality, or else as enhancement. And, of course, there is the example of plastic surgery, which is used both for treatment, such as repair of congenital defects and reconstruction after burn or trauma, and for enhancement of beauty and self-esteem. A mood brightener would presumably be handled similarly: it would be used both for treatment (of depression, in which case it would be covered by insurance) and enhancement (of normal people's mood, in which case it would not). Both uses, like both uses of plastic surgery, would be culturally sanctioned as "medical."

The treatment of undesired nonpathologic conditions is common in medicine. Estrogen used to combat the normal effects of menopause is controversial in terms of its risk and benefits, but not its morality. Treatment, with sedatives, of the normal decreased sleep in the elderly arouses technical objections (used chronically, sedatives do more harm than good), but no moral objections.

Closer to the point, psychiatrists use psychotherapy for an impossibly wide range of indications, from cure of illness to enhancement of "human potential." Psychotherapy defies conservation of mood—that is, no one believes that improving mood via psychotherapy leads inexorably to later deterioration of mood; on the contrary, psychotherapy's great selling point is that, in addition to being ameliorative, it is prophylactic. Psychiatrists who practice psychotherapy should be adept in managing the shaky boundary between health and illness and in applying judgment in using professional interventions—whether medication or talking and listening—for conditions on both sides of the line.

Perhaps most important, contemporary models of mental disorder—models Prozac has helped to legitimize—blur the line between illness and health. Minor depressive states—melancholic temperament—are normal variants, but they can also be seen, from the vantage of cellular biology, as early stages of kindled depression or, from the vantage of sociobiology, as risk factors, in a hostile culture, for the development of depression. New medicines create new challenges, but they do so in a context that is itself new.

●   ●   ●

In short, I think traditional medical ethics fails to pinpoint what it is about Prozac that makes us uneasy. Part of the problem lies in the phrase "mood brightener," which captures one aspect of Prozac's potential but at the same time mistakes the character of the drug. When we imagine a hypothetical mood brightener, we model the image on an actual drug, one that already exists. The tradition of medical ethics in the area of mood is to worry about heroin and cocaine; the antidepressants are different. The issue of mood enhancement really concerns hedonism—should we use drugs for pleasure? But the word "hedonism" contains the same ambiguity as the phrase "mood brightener." Stimulants, opiates, and antidepressants are all hedonic but in different ways.

Philosophers have long debated the nature of pleasure. Is it inherent in pleasurable acts, or is it a separable result of certain acts? The discovery ten years ago of endorphin receptors in the brain seemed to support the latter alternative, what the philosopher Dan Brock has called "the property-of-conscious-experience theory," of pleasure.

According to this theory (which I will call "separability"), we engage in actions for the pleasure they bring. Pleasure is a state of the brain neurons—satiety or excitation, for example—that is separable from the actions people undertake to make themselves happy. Opiates and amphetamines shortcut the hedonic process: they allow us to have the pleasure without the pleasurable acts, and thereby cut us off from the realities of the world. "Mood brightener" implies a substance that makes people happy when they haven't done anything to earn happiness.

Separability is the basis of the usual argument not only against psychotropic drugs but against hedonism altogether. The concern is that people will pursue pleasure directly—orgies are the usual sin of hedonists—rather than achieve pleasure through "distinctly human"—intellectual, altruistic, planful—efforts for which pleasure is the reward. This case against pleasure as the direct goal in life is sometimes called the "swine objection," from John Stuart Mill's contention that hedonism is a doctrine "fit only for swine."

Just as the endorphin receptor revived interest in the idea that pleasure is separable from pleasurable acts, I expect Prozac to refocus attention on an alternative theory: that pleasure is to be found throughout (and not separable from) certain activities such as reading a book. There is no receptor that corresponds to the pleasure of reading a book, and no single state of the neurons. By this understanding, pleasure is a matter of preference among experiences. Though generally not used in connection with illicit drugs, what Brock calls the preference theory of pleasure could well apply. For instance, marijuana not only gives pleasure directly (separability); it also may enhance, or allow an anhedonic uptight person to enjoy, the inherent pleasure of a walk through the countryside.

The swine objection to hedonic drugs seems irrelevant in the face of drugs that draw people *toward* ordinary and even noble human activities. My sense is that the preference theory of pleasure has received little attention because the usual experience-enhancing mood altering drugs, like marijuana or LSD, encourage self-absorption. The experience they enhance is most often autistic. Prozac is different. It induces pleasure in part by freeing people to enjoy activities that are social and productive. And, unlike marijuana or LSD or even alcohol, it does so without being experienced as pleasurable in itself and without inducing distortions of perception. Prozac simply gives anhedonic people access to pleasures identical to those enjoyed by other normal people in their ordinary social pursuits.

My impression is that Prozac, because it gives pleasure indirectly, by enhancing hedonic capacity and lowering barriers to ordinary social intercourse, generally increases personal autonomy. Aranow and his colleagues have argued to the contrary, using a fascinating example to make their point.

They describe a woman, Ms. B., prescribed Prozac for trichotillomania, a syndrome in which a person cannot resist the impulse to pull out her own hair. Hair-pulling in moderation is a sign of anxiety; but the need to pull hair relentlessly, to the point of disfigurement, is recognized as an illness, related to obsessive-compulsive disorder. Besides hair-pulling, Ms. B. has a second concern: she is unmarried at age thirty-six, despite her "appropriate, if somewhat strenuous efforts to meet eligible men." On Prozac, Ms. B.'s hair-pulling diminishes, but so does her feeling of urgency about meeting men. Ms. B. does not isolate herself: on the contrary, she now enjoys time spent with people, such as her parents, with whom she argued in the past. She is more content with life, more reconciled to the possibility of never marrying, and, though still interested in men, is no longer driven.

Regarding Ms. B.'s social behavior on Prozac, Aranow and his colleagues ask whether she has been opiated into a cocoon. Aranow puts forth drivenness as a desirable human quality that produces, if not happiness, certain admirable accomplishments on which the species thrives.

The notion that Prozac diminishes autonomy because it diminishes drive is an important one: it echoes Walker Percy's concern about "not worrying the same old bone." But Ms. B.'s case is unusual, and not only because she has a rare illness. Heretofore, we have seen nothing but examples in which Prozac moves people toward courtship activity. In this story, it moves someone away.

I think we can dismiss the concern that Prozac diminishes social intercourse: the usual complaint against Prozac is that it leaves people too social, too little in touch with their solitary core. Even Ms. B. seems to arrive at a more comfortable relationship with her social strengths and possibilities. The story as told implies that her drive produced strenuous social efforts that were ineffectual; her measured approach on medication might well work better.

Inner drive can lead to great accomplishments. But often "being driven" indicates compromised autonomy (as indicated by our use of the passive participle, "driven," as if by an alien force). To be opiated into a cocoon is one thing, but to be granted peace where once you were neurotically compelled is quite another: there are instances in which contentment contains more autonomy than drive.

It happens that the psychiatrist who treated Ms. B. has also given an account of her recovery. He is Ronald Winchel, who introduced the theory that an "aloneness affect" spurs primates to affiliate. Winchel describes himself as having been surprised when he learned that his hair-pulling patient, who had for so long engaged in "mildly agitated spouse-pursuit," socialized less on medication:

> . . . For the first time in her memory she felt perfectly relaxed and happy sitting at home reading books or listening to music and felt less of the free-floating anxiety that was previously quelled by going out. She then mentioned, parenthetically, that for the first time in her adult life, she considered that maybe marriage wasn't in her future—but, she felt, that was

not necessarily bad. She would make her life happy, she considered, in other ways.

Off Prozac, Ms. B. bar-hopped in search of men. Prozac moderated her sense of aloneness and allowed her to enjoy a variety of social settings. In Winchel's account, Ms. B. is not opiated, merely spared the pain of social desperation.

If Ms. B.'s story is disturbing, it is because she took medication to treat one problem, hair-pulling, and found a change in a quite separate area, courtship. For her, mood brightening is something like a side effect, one about which an ethically punctilious clinician might warn: We can diminish your hair pulling, but I must warn you, you may feel more contented.

If Ms. B. had taken Prozac as a mood brightener—more precisely, if she had taken it because she felt she was overanxious about men —we would see the drug as a useful tool toward a desired end. The vignette illustrates an important quality of Prozac—namely, that it often surprises us. Sometimes it will change only one trait in the person under treatment; but often it goes far beyond a single intended effect. You take it to treat a symptom, and it transforms your sense of self.

The medical ethicists approach Prozac as if it were a case of dull or bright, down or up. Unlike amphetamine, Prozac is not a case of down or up but of same or other. Prozac has the power to transform the whole person—illness and temperament, drive to pull hair and drive to affiliate, anxiety and hedonic capacity. When you take it, you risk widespread change.

The story of Ms. B. made me realize that the concept of mood brightener just will not do—it arises from the limited idea of an "antidepressant," when what we are dealing with is a thymoleptic, a drug that acts on personality. Instead of looking at mood and being surprised to discover that Prozac affects other areas, why not begin with the understanding that Prozac can induce the sort of widespread change ordinarily brought about by psychotherapy? There really is no way to assess Prozac without confronting transformation.

The idea of transformation leads us to address a new set of ethical issues. Who is Ms. B.? The change Prozac brings about in her is so profound that there are almost two different persons in the story, one discontented and driven, the other contented and complacent. Whose autonomy are we out to preserve?

Instinctively, we might want to say that the unmedicated woman has priority; this is the stance the ethicists take when they worry whether the patient has been opiated into a cocoon. But consider circumstances that might make us change our mind. If medication were not an issue, if Ms. B. had spontaneous mood swings, would we attend to her more closely in her driven or in her contented state? How would we see the matter if we considered her drivenness to be the result of a deficiency state—if we believed she "needed" more serotonin in the brain the way some people need vitamins or insulin or thyroid hormone? In that case, we would associate personhood with the medicated self. How would we understand Ms. B. if she were, like Sam, to "discover" on Prozac that her man-chasing had been compulsive? Or if she were, like Tess, to say she felt "like myself at last" on Prozac? Perhaps the most interesting case would arise if she reported she felt fully herself both on and off medication, so that the personality she chose would be purely a matter of preference.

There are many perspectives from which we might say that denial of medication would injure Ms. B.'s autonomy, precisely because we accept that Ms. B. as she is when medicated has the standing of personhood. If we believe that she is in fact transformed—one person when driven and one when contented—then we must determine how to choose between the autonomy of two distinct "persons," each fully human and deserving of autonomy. If Prozac has brought about a break between an individual and her humanity, the break may be so substantial that we are left asking, whose humanity is it?

My guess is that medical ethicists writing about Prozac have ignored the issue of personhood because they are hesitant to see in a medication this power to transform—and who can blame them? The idea is unlikely and uncomfortable.

Part of what may bother us is the nature of the changes that Prozac can accomplish. Michael McGuire hypothesized that low mood in dysthymic women results from a mismatch between the personality with which they enter adulthood and the one their culture rewards. It follows that a mood elevator for dysthymics, at least one that works through altering temperament, will necessarily be a drug that induces "conformity." I put "conformity" in quotation marks because here it means conformity to traits that society rewards, which might well be rebelliousness, egocentricity, radical self-confidence, or other qualities that lead to behaviors we ordinarily call nonconformist. (The evolutionary model entails certain paradoxes. It holds that in a given society an "antidepressant" is any chemical that leads to a rewarded personality—different cultures may have quite different antidepressants. In a culture that rewards caution, a compulsiveness-inducing drug might produce the temperament that leads to social rewards and thus brightened mood.) What are the implications of a drug that makes a person better loved, richer, and less constrained—because her personality conforms better to a societal ideal? These moral concerns seem at least as complex as those attending a drug that just inherently makes a person happy. In terms of its interaction with cultural norms, a transforming drug might be even more ethically troubling than a mood brightener.

•   •   •

Consider the Greek widow who over the course of five years is given a chance to allow her feelings to attenuate. She lives in an affect-tolerant culture, though she may be far from affect-tolerant: the widow may be rejection-sensitive and for that reason in need of an especially long time to recover after the death of a husband. Perhaps rural Greek society is organized precisely to allow widows with low affect tolerance to recover at their own pace. In an affect-tolerant traditional culture, rejection-sensitivity might be an adaptive trait. A more assertive widow, or one quicker to heal, would find the society stifling and infuriating: she might be happier in a less affect-tolerant culture, and indeed might find that rural Greek society makes impossible demands that she is temperamentally ill-equipped to meet.

To say that our society is less affect-tolerant is to say that it favors different temperaments. The Greek society is not preferable, just more comfortable for certain people. But it may be in our society that what doctors do when they treat mourning with medication goes far beyond elevating mood: they are asking a fragile widow to adopt a new temperament—to be someone she is not.

Prozac highlights our culture's preference for certain personality types. Vivacious women's attractiveness to men, the contemporary scorn of fastidiousness, men's discomfort with anhedonia in women, the business advantage conferred by mental quickness—all these examples point to a consistent social prejudice. The ways in which our culture favors one style over another go far beyond impatience with grief.

A certain sort of woman, socially favored in other eras, does poorly today. Victorian culture valued women who were emotionally sensitive, socially retiring, loyally devoted to one man, languorous and melancholic, fastidious in dress and sensibility, and histrionic in response to perceived neglect. We are less likely to reward such women today, nor are they proud of their traits.

We admire and reward a quite different sort of femininity, which, though it has its representations in heroines of novelists from Jane Austen to Fay Weldon, contains attributes traditionally considered masculine: resilience, energy, assertiveness, an enjoyment of give-and-take. Prozac does not just brighten mood; it allows a woman with the traits we now consider "overly feminine," in the sense of passivity and a tendency to histrionics, to opt, if she is a good responder, for a spunkier persona.

The Mexican poet and essayist Octavio Paz has put the issue of American expectations of women in the context of our form of economic organization: "Capitalism exalts the activities and behavior patterns traditionally called virile: aggressiveness, the spirit of competition and emulation, combativeness. American society made these values its own." Paz acknowledges that the position of women under American capitalism is legally and politically superior to that of women under Mexican traditionalism. But American social equality, Paz contends, comes in the context of a masculine society, in terms of values and expectations; Mexican society, though deplorable in the way it treats women, is more open to values Paz calls feminine.

Does Prozac's ability to transform temperament foster a certain sort of social conformity, one dominated in this case by "masculine" capitalist values? Thymoleptics are feminist drugs, in that they free women from the inhibiting consequences of trauma. But the argument can be made that, in "curing" women of traditional, passive feminine traits and instilling in good responders the attributes of a more robust feminine ideal, Prozac reinforces the cultural expectations of a particularly exigent form of economic organization.

This issue of conformity and psychotropic medication is an old and fascinating one. Consider opium. In the romantic imagination—I am thinking of Thomas De Quincey's *Confessions of an English Opium Eater,* and Coleridge's "Kubla Khan"—opium is an instrument of nonconformity, a source of sustenance for the individual imagination. But in Marx's metaphor for religion, "the opiate of the masses," opium is an instrument of conformity, a substance that deadens mind and body to pain or injustice against which one ought properly to rebel.

On the one hand, Prozac supports social stasis by allowing people to move toward a cultural ideal—the flexible, contented, energetic, pleasure-driven consumer. In the popular imagination, Prozac can serve as a modern opiate, seducing the citizenry into political conformity. The poet James Merrill writes of "The stick / Figures on Capitol Hill. Their rhetoric, / Gladly—no rapturously (on Prozac) suffered!" On the other hand, Prozac lends, or creates, confidence. It catalyzes the vitality and sense of self that allow people to leave abusive relationships or stand up to overbearing bosses. The impact of such a medicine remains unclear: perhaps the apparent liberation it offers is merely the freedom to be hyperthymic, that is, to embody a cultural ideal; or perhaps it allows formerly inhibited people to exercise power in social or political arenas that previously made them uncomfortable, where they may be disruptive of the status quo.

Early in this century, psychotherapy was criticized for inducing adaptation to the dominant culture; even if it contained a radical critique of that culture, psychotherapy was ultimately an agent of stasis. This argument applies well to Prozac. The counterargument is that Prozac, like psychotherapy, emboldens the inhibited and the injured. My own sense is that psychotherapy has been on balance a progressive force, and I suspect the same will prove true of Prozac.

The concern that Prozac raises regarding social coercion is that, once a transforming drug is available, people might be forced to take on new personalities. I am not thinking of drugs in the hands of a totalitarian state, though the interaction of psychotropic drugs and totalitarianism is always terrifying, but of the benign coercion that pervades all mass societies.

The ethics of drugs and social coercion have been most thoroughly addressed around the issue of steroids in competitive sports. We might say that a mentally competent adult athlete should be free to choose to take steroids even if they harm his body and mind; the drugs are not being used for mere pleasure but to increase excellence, a socially valued goal. But this choice has an impact on other athletes. Ethicists have argued against enhancing athletic performance with steroids because drugs diminish fairness in sport and because medical inventions ought not to be put to such a nonmedical use. But the strongest reason for banning steroids in competition has to do with coercion, or, more precisely, "free choice under pressure," as Thomas H. Murray puts it in his essay "Drugs, Sports, and Ethics." Once a few athletes take steroids, others remain free not to do so, but only at the cost of forsaking goals to which they have devoted many years of painful effort. The choice not to take drugs (with their attendant risks) has been diminished.

A parallel example is cosmetic surgery for breast enhancement among female fashion models. No one coerces women to have breast implants, but, according to media reports, only women with enlarged breasts receive the desirable and lucrative assignments in television and print advertising. For aspiring models, the decision whether to undergo surgery is free choice under pressure. What once was (arguably) a social good—allowing a woman to gain the appearance that gives her a sense of well-being—becomes a clear social ill, the requirement, putting it in the severest terms, that a woman undergo mutilating surgery in order to pursue her chosen career.

The possibility of chemical "enhancement" of a variety of psychological traits—social ease, flexibility, mental agility, affective stability—could be similarly coercive. In the science-fiction horror-story version of the interplay of drug and culture, a boss says, "Why such a long face? Can't you take a MoodStim before work?" A family doctor warns the widow, "If you won't try AntiGrief, we'll have to consider hospitalization." And a parent urges the pediatrician to put a socially anxious child on AntiWallflower Compound. (Parents tend to want their children to be leaders—but how does a troop of monkeys or a classroom of children function when every member has high levels of serotonin?) Only slightly less nightmarish is the prospect of free choice under pressure. There is always a Prozac-taking hyperthymic waiting to do your job, so, if you want to compete, you had better take Prozac, too. Either way, a socially desirable drug turns from boon to bane because it subjects healthy people to demands that they chemically alter their temperament.

————

Such an outcome would clearly be bad, but it also seems unlikely, not least because of our society's aversion to prescribed medication —our "pharmacological Calvinism." That phrase was coined over twenty years ago by the late Gerald Klerman, a pioneering researcher into the outcomes of both drug treatments and psychotherapy. Thinking about psychotropics in the late sixties and early seventies inevitably was influenced by the mushrooming use of street drugs in conjunction with a variety of forms of social ferment. Klerman characterized the contrasting reactions as psychotropic hedonism and pharmacological Calvinism. He defined the latter as "a general distrust of drugs used for nontherapeutic purposes and a conviction that if a drug 'makes you feel good, it must be morally bad.'"

Study after study has shown that, when it comes to prescribed drugs, Americans are conservative. Doctors tend to underprescribe (relative to the recommendations of academic psychiatrists) for mental conditions, and patients tend to take less medicine than doctors prescribe. This appears to have been true in the "mother's little helper" period, during which Klerman formulated his dialectic, and it is true today. Relative to the practice in other industrialized countries, prescribing in the United States is moderate.

Past experience suggests that we can count on our pharmacological Calvinism to save us from coercion. On the other hand, pharmacological Calvinism may be flimsy protection against the allure of medication. Do we feel secure in counting on our irrationality—our antiscientific prejudice—to save us from the ubiquitous cultural pressures for enhancement? Perhaps the widespread use of new medication will erode our "Calvinism," and then a myriad of private decisions, each appropriate for the individual making them, will result in our becoming a tribe in which each member has a serotonin level consonant with dominance.

But the pressure to engage in hyperthymic, high-serotonin behavior precedes the availability of the relevant drugs. The business world already favors the quick over the fastidious. In the social realm, an excess of timidity can lead to isolation. Those environmental pressures leave certain people difficult options: they can suffer, or they can change. Seen from this perspective, thymoleptics offer people an additional avenue of response to social imperatives whose origins have nothing to do with progress in pharmacology.

•   •   •

One aspect of pharmacological Calvinism is the belief that pain is a privileged state, a view inherent in the arguments concerning affect tolerance and the adaptive value of sadness. It is also at the heart of Walker Percy's concerns over Heavy Sodium. Better even than the ethicists who responded directly to Prozac, Percy both depicts and personifies the objection to technological attenuation of ordinary suffering.

Percy was a man to whom ailments proved precious. His father committed suicide when Percy was thirteen; his mother died in a traffic accident two years later. Percy, who had chosen medicine as a career, fell prey to tuberculosis during his internship year while performing autopsies at Bellevue Hospital. Calling tuberculosis "the best thing that ever happened to me," Percy spent two years recuperating at Saranac Lake, devoting this time to reading literature and philosophy. Upon his recovery, Percy traveled to the New Mexico desert for further self-exploration. He married and, after another year of self-examination, converted to Catholicism. For Percy, as for many of his protagonists, illness and solitude were transforming. Percy turned from medical pathology to a novelist's examination of the pathology of contemporary society. He found a central flaw to be precisely a lack of respect for symptoms: fear, pain, depression, anxiety. Had he been given Prozac (or iproniazid) along with the rest and exercise that were prescribed him, would Percy the seeker have emerged?

In his characterization of "a housebound Emily Dickinson," Percy implicitly alludes to the relationship between suffering (or neurosis) and art. This subject was best captured, to my mind, in a wonderful literary debate between Edmund Wilson and Lionel Trilling. Wilson, writing about Sophocles' *Philoctetes,* takes as his theme "the wound and the bow." Philoctetes is possessed of both a godly bow that never misses its mark and a suppurating, never-healing snakebite that causes him constant pain and makes him disgusting to others. Wilson traces the Philoctetes theme through contemporary drama, where wounds tend to be psychic, and he attributes to Sophocles "some special insight into morbid psychology." You cannot get Philoctetes the astonishing marksman without Philoctetes the loathsome invalid.

Lionel Trilling rebutted Wilson in an essay "Art and Neurosis." He concedes that numerous authors believed their wounds were what gave them insight: "Zola, in the interests of science, submitted himself to examination by fifteen psychiatrists and agreed with their conclusion that his genius had its source in the neurotic elements of his temperament." But Trilling argues that the wounds of most artists are mild—artists are ill only in the Freudian sense that "we are all ill"—and that art grows out of suffering no more than do all human activities, successful and unsuccessful. Trilling counters the Philoctetes myth with those of Pan, Dionysius, Apollo, and Hermes, in which art is associated with the antithesis of neurosis: superabundant energy and power. We might say, in the language of psychobiology, that there is hyperthymic as well as dysthymic art.

Surely Trilling is right. There are many founts of creativity; not all artists suffer. There is also the issue of whether an artist who does suffer denies the muse if he or she chooses relief from pain. The wound-and-bow argument applies equally to psychotherapy, a point made by the Peter Shaffer play *Equus,* in which a boy's unique visions succumb to psychoanalysis. Does relieving suffering amount to stifling art? Psychiatrists have claimed that manic depression is correlated with creativity, but there is no evidence that lithium or psychotherapy destroys creativity in manic-depressives. My own sense is that antidepressants improve artistic creativity in certain people. Indeed, it is a practice in certain segments of the artistic community to "chip" antidepressants, taking small doses in the hopes of treating low-level depression or creative inhibition.

Percy's concerns are not limited to art but extend to transcendence. His central metaphor is the quest. I suspect much of what draws me to Percy's work is my own predilection for quest in myself and in my patients—my agreement with Percy's definition of what gives man worth. The issue in judging Prozac or Heavy Sodium on Percy's terms concerns the role of discomfort as a stimulus to the quest that is man's proper pursuit.

To Percy, guilt and self-consciousness, as well as sadness, are important signals of what is wrong with us, signposts in the quest. Shame, Percy implies, links us to awareness of original sin. Anxiety is our visceral understanding of the ways in which the world is out of joint. Symptoms signify the human condition; they are mysteries to probe and savor. Percy's understanding of the quest is religious, but there is also an important secular tradition—the dominant tradition in psychology for a century—that considers anxiety and heightened self-consciousness to be intimate signs of inner disturbance, signs that ought not to be altered except through journeys of self-discovery.

According to psychoanalysis, to lose pain without quest or struggle is to lose self. Klerman mocked a simplistic form of this view: "Thus if a drug makes you feel good, it not only represents a secondary form of salvation but somehow it is morally wrong and the user is likely to suffer retribution with . . . medical-theological damnation." But the preciousness of suffering has always had a respectable place in intellectual life.

For Percy, the problem is not merely that the artist loses his art when he takes a pill, but that he loses his art because of the greater loss of what is distinctly human. Percy argued this case throughout his career, beginning as far back as the fifties. By attending to the biological, psychiatry becomes "*unable* to take account of the predicament of modern man." Percy favors Erich Fromm's formulation that anxiety among the affluent—that is, both the potential consumers of mother's little helpers and the heroes of Percy's novels—is the sign and symptom of alienation from the self, an appropriate reaction to the accurate feeling that life runs through our hands like sand. To Percy, the person who is anxious and confused is less pathological than the one who is complacent and tranquilized. Anxiety is "a summons to authentic existence, to be heeded at any cost."

Percy's argument successfully expresses the underpinnings of our unease with drugs. But I find that his case for transcendence becomes obscure in the face of actual patients and the research they call to mind. Here is Paul, the Renaissance historian who, off medication, could only imagine his feelings in childhood; on medication, he recaptures his past with all its richness of emotion, not least its pain. Here is Allison, the woman who, off medicine, continually checks the mirror to see who is in the driver's seat of the car she is driving; on medicine, she can see herself at last. In my experience, many patients, including some who may never have had a diagnosable mental illness, are better able to explore both their past and their current circumstances while they are taking Prozac. For these people, to whom medication constitutes help in recovery from childhood trauma or protection from the threat of terrible decompensation, the drug seems to aid rather than inhibit the struggle to locate the self.

There are cases that result in precisely what Percy fears: Julia stops struggling with her husband; Gail buys clothes with less guilt and fights for promotions; Tess distances herself from her needy mother; Hillary feels a loss of moral sensibility. These are affluent, or fairly affluent, consumers made more socially comfortable and less angst-ridden by medication. But are they really robbed of their life's meaning? Are they distanced from the existential dilemma?

Percy quotes approvingly Fromm's assertion that "there are no physiological substrata to the needs of relatedness and transcendence." Today, the first half of this statement seems false: lower animals have needs for relatedness (remember Winchel's serotonin-mediated "aloneness affect" in primates); and our own degree of inhibition or gregariousness seems to have biological underpinnings. To accept the second half of the statement, we must conclude that phenomena that respond to medication, from sensitivity to self-esteem, are not essential to transcendence.

In 1959, almost thirty years before he wrote *The Thanatos Syndrome,* Percy explored the connection between uncomfortable affect and quest in his celebrated essay "The Message in the Bottle." He begins by asking us to imagine a man, with no memory of where he came from, who finds himself cast upon the beach of an island with highly developed social institutions. The man becomes a member of the local community. But as he walks on the beach each morning, "he regularly comes upon bottles which have been washed up by the waves."

Initially, Percy uses this thought experiment to examine practical linguistics. He lists twenty-odd messages, such as "Lead melts at 330 degrees," "In 1943 the Russians murdered 10,000 Polish officers in the Katyn forest," "If water John brick is," and "There is fresh water in the next cove." Percy considers ways of grouping these messages. Some messages are sensible and some nonsensical. Some refer to repeatable events and some to unique historical events. But Percy is most interested in a division between *Wissenschaft* (professional knowledge, expressed perhaps in the language of physics, psychoanalysis, or literary criticism) and news (information, like the location of fresh water, that the islander can use now).

Whether a sentence is knowledge or news is not a function of anything a linguist can specify. It is not determined by the types of words the sentence contains or its grammatical structure. The posture of the reader makes a difference, as do the potential significance of the information and the reader's criteria for believing the truth of the message. What is news to one man will be a matter of indifference to another: "In summary, the hearer of news is a man who finds himself in a predicament. News is precisely that communication which has bearing on his predicament. . . ." If a man is searching for water, and another, seemingly reliable, man says, "Come! I know your need. I will take you to water," then the searcher will consider the speaker a bearer of news.

Percy next posits two commuters on a train. One is "fat, dumb, and happy." The other commuter "feels lost to himself: He knows that something is dreadfully wrong. More than that, he is in anxiety; he suffers acutely, yet he does not know why. What is wrong? Does he not have all the goods of life?" A stranger approaches each of the commuters and says, "My friend, I know your predicament; come with me; I have news of the utmost importance for you." To the happy commuter, the stranger's speech sounds nonsensical. But the lost and anxious commuter who needs help might well follow the stranger.

The preconditions for questing are the same as the preconditions for accepting a message as news: predicament, and hope or faith. What interests Percy is not the search for water (what Percy here calls "island news") but the search for transcendence. The news that matters to a castaway is not news of the island but news from across the seas—where he comes from and what he is to do. But the castaway can be ready for news from across the seas only if he faces the truth that he is a castaway: "To be a castaway is to be in a great predicament and this is not a happy state of affairs. But it is very much happier than being a castaway and pretending one is not." Forms of pretending, in response to our existential anxiety, are the resort to psychotherapy or to drugs. These alternatives may assuage anxiety or loneliness, but they allow the castaway to deceive himself as to the cause and meaning of his symptoms, so that, "even if his symptoms are better, he is worse off than he was." The proper response to symptoms is not to seek to allay them, but to use them as the stimulus for a search.

Percy's search leads him to apostolic Christianity—that is, the attempt to promulgate a particular call from across the seas. He groups drugs and psychotherapy as false friends. Less religious existential philosophers might allow psychotherapy as a proper form of quest—

here the news from across the seas is news from the repressed unconscious. In either case, it is a grave error to understand symptoms as mere cries of the body. Percy, I think, would grant that there are instances of discrete mental illness for which drugs are appropriate. But in the case of the healthy person who feels out of touch or limited in some way—whether an anxious castaway or a housebound Emily Dickinson—medication is, to Percy, a soul-deadening distraction.

I suspect that the ways in which we see Percy's housebound Emily Dickinson and his anxious castaway have changed, over the course of a very few years. The issue is not whether man should strive for transcendence, but how often his disturbed affect is distinctively human, how often it is best seen as a stimulus for a quest. Here we return to the issue of personhood: Is the formerly inhibited and driven patient on Prozac pretending not to be a castaway? Or has she—beyond the need for pretense—found home?

If I were to rewrite Percy's thought experiment today, I would have us imagine a woman—one who finds herself a castaway, always feeling like an outsider, somewhat sad, compulsive in ways that seem alien to her, quirky in ways that are only partly comfortable, oversensitive to slights, limited in her capacity to enjoy the fruits of the island, a bit vague in her thought, listless, doubtful of her worth. She has struggled to ascertain the roots of her unease and perhaps has come a certain distance toward that goal, having made herself aware of difficult experiences in her childhood. But her mood and social circumstances remain unchanged, and so her search continues. Now let us imagine that as she walks along the beach she finds a bottle containing not a slip of paper but a number of green-and-off-white capsules filled with a white powder. Questing and desperate, she decides to take the capsules, one each day, and in time she feels bolder and less troubled, more at ease with herself, keener of thought, energized, more open to ordinary pleasure. Is there a message after all, a message in the capsule?

Certainly patients draw conclusions from their responses to medication. We began with one such new understanding, Sam's inference that a valued idiosyncrasy was actually a biological compulsion. But the conclusions our discontented beachcomber draws might be broader. In discovering that self-esteem can be turned on and off like a switch, that without her seriousness she feels very much "like myself," that social inhibition can be laid down like a soldier's impedimenta, leaving the self light and unencumbered, she may arrive at a number of new understandings about what constitutes news and about the nature of her (human) nature.

Her startling transformation will make her seek out a fresh explanation for her old discomfort. Discarding her old beliefs—that she is self-undermining, defensive, and resistant to self-awareness— she may find herself attending to categories of analysis that might once have seemed quite foreign: rejection-sensitivity, social and affective temperament, hedonic capacity, kindled depression, and so forth. Given the physiological nature of her makeover, she may attend with more interest to a new range of inquiries, from cellular biology to animal ethology. What once seemed *Wissenschaft* may now seem news, and not just island news but news about the essence of the self.

Since she is inquisitive, our castaway may undergo a metamorphosis that reaches far beyond the mere effect of new chemicals on her neurons. Having pondered her response to the capsules from over the seas, our castaway may relate differently to her anxiety, guilt, shame, timidity, depression, and low self-worth, experiencing them no longer as uniquely human or preferentially responsive to insight and self-understanding. If so, she will attend to them in a new way, reading them not exclusively as signs of and stimuli to transcendence, but in part as scars of old injuries, in part as her family's physical heritage, burdens it would not be shameful to modify chemically. Or, noting a certain mismatch between her propensities and the demands of island culture, she may strive to create a culture that values her temperament. And if she spreads the news, a changed way of understanding melancholy and angst may spread throughout the island.

Do we imagine that our castaway will be so contented that she no longer seeks a wider meaning in life? Does man's quest for transcendence rely for its motive force on anxiety and sadness? Perhaps, if she values self-understanding, the castaway will discover she has access to a richer store of memories, to long-suppressed feelings she is now unafraid to experience. Perhaps she will find the energy to pursue good works or to fulfill her creative potential. Or perhaps she will feel herself less morally driven, and then she will have to ask whether the pills have caused her to betray her self or to discover her self, whether her old drive—her tendency to worry the same old bone—was inspired, divinely or through wise forces of evolution, or only compelled, in a way that deprived her of autonomy.

The castaway, if she seeks out the professional knowledge, will discover that it is imperfect. Biologists do not know what depression is. The reigning model at the cellular and chemical level, the biogenic-amine hypothesis, is demonstrably false or incomplete. Understanding of minor mood disorders, or normal variants, is even more primitive. Though the kindling model of depression has its appeal, it constitutes argument by analogy. About affective and social temperament, the experts know least of all. Social inhibition may be a persistent trait in children, but how it relates to anxiety in adults is uncertain, its relevance to minor depression is wholly speculative, and its implications for other domains of personality theory are unknown. Animal studies remain a highly imperfect way to explore human behavior, especially such deeply human traits as valuation of the self. And about a most important issue, whether anatomically encoded injuries can be repaired or only compensated for, the professionals know nothing at all.

The biological study of the self is so primitive as to be laughable. And yet the experience of taking the pill will lead our castaway to look to biology for answers about the construction of personality and particular personality traits. The message in the capsule is "Dig here," in physiology, as well as there, where she had previously preferred to dig, in the territory of the mind.

Our castaway will avoid biological reductionism, because she thinks complexly. She will note that the experts whose work is of interest have been curious about social forces and social experiences, not just physiology. Jerome Kagan, in studying inborn temperament, wonders about the role of hostile siblings in a shy child's development. Michael McGuire leaves his monkey colonies to examine the way dysthymic women spend their lunch hours, at the end of a long line at the bank. Far from the laboratory bench, Robert Post sits with families of rapid cyclers, mapping out the history of his patients' illness in the manner of a turn-of-the-century German descriptive psychiatrist. Donald Klein asks about the inculcation of images of femininity in young girls. Even if certain aspects of mood and personality now seem "biological" or "functionally autonomous," the mind maintains a role in assessing the environment: ultimately it is the imagination that defines the scope of "home" for the person with panic anxiety, of "loss" for the rejection-sensitive, of "novelty" for the socially reactive.

Our castaway may choose to dismiss the new perspectives on mind and brain. Conceding that her self has an animal aspect, she may argue that what makes her human is the way she applies her animal capabilities to higher purposes. A traumatized ape is uneasy when it feels far from the familiar; but only men and women can be alienated from the self. Only a person can say that the familiar—marriage, television shows, the political environment—is slightly askew and therefore "novel" or "not home." Only a person can feel lost in the cosmos.

This response is entirely reasonable: were he alive, Walker Percy might argue along these lines. But if our castaway is at all like the patients we have met, she will no longer experience her angst and melancholy as privileged, guiding, sentinel emotions. Even if she avoids reductionism, she will likely turn to new models to understand the formation of her personality and the meaning—or lack of meaning—of her emotional state. Those models will give biology, both cellular and evolutionary, a much-expanded role.

•   •   •

This change is not just a matter of "taking biology into account," as if one can maintain old ideas about behavior and personality and tack on a separate biological point of view. Medication has a pervasive influence, changing the way we see people and understand their predicaments. Its impact is especially apparent in the work of psychotherapists.

After I had seen a number of rejection-sensitive patients respond to Prozac, I was consulted by a woman regarding unhappiness in her marriage. Susan had discussed the marriage in a psychotherapy that ended two years earlier, and she had concluded that she should leave her husband. He had disappointed her in different ways, and she believed that the constraints he placed on her stunted her growth. But something prevented her from separating.

Before Prozac, I might well have taken up where the former therapist had left off, exploring the possibility that unconscious wishes to remain in the marriage opposed Susan's expressed intention to leave. I would have begun with the assumption that clarifying the ambivalence—making her aware of unconscious conflict—would free her to act on whatever choice she made. Respecting a time-honored principle of psychotherapy called neutrality, I would have taken especial care not to side with Susan in her complaints about her husband.

But Susan seemed quite clear about the marriage—she had done her work in the previous therapy, understood her tendency to make certain sorts of bad choices. And she gave me abundant evidence of an extreme reactivity to loss. Since childhood, she had been sensitive to the disruption of even small attachments, as had her parents. In Susan, this pattern seemed relatively autonomous: it persisted despite her rather sophisticated self-understanding and her high degree of maturity in other aspects of her life.

I saw this woman differently than I would have before my exposure to Prozac. I did not perceive her as ambivalent, or at least I did not imagine that mixed feelings toward her husband were the main contributor to her current paralysis. I saw someone who wanted a divorce but could not make the move because of the overwhelming feelings of pain and disorganization she anticipated from separation.

Susan did not want to take medication, and I felt no need to press her to do so. But I did take her reactivity to loss—a mixture of rejection-sensitivity and separation anxiety—into account in the therapy. I supported her in her wish to leave her husband, something that in the past I would never have done so early in a therapy. And this choice worked out well for Susan. As she and I had both predicted, she became anxious and apathetic at each of the stages of separation, but once she had restabilized, she felt freer and happier, and she felt she had grown psychologically. My belief was that a relatively fixed trait of personality, one related to a biological reactivity to loss, had arbitrarily limited Susan's ability to carry out her own wishes, so that siding with her in her decision to divorce best supported her autonomy.

In the course of psychotherapy, Susan and I discussed both her personality structure—her difficulty letting go, her demands for admiration—and the reasons, based on her family history, that she had formed strong ties to the particular man she had married. But for the most part, in my role as psychotherapist, I acted like a medication—like Prozac—helping to mitigate my patient's sensitivity to loss. Soon we may be able to go further and say that the therapy mimicked medication more closely—that it altered Susan's serotonin levels—but that speculation is as yet a barely tested notion.

My brief account of this case serves as an example of an interaction of pharmacotherapy and psychotherapy that can take place even when no medication is prescribed. Taking biology into account entails attending to a new set of categories of analysis (such as reactivity to loss), and that new perspective leads to radical changes in the therapy—in this case, abandoning neutrality, de-emphasizing ambivalence, and giving the patient open support in her decision to divorce.

In traditional psychodynamic psychotherapy—my usual approach to patients—cure comes from within the patient through self-understanding. Here, in my work with a woman who was quite capable of self-examination, I opted instead to work through support for a concrete choice. I did so in part because I believed that Susan's reactivity—which I saw as a relatively fixed biological instability of mood in reaction to loss—would respond slowly, if at all, to psychotherapy; instead, I hoped a change in social circumstances would enhance her sense of her own status and her self-esteem.

My treatment of Susan was relatively simple, because she had already undertaken a course of self-examination that made her aware of her self-destructive impulses. A more complicated psychotherapy might address both ambivalence and reactivity. But in any case, seeing who people are, in the psychopharmacologic era, entails attending to their temperament and their functionally autonomous emotional responses.

Even at rather traditional institutions, psychoanalysis, the most conservative of psychotherapies, is changing in response to the perspective medication brings. A group of psychoanalysts at the Payne Whitney Clinic in New York, including a past president of the American Psychoanalytic Association, is constructing models for the treatment of panic disorder that integrate concepts drawn from biological psychiatry into psychoanalysis.

Though they do not accept Donald Klein's assertion that panic attacks "emerge 'out of the blue,' " the analysts' understanding of their patients has been influenced by the theories of Klein and other psychopharmacologists. The Payne Whitney analysts see panic as arising from a "bad fit" between a temperamentally inhibited or reactive child and a parent who cannot assuage the child's fear of novelty. (This new starting point is remarkable in itself: traditional psychoanalysis overlooks temperament in favor of a focus on the universal Oedipus complex.) The less empathic the parent is, the more dependent the child becomes. Rather than feel the humiliation of attributing the dependency to himself, the child projects dependency needs onto the parent, who is experienced as smothering. The parent is alternately experienced as overinvolved (smothering) and underinvolved (rejecting). In the words of the Payne Whitney group, "One result of this pattern can be heightened separation anxiety, in which the child clings to the parent in an attempt to ensure the child's and the parent's safety, and this clinging may in turn precipitate suffocation fears related to the parent's smothering presence."

What fascinates me is how brazenly this psychoanalytic model of panic borrows from psychopharmacology. The focus on smothering and rejection exactly parallels Klein's biological theories regarding the genesis of panic. Klein believes that the physiological problem in people prone to panic is either hypersensitivity of the carbon-dioxide receptor (the false-suffocation alarm) or a recrudescence in the adult of infantile separation anxiety (a failure of the adult brain to suppress a primitive, age-inappropriate, neurological function). In parallel fashion, the analysts trace panic anxiety to the patient's fears of suffocation and separation. Psychoanalysis, which in Freud's day leaned on physics for its metaphors—conservation of psychic energy, the hydraulic theory of repression—is now looking to psychopharmacology for its imagery.

Descriptive psychiatry—the diagnosis-centered discipline that traces its roots to Kraepelin's differentiation of schizophrenia from manic depression—is also undergoing changes in response to the observation that patients with widely differing conditions respond to the same medications.

Descriptive psychiatry today has two linked problems. On one hand, it is impossibly complex and overly specific. On the other, it contains no appropriate niche for a high percentage of patients who arrive at doctors' offices with serious psychological complaints. Perhaps 25 or even 35 percent of these patients are undiagnosable according to current criteria. Most of these undiagnosable patients have mixed forms of depression and anxiety. These figures do not include the much larger group of people, not disturbed enough to be counted "mentally ill but undiagnosable" in the studies, who also complain of depression, anxiety, and related symptoms.

The fact that a variety of people respond to medicines like Prozac—patients with specific diagnoses, patients without specific diagnoses, and nonpatients—presents a serious challenge to descriptive psychiatry. In the past, psychiatry has multiplied diagnoses—there are now over two hundred—in order to encompass new groups of distressed people. I believe that this strategy has failed, especially as regards minor disorders, prime evidence of this failure being the efficacy of both psychotherapy and Prozac (or other thymoleptics) for a wide range of these ostensibly distinct conditions. It is hard to know just how descriptive psychiatry will address the diverse syndromes that respond to new medications, but I think a good case can be made for the return of "neurosis," a catchall category for serious minor discomfort related to depression and anxiety.

The term will not mean what it meant in the 1950s. Neurosis then entailed trouble related to the "unanalyzed self," a self subject to the vicissitudes of castration anxiety, Oedipal conflict, and repressed sexuality. Neurosis of the twenty-first century will be a disorder that encompasses the effects of heredity and trauma—risk and stress—on a variety of neuropsychological functions encoded in neuroanatomy and the states of the neurotransmitters. The coalescing of diagnoses would then require descriptive psychiatrists to take into account the data of psychotherapy—parent-child interactions, significant losses, patterns of social relationships, quality of self-esteem. In other words, the success of medication is changing both mind-centered and biological psychiatry and moving them closer to each other.

The ideal modern psychiatrist will be one who can use drugs intimately and help patients to grow in self-understanding. Woody Allen has given us an image of such a healer: Dr. Yang, the all-knowing herbalist in Allen's fantasy *Alice*. The film tells the story of Alice Tait, a hypochondriacal, directionless wife and mother. Yang provides her with an herbal infusion that proves to be a sort of instant super-Prozac. Under its influence, the ordinarily shy and insecure heroine propositions a saxophonist in a dialogue that finds her mistress of both a seductive manner and an inexplicable fluency with jazz history and lingo. Like psychiatrists who have observed the effects of Prozac, Allen appreciates that a change in mood state can reveal hidden social skills.

Yang combines ever more fantastic potions with parsimonious interpretations, sending Alice on journeys of exploration that leave her "ten feet tall": confident, independent, able to sever ties with her husband and act with new moral decisiveness. Yang's herbs allow his patient to experience the world differently—to see husband, lovers, parents, siblings, and children in a new light—and then to bear the possibility of loss inherent in that fresh vision. Yang's magic is as much in his judgment as his pharmacopeia. His drugs only potentiate change; ultimately, it is Alice's quest that transforms.

The Dr. Yang fantasy is the fantasy of psychotherapy saved and redeemed by medication, where drugs do not cure patients but liberate them. Used properly, this new freedom can open people to insights that then shape the new self. Allen, so long inspired by psychoanalysis, creates in Dr. Yang a pharmacologist whose stock-in-trade is not science but wisdom. That is, Allen has imagined the ideal psychiatrist of the future, one who can use drugs, in the deepest sense, psychotherapeutically.

Dr. Yang stands in strong contrast to Walker Percy's selfish apes, who put Heavy Sodium in the water supply. These two fables, Allen's and Percy's, represent dialectical views of the potential of pharmacology: medication, in the wrong hands, as thief of the self; medication, in the right hands, as restorer of the self.

• • •

Our theme has been the significance of Prozac's transformative powers—its effects when it works well—for the modern view of the self. I have therefore had little occasion to discuss bad reactions to Prozac, a topic I broach in an appendix. But there is one negative response that has obvious bearing on whether Prozac is a good thing—on whether it is more like Heavy Sodium or more like Dr. Yang's herbs—and that is the feeling, reported by Hillary and Tess, of the numbing of moral sensibility.

I have treated other patients who, even if their depressed mood or social inhibition decreases on Prozac, complain that they feel uncomfortable, as if they have been deprived of a feeling state or a sense of urgency that is vital to them. In each case, I have tried to understand what this discomfort means.

I worked with an undergraduate whose constant complaint in psychotherapy was the series of humiliations he had suffered at the hands of his parents. Philip was moderately depressed and isolated from classmates, whom he scorned. But his moodiness and irritability were comfortable to him, because they represented his legitimate suffering and rage. Quite early in our time together, Philip's depression worsened to the point where he did not care whether he lived or died, and I suggested he take Prozac.

He was a "good responder." On Prozac, Philip felt better than well, and he hated it. He had been prematurely robbed of his disdain, his hatred, his alienation. His acute episode of depression had been frightening, and I urged him to stay on the Prozac for six months, in order to prevent a recurrence. He took my advice, but the six months of feeling fine were hell for Philip. He felt phony; he did not trust himself. He was truly relieved to stop the medicine and resume his bitterness, although in truth it did not return with its former vehemence.

———

The patients I medicate with Prozac tend first to have undergone extensive courses of psychotherapy. Philip had not, and one way to see his discomfort on Prozac is to say that he was not prepared to be well. I like this understanding of what occurred—the sense that there needs to be a readiness for Prozac, that Prozac works best in patients whose conflicts are resolved but whose biologically autonomous handicaps remain.

Philip's uncomfortable response to Prozac warns against a potentially unfortunate interaction between medication and another societal force: the focus on cost, rather than quality, in medicine. The patients we have met here almost all underwent treatments that entailed effort, time, and expense. If, at the start of those treatments, these patients had just been given Prozac, they would have felt some relief, and in some cases that intervention might have been enough; but I suspect it most often would not.

To my mind, psychotherapy remains the single most helpful technology for the treatment of minor depression and anxiety. Medication can speed treatment, and sometimes it can bring about remarkable transformation on its own. Certainly medication has had a profound influence on psychotherapy, and any psychotherapy today should include awareness of biological influences on mood and behavior. But the belief—espoused not infrequently by health-care cost-cutters in the "managed care" industry—that medication can obviate psychotherapy conceals, I believe, a cynical willingness to let people suffer. If medication does interfere with self-examination, it may be in this concrete and practical way—that it serves as a pretext for denying patients psychotherapy.

Philip's angry feelings were his problem to solve—his impetus to quest—and it was a hardship to be relieved of them prematurely. As regards Philip, Walker Percy is right: not worrying the same old bone is inherently self-alienating. For Hillary and Tess, the moral calculus seems different. Hillary—the laziest gal in town—wondered, when she recovered from anhedonia, whether she had lost a degree of moral urgency. On Prozac, Tess found herself less "serious"—less preoccupied with the needs of her mother, her siblings, and her boyfriends. But each patient went on to approach her dilemmas with new perspective and energy.

Moral urgency can be seen in clinical terms: Prozac tempered a compulsive trait in these women—affiliative neediness, or aloneness affect, or rejection-sensitivity, or the drive that forms part of the melancholic temperament. To the extent that biologically driven compulsion supported Hillary's and Tess's moral sensibility, Prozac diminished that sensibility. The dysthymic's critical appraisal of right and wrong has been replaced by the hyperthymic's easygoing acceptance of the world as it is.

Working with Prozac has heightened my awareness of the extent to which compulsion is a basis for moral action. Is it a sound basis? Surely one could make the case that what is compelled is inherently amoral; what characterizes moral action is choice. Still, in addressing this effect of Prozac, we face the least irrational, most cogent aspect of pharmacological Calvinism: perhaps diminishing pain can dull the soul.

In discussing evolutionary adaptation, I argued that, insofar as Prozac only makes Hillary and Tess as free of compulsiveness and aloneness as many other people, its effect on fitness is unexceptionable. We do not want to say that ordinarily flexible people are adaptively unfit. I am not sure whether the same approach answers the apprehensions apparent in Walker Percy's novels and essays. Perhaps Percy would see certain "good responders" to Prozac as happy, and therefore uninteresting, commuters; one gets the sense that he finds commuters who know something is dreadfully wrong to be more humanly complete. Presumably Percy's own quest, an enormously productive one, arose from his sense of unease, his feeling of being a castaway stranded in contemporary culture.

I find myself caught between paradigms. I agree with Percy that what distinguishes and dignifies humanity is the quest for transcendence, attentiveness to news from across the seas. But listening to Prozac has made me so attentive to the phylogenetic origins and biological underpinnings of free-floating anxiety and melancholy that I have trouble understanding them as special communications that make humans distinct from beasts. This posture arises from my observation of patients: I think of Allison, who had the most concrete form of alienation of self—an inability to find the self at all—and whose condition responded dramatically to medication. Her 'self-alienation added nothing to her life; medication freed her to pursue her quest.

One can hardly deny the cogency of Percy's observations about our culture—its lack of direction, its preference for stimulation over contemplation, its denigration of solitude. Percy was one of the keenest, most clear-eyed critics of American social mores. Still, what are we to make of patients who navigate that culture more effectively—and achieve self-realization—on medication? Once we see driven patients conduct their lives in free and complex ways on medication, and once we have looked at the evidence that emotional patterns much like the ones that handicapped them occur in lower animals in response to simple traumas, the connection between uncomfortable affect and transcendence becomes less self-evident. The question is not whether our culture undermines efforts at transcendence—surely it often does—but whether medication is a proper metaphor for those self-alienating social forces, and, more centrally, whether hurt, anxiety, melancholy, and inhibition—the whole range of affect states from which Prozac and Heavy Sodium free people—are privileged signals about man's condition.

The relationship between affective and moral sensibility is complex. When depressed, many people lose their interest in outside causes and become preoccupied with themselves; manics often seem sociopathic in their indifference to the consequences of their acts. In these patients, treatment of the mood disorder can turn a morally unattractive person into an admirable one. Other depressed patients are fascinating in their ethical ruminations or punctiliousness, and on recovery they may seem disappointingly ordinary in their moral focus.

Similar associations between mood and moral sensibility exist in the minor disorders, so that a movement along the spectrum from dysthymia to hyperthymia can be accompanied by a change in level of ethical sensitivity and profundity, although in different directions for different people. Some, who have been obsessed with moral concerns, may become less preoccupied; others, who have been self-centered, may find the emotional flexibility to attend to ethical concerns.

My own belief is that the moral sensibility can arise in the company of a variety of affect states. Perhaps even the fat, dumb, and happy commuter has his quest. The drive that results from inborn compulsiveness and pain experienced in childhood is only one reason to search for transcendence, and if lessening that drive ruins us morally, then our moral predicament is sad indeed. Still, the specter of Heavy Sodium is powerful. We cannot entirely escape the fear that a drug that makes people optimistic and confident will rob them of the morally beneficial effects of melancholy and angst.

● ● ●

We are, it seems to me, denizens of an island whose castaways have been receiving capsules rather than notes. What is most disturbing about those capsules is how they affect even those who never take medication. Castaway or not, in the psychopharmacologic era, when we look at our children, we will attend more to their constitution. At the same time, we will worry about losses children suffer, about our failures in empathy toward them, about the myriad of pains that can elevate stress hormones and stimulate dysfunctional neuronal sprouting.

Certain people we may tolerate better, or dismiss more readily, because their struggles are so transparently responses to functionally autonomous anxiety or depression, problems in regulation of mood that they ought really to get tended to, one way or another. Where once we might have sat with a friend, puzzling over her social dilemmas, now we will smile knowingly, wondering which subculture will best tolerate her quirks, or which medicine might enhance her appeal or her social skills.

We may become more aware of our own feelings of confidence or despondency, noting how they respond to our social circumstances—how applause is a tonic for us, how loss devastates. We will no doubt worry over our depressions as once we worried over carcinogens: are they causing covert damage? An unreliable lover enrages us—he is doing not just psychic but physical harm; we assume the two are much the same. Or we see our spouse as a sort of first neurotransmitter in a cascade of chemicals, one who keeps our serotonin levels high. We are keenly aware of our temperament, our psychic scars, our animal nature. Assessing both ourselves and others, we find ourselves attending to strange categories: reactivity, aloneness, risk and stress, spectrum traits, dysthymic and hyperthymic personality. We understand that our reliance on biological categories has run far ahead of the evidence, but we are scarcely able to help ourselves.

Or perhaps our transformation has been less thorough. Perhaps we are, like certain patients on Prozac, altered by our encounter with medication but still aware of the persons we were before. We stand between worlds, uneasy about the rapidity with which we have dropped old concerns.

Having seen people not unlike ourselves respond to medicine, we experience angst and melancholy differently—our own and others'. Perhaps what Camus's Stranger suffered—his anhedonia, his sense of anomie—was a disorder of serotonin. Kierkegaard's fear and trembling and sickness unto death are at once spiritually significant and phenomenologically unremarkable, quite ordinary spectrum traits of mammals, affects whose interpretation in metaphysical terms is wholly arbitrary.

This change in our sensibility may disconcert us. Yet we know models of the relationship between affect and morality change in each era. The romantic decadence that once swept Europe—the self-absorption of Goethe's Werther and Chateaubriand's René—now seems jejune. A few decades after he proposed it, Sartre's notion of nausea as the most basic of human emotions is dismissed by most psychologists and philosophers. It should not surprise us if today we understand "existential anxiety" and even "self-alienation" to relate not only to our loss of moral guideposts but also to our animal heritage.

Perhaps it is best to imagine that we are in a transitional phase. Our free-floating angst and melancholy feel less and less like signals of our existential dilemma. But nothing we learn about our neurophysiology or our animal nature will deny the possibility of man's transcendence. We remain cast away, perhaps more lost than ever, precisely because we are less able to experience our affect as a guide to our moral state. We must look elsewhere for signs. Despite our sense of its limitations, we may turn more then ever to psychotherapy, or introspection, or even spirituality.

Observing responses to Prozac, we learn not only about ourselves but about our island's culture. Certain intellectuals at mid-century—those who tried to combine the thoughts of Karl Marx and Freud, such as Erich Fromm and the literary critic Norman O. Brown—believed that industrial capitalist society instilled and rewarded the "anal character," a style marked by dampened enthusiasms, compulsive control, and conformist rigidity. The success of Prozac says that today's high-tech capitalism values a very different temperament. Confidence, flexibility, quickness, and energy—the positive aspects of hyperthymia—are at a premium.

Copernicus wrenched the earth from the center of the universe. Darwin undercut the human race's uniqueness among God's creations. Freud made the conscious mind less special. Modern biology attacks the centrality of mind altogether, highlighting the roles of brain and body. Psychiatrists used to concede that mind and brain were one, where the concession entailed letting a little biology creep into a mind-dominated discussion. Today, an exclusively mind-centered psychology would have trouble finding a seat at the table. There is no privileged sphere of the mind, no set of problems that is the exclusive domain of self-understanding. We are not formed of experience alone, and those elements in us that have been shaped by experience are not infinitely plastic.

That there are limits to human malleability is disturbing to our political tenets. All men are created equal—at least in our political and moral ideal—but they are created biologically heterogeneous, in temperament, and in predisposition to a variety of specific traits that relate to temperament. By the time they reach adulthood, people also differ biologically according to their good or bad fortune in periods of critical development. Psychotherapeutic medication is both instructive and problematic for a liberal society. It leads us to focus on biological difference, whereas for years our culture has chosen to ignore biologically based characteristics that, in Carl Degler's words, "might serve as an obstacle to an individual's self-realization." Emphasis on temperament can be divisive and oppressive, if a culture too strongly favors one temperament over another—traditionally masculine over traditionally feminine traits, for example. Or awareness of temperament can be inspiring, leading perhaps to efforts to minimize psychological harm to children, or to foster a social environment welcoming to constitutionally diverse adults.

To the extent that medications are important agents of personal transformation, change becomes ever less a matter of self-understanding and ever more a matter of being understood by an expert. If what is wrong with us is explained on a physiological basis, it lies in a sphere with which we are unfamiliar and with whose manipulation we are inept. As modern men and women, we may already be uncomfortable with the extent to which our surroundings, in the form of complex equipment, are beyond our ken. Now we are faced with the likelihood that introspection alone will not explain us to ourselves.

The personality-altering pill is high technology, something unknowable, foreign, perhaps even hostile. Prozac arises from the science of twenty years ago; even that science is so complex it is beyond the reach not just of lay people but of most practicing doctors. Psychoanalysis was criticized for creating a cult of expertise, but analysis is at least a joint effort, a journey of self-exploration for the patient, with feeling, insight, and intuition as guides. In this context, pharmacology may be experienced as self-alienating even when, in particular instances, it restores people to themselves. Having diminished the power of psychoanalysis, we are all the more at the mercy of professional knowledge.

In this regard, we may recognize in ourselves a certain prejudice, in favor of humanism (narrowly taken) and against science. For centuries, people were comfortable with the belief that they were governed by humors whose workings were mysterious. Why should we be less comfortable with the neurohumors, substances about which, after all, our experts do know something?

None of the ethical concerns about Prozac—its influence on affect tolerance, autonomy and coercion, cultural expectations, evolutionary fitness, transcendence—has disappeared. But once we have lived with Prozac for a while, once we have taken the measure of the drug, and once it has worked on us, those worries may seem less urgent. Our worst fear—Walker Percy's fear, the fear of the medical ethicists and evolutionary biologists, my own fear when I first saw patients respond to Prozac—was that medication would rob us of what is uniquely human: anxiety, guilt, shame, grief, self-consciousness. Instead, medication may have convinced us that those affects are not uniquely human, although how we use or respond to them surely is.

In the end, I suspect that the moral implications of Prozac are difficult to specify not only because the drug is new but because we are new as well. Like so many of the "good responders" to Prozac, we are two persons, with two senses of self. What is threatening to the old self is already comfortable, perhaps eagerly sought after, by the new. Here, I think, is Prozac's most profound moral consequence, in changing the sort of evidence we attend to, in changing our sense of constraints on human behavior, in changing the observing self.

Is Prozac a good thing? By now, asking about the virtue of Prozac—and I am referring here not to its use in severely depressed patients but, rather, to its availability to alter personality—may seem like asking whether it was a good thing for Freud to have discovered the unconscious. Once we are aware of the unconscious, once we have witnessed the effects of Prozac, it is impossible to imagine the modern world without them. Like psychoanalysis, Prozac exerts influence not only in its interaction with individual patients, but through its effect on contemporary thought. In time, I suspect we will come to discover that modern psychopharmacology has become, like Freud in his day, a whole climate of opinion under which we conduct our different lives.

Appendix:
Violence

Though Prozac has been of remarkable help to millions of patients, a cloud hangs over the drug—accusations that its effects on a few patients have been devastating. These patients, or their families, believe that Prozac has caused them to attempt suicide or commit violent acts. The issue of dramatic negative effects—whether Prozac can arouse in certain people obsessional impulses to do terrible things that are otherwise alien to them—began as a scientific concern and rapidly became a media three-ring circus. The stories of many of the patients who appeared on television have been convincingly debunked, but the question of Prozac's dark side raises fascinating issues that relate to topics we have already discussed.

When it emerged in 1990, the allegation that Prozac could cause violent acts surprised scientists. To understand why, it is necessary to know something about studies of the relationship between serotonin and aggression, both in man and in monkeys.

The monkey research is of special interest. A variety of evidence—from blood serotonin levels in wild monkeys to medication responses of monkeys in captivity—points to a correlation between high serotonin levels and dominance. But dominance is quite different from aggression.

Dominant monkeys are almost never impulsively violent. On the contrary, they tend to be purposeful in their behavior; when challenged, they win the encounters they engage in, but they do not seek fights. Dominant, high-serotonin monkeys tend to be well integrated socially and to engage in a high level of affiliative activities, both with other males and with members of the opposite sex. Indeed, winning affiliation with females is part of the sequence that leads to and maintains dominance. Fighting with females is a sign of low hierarchy.

It is when they have low serotonin levels that monkeys become maladaptively aggressive and, at the same time, less socially competent. Low-serotonin monkeys tend to be socially deviant and ostracized; and socially deviant and ostracized monkeys tend to have low serotonin levels.

Drugs, like Prozac, that increase brain-serotonin transmission decrease aggression and impulsivity in low-serotonin animals. The most specific effect may be on what has been called "affective aggression"—that is, aggression against other members of the same species, marked by arousal and vocalization, as opposed to "predatory aggression," a more controlled form of aggression directed against other species. Affective aggression is thought to be a model for violence against the self or family members in humans.

The relationship between serotonin and aggression—as opposed to dominance—also has been studied in monkeys in their natural habitat. Because rhesus monkeys are naturally aggressive within the species, they were chosen for a large-scale correlational study. Scientists corralled small groups of free-ranging adolescent monkeys and rated them according to observed aggression, fight wounds, and old scars. The monkeys' spinal fluid was tested for levels of a serotonin-breakdown product, or metabolite. High aggressivity correlated with low levels of the metabolite, a sign of low brain-serotonin levels.

Studies indicate that humans are similar to monkeys in this regard. In human children and adolescents, low levels of a serotonin metabolite in the spinal fluid predict the severity of physical aggression on follow-up two and a half years later. Similarly, low levels of the same metabolite in spinal fluid correlate with highly planned suicide attempts—violence against the self—in hospitalized adults.

And research indicates that violent tendencies in aggressive and impulsive humans and other animals can be diminished with serotonin-enhancing drugs. Serotonin-elevating drugs, on the basis of this use, are sometimes called "serenics." BuSpar, a medication that acts on nerves that respond to a particular subtype of serotonin, has gained widespread use in the treatment of violence in retarded or brain-damaged patients; this usage qualifies BuSpar as a serenic. Prozac is also a serenic. In a study of depressed patients, some of whom were prone to impulsive anger, treatment with Prozac resulted in a marked decline in hostility and a decrease in the expression of anger.

Advocates of "assertiveness training" seem to be right when they say that assertiveness is different from aggression. Assertiveness gets you what you need, and it correlates with high brain-serotonin levels. Aggression—uncontrolled or rageful violence, whether against self or others—is unassertive, disruptive, and generally ineffectual, and it correlates with low brain-serotonin levels. Animal studies resulted in what might be called an ethological dissection between assertiveness and aggression, one that has had influence far beyond psychiatry, on the intellectual understanding of violence. Raising serotonin levels makes for assertiveness, not aggression. The notion of serotonin-enhancing drugs as serenity-inducing makes the purported association between Prozac and violence all the more puzzling.

Biochemically, suicide looks a good deal like aggression. A variety of postmortem studies have compared the brains of otherwise physically healthy people who died from suicide with those who died as accident victims. What distinguishes the suicides is low levels of brain serotonin. In other words, scientists had every reason to believe that a drug like Prozac, which enhances serotonergic transmission, would *decrease* aggression and suicidality.

The issue of Prozac and suicide—the beginning of wider concern about Prozac and violence—was first raised in a group of cases reported in the *American Journal of Psychiatry* in February 1990. Martin Teicher and two colleagues at McLean Hospital, part of the Harvard teaching system, had observed six depressed patients who developed "intense, violent suicidal preoccupations" after between two and seven weeks of treatment with Prozac. These patients were, by the authors' own description, "complex." Almost all had very extensive histories of depression and had failed to respond to a long series of prior drugs or even to electroshock treatment. Five had considered killing themselves in the past, and three had actually made prior attempts. Some were taking other psychotherapeutic medications along with Prozac; in one case, Prozac was the sixth medication in the regimen.

Still, in each of these patients, Teicher and his colleagues noted a distinct and surprising change: the emergence on Prozac of urgent, obsessional suicidal preoccupations. These preoccupations disappeared after discontinuation of Prozac, though often not for some weeks. Interestingly, two patients in whom a careful assessment was made (using standardized depression-rating scales) were found not to have gotten more depressed on Prozac, only more suicidal; and in some patients, when Prozac was withdrawn the self-destructive preoccupations diminished even though the depression did not. The suicidal thoughts seemed independent of the level of depression.

The Teicher report had certain flaws. Some of the studied patients were quite seriously depressed, and their deterioration and emerging suicidality might have represented the natural course of their depression, a failure of Prozac but not a side effect. Only one of the patients had the sort of minor disorder we have discussed here, and his story had a complication that makes the role of Prozac hard to interpret.

Mr. B was a successful professional who had been treated intermittently with psychotherapy over a twenty-one-year history of minor depression. His dysthymia deteriorated into depression after a divorce. What makes Mr. B's story distinctive is that he responded to a monoamine-oxidase inhibitor (MAOI), but then his depression re-emerged, while he was still taking the MAOI.

This phenomenon is called tolerance. When applied to antidepressants, tolerance refers to cases in which a medicine at first suppresses depression but then—while the patient is still on the same dose of the same medicine—the depression "breaks through" full-force. Tolerance has been most widely reported with MAOIs (it also occurs with lithium and, it now appears, Prozac), and tolerance to MAOIs is a difficult, disturbing phenomenon. Patients who become tolerant to MAOIs often suffer a quite vicious deteriorating course, one that does not respond to other medication treatment.

Mr. B was withdrawn from the MAOI. Two weeks later, he was placed on Prozac, and then Prozac and lithium, during which time he continued to deteriorate. In particular, his suicidal ideation, which had been present on the MAOI, became an alarming preoccupation. The worsening suicidality was, however, only one of many new symptoms, and might not ordinarily have been considered remarkable following the development of tolerance to an MAOI. Over the next three months, Mr. B failed to respond to—and remained suicidal on—imipramine, a second tricyclic antidepressant (doxepin), and a stimulant. Only when placed back on an MAOI did he recover, as patients sometimes do upon re-exposure to a drug to which they were once "tolerant." It is not at all clear that what Mr. B suffered was Prozac-induced suicidality.

Whatever its shortcomings, the Teicher report aroused great interest. The emergence of suicidal thoughts in patients on Prozac was noteworthy because it flew in the face of what is known about the relationship between serotonin and suicide. Prozac increases serotonin levels, so it should decrease suicidality. Indeed, there is evidence from certain research centers that Prozac and related drugs act faster than other antidepressants in decreasing suicidality, and even that Prozac might be preferentially effective in patients with past histories of suicide attempts. And Prozac is known to decrease obsessionality. If what Teicher and his colleagues observed is real, it is, as they themselves put it, a paradoxical effect.

The Teicher report gave rise to a flurry of research regarding Prozac and suicide. These subsequent studies showed that Prozac is a remarkably safe drug, perhaps safer than other antidepressants in terms of any tendency to induce suicidality. Review after review found as few suicide attempts on Prozac as on other antidepressants, or fewer; in one study, it seemed there might also be less frequent emergence of suicidal ideas on Prozac.

However, survey research does not address the individual case. If the Teicher report is right—that Prozac has a special effect in eliciting suicidal ideation—what is happening may be this: Prozac induces suicidality in a few patients who would otherwise not have been suicidal; but because Prozac is simultaneously more effective than other antidepressants in treating suicidality, in survey data those few patients who deteriorate are swamped by the much larger number of patients who improve. As one group of researchers put it, "Examining large, placebo-controlled databases for treatment-emergent suicidal ideation is not likely to be instructive because the active treatment, even if it causes suicidal ideation in a subgroup, also *suppresses* it. As long as the treatment (fluoxetine) suppresses more suicidal ideation than it induces, it will compare favorably with the placebo group."

The reviews responding to the Teicher report serve as a reminder that suicidal ideas emerge frequently in depression and that they emerge on all antidepressants. The most extensive surveys estimated that a small but substantial number of depressed patients, under 5 percent and probably closer to 1 percent, experience a paradoxical worsening of suicidal thoughts on any antidepressant. The percentage is likely much lower for the healthier patients we have discussed here.

There are many reasons why patients worsen on medication: the drug may not be working, certain side effects may be intolerable, the energizing effects of the drugs may cause people to consider acting on fantasies they had earlier not expressed or formulated. But it is also possible that antidepressants, for unknown reasons, make certain people more depressed directly, through unintended changes for the worse in neurotransmission.

Teicher's group and others have raised the possibility that the induction of suicidality by Prozac, if and when it occurs, is due to an infrequent medication side effect. Prozac and many other psychotherapeutic medications can cause akathisia, a sense of physical restlessness that makes people pace or otherwise try to remain in constant motion. This side effect can be extremely unpleasant and disturbing. An alternative hypothesis posits an idiosyncratic response to Prozac that involves a lowering of serotonin levels. No one has measured such an effect, and no one knows whether it occurs.

The most extensive review article on antidepressants and worsening suicidality concludes: "Because patients seek treatment at different points during illness and a significant number do not respond to treatment, the appearance or worsening of suicidality in a small number of patients is not sufficient to implicate the medication as the cause. . . . If the association between an antidepressant drug and worsening suicidality is established, the question of the mechanism becomes relevant. Given the reported infrequency of this effect . . . it is likely that each case results from an interaction between a drug effect and a specific patient-related vulnerability."

The Teicher report, by respected clinician-researchers, remains the single most cogent piece of evidence linking Prozac to suicide, impulsivity, or violence. The association between Prozac and suicidal ideation is speculative, based on doctors' and nurses' observation of a few cases—like some of the conjecture I have engaged in elsewhere in this book.

I have had one patient attempt suicide while on Prozac. His chief complaint—the main reason he consulted me—was persistent, intrusive thoughts of suicide, and he had attempted suicide in the past. I had put him on Prozac in part because it seemed to me that he was becoming increasingly suicidal. His attempt, when he made it, was quite serious—he was discovered and rescued only by chance. Despite the differences between this case and those reported by the McLean group—though their patients had a history of suicidal thoughts, they were not suicidally obsessed when drug treatment began—I did consider the possibility that Prozac had made things worse. This patient ultimately did better on an MAOI.

My own impression is that the risk that Prozac will induce suicidal thoughts is small. On the basis of stories I have heard from colleagues and the report of the McLean group, whose observations I respect, I would say that Prozac may, in rare cases, stimulate or worsen suicidal thoughts and impulses, probably not just idiosyncratically but on some common basis, perhaps a paradoxical lowering of serotonin-based transmission. The public worry about this possibility is, however, so exaggerated as to be dangerous, because it tends to discourage people from taking Prozac even where it is very likely to do them good and very unlikely to cause harm.

Hard upon the Teicher article, there emerged a series of lawsuits involving Prozac. Soon there were claims that Prozac had caused not just suicide but violence against others. Two of these cases received national attention.

On September 14, 1989, a former employee named Joseph Wesbecker entered the Standard Gravure printing plant in Louisville, Kentucky, carrying several semi-automatic weapons. He killed eight workers, wounded twelve, and then killed himself. Wesbecker had taken Prozac for a short time—it had recently been discontinued by his physician. At autopsy, Wesbecker was found to have in his bloodstream therapeutic concentrations of Prozac and lithium and low concentrations of two or three other antidepressants and a sedative.

In the wake of Teicher's report, a lawyer named Leonard Finz filed suit against Prozac's manufacturer, on behalf of Wesbecker's family and victims. Two sons, Jim and Kevin Wesbecker, went on "Larry King Live." Jim Wesbecker said that none of his father's psychiatrists had noted "any kind of violent behavior, any kind of violent reactions of any kind in his behavior," before the father took

Prozac. Finz said he planned to file dozens of lawsuits based on the "300 to 400" reports he had received of violence, death, and suicide related to Prozac. One of Wesbecker's victims and former co-workers, again in the company of Leonard Finz, went on "Donahue" (the show was titled "Prozac—Medication That Makes You Kill"), where she said that, except for a single episode of suicidality, Wesbecker had never in the ten years she knew him shown any violent tendencies. "Everyone who know him, knew him to be just your average nice Joe." The impression given the public was that Prozac can turn average Joes into homicidal maniacs.

The local press in Louisville provided a different picture. They concluded that the slaughter in the Standard Gravure plant was the culmination of a "lifelong journey of disintegration" of a disturbed man with a substantial history of violence against himself and threats of violence against others.

Wesbecker's story appears to be one of chronic insecurity complicated by hypochondriasis, social awkwardness, a short temper, mood disorder, and finally paranoia. He was hospitalized for mental disorder in 1978, 1984, and 1987. The more serious deterioration began in 1984, after which Wesbecker tried to commit suicide three times and began threatening to kill himself with a gun; by the time of his 1987 hospitalization, he had attempted suicide twelve to fifteen times.

Four psychiatrists who treated Wesbecker over the years found him to have a variant of manic-depressive illness with paranoia. He had told one psychiatrist by 1987, and perhaps as early as 1984, that he might like to harm his foreman. He brought a gun to Standard Gravure and talked about killing a supervisor with it as early as 1986. A year before the actual shooting, Wesbecker told his ex-wife he would like to go to the plant and "shoot a bunch of people." He saved a January 1989 *Time* magazine with a cover story about a mass shooting. In May 1989, before he was prescribed Prozac, Wesbecker bought the AK-47. He was apparently prescribed Prozac late that summer.

Wesbecker was hardly your average Joe before the summer of 1989. He may have been made manic or agitated by Prozac; any antidepressant can "switch" depression to mania in a patient with pre-existing manic-depressive illness. There are other possibilities: Wesbecker may have been disinhibited by the sedative he took; the six drugs in his system may have had an idiosyncratic effect in combination; his illness may have progressed independent of medication. But one thing is clear: this was not an episode of Prozac's causing an obsession that had not previously existed. According to press reports, none of the doctors who treated Wesbecker believed that Prozac played a role in his behavior; certainly there is no indication that it played a special role related to the phenomenon described by Teicher and his colleagues.

The other highly publicized case—that of Rebecca McStoots—also involved a hidden history of prior difficulty. In March 1990, McStoots shot her doctor, John Tapp, in the neck. She was convicted by a jury and sentenced to ten years in prison for first-degree assault, but she turned around and sued Eli Lilly, Prozac's manufacturer, alleging that she had had no prior history of violence or depression. In March 1991, McStoots joined "Larry King Live" by phone from jail in Bowling Green, Kentucky. It appears she had taken Prozac some six months before the shooting and then on her own resumed taking it for a week before pulling the gun on Dr. Tapp. McStoots said she had been taking Prozac for back strain, although on further questioning she admitted to depression, past suicidal thoughts, and a suicide attempt. McStoots also appeared on "Prime Time Live" with a denial of past difficulties. In court, Eli Lilly introduced evidence that McStoots had been violent long before taking Prozac, saying she had told doctors she had shot a former husband in New Mexico and later stabbed a woman in California. A judge dismissed McStoots's suit, as well as her claim that Lilly had slandered her and interfered in her criminal trial.

Many other cases have been publicized in which people claim to have been made newly suicidal or violent on Prozac. I am not familiar with every episode, but those I have seen resemble the Wesbecker and McStoots stories. In general, the people who claim never to have been suicidal before taking Prozac turn out to have been suicidal in the past, and those who claim never to have been violent turn out to have histories of prior violent threats or acts. I have not seen a publicized case associated with Prozac that is convincing as an example of the new onset of violent obsessions. Much of the publicity regarding a link between Prozac and suicide or violence was fomented by the Citizens Commission on Human Rights, a group affiliated with the Church of Scientology, which opposes psychiatry in general.

The publicity attendant on stories of Prozac's violent dark side is intriguing. It represents, I think, our cultural conviction that there is no averting conservation of mood, that what goes up must come down. Because Prozac has done great good, we are ready to believe it can do great harm.

Prozac does have side effects, as do all drugs. It is not Heavy Sodium; you could not put it in the water supply without making some people sick. Prozac not uncommonly causes nausea, loss of appetite, nervousness, insomnia, drowsiness, fatigue, sweating, rash, dizziness, and headache. More rarely, it has been associated with damage of one sort or another to almost every body system and organ—from arrhythmia of the heart to inflammation of the liver to dysfunction of the thyroid gland. As antidepressants go, Prozac is relatively safe, but no drug is risk-free.

Part of what makes people uneasy about Prozac is precisely that it works so well and has so few side effects. Prozac is enormously seductive. It is not addictive—patients do not crave Prozac, and there is no known withdrawal syndrome—but people who have experienced a good response to it are often leery about coming off medication, out of fear that they will return to their old way of feeling and behaving. Since we continue to believe in conservation of mood, we are suspicious of a drug that is so pleasant to take.

This seduction is legitimately worrisome because we know that some drugs, especially those that are taken chronically, will have unknown or even late-appearing (tardive) side effects. Psychotherapeutic drugs can sometimes cause tardive neurological disorders, which may appear years after a drug is discontinued; and questions have already been raised whether Prozac can cause such syndromes. Recently a small, preliminary study in rats has raised concern—quite prematurely, according to oncologists—over whether antidepressants, Prozac among them, can promote tumor growth in patients with cancer. Concern over unforeseen or tardive effects is realistic, because Prozac has been around too briefly for anyone to know its long-term effects.

But the panic about Prozac and violence seems to me to have gone beyond rational fear—to be what psychoanalysts call "overdetermined," that is, welcome because of the way it corresponds to our fantasies. The reports about Prozac and violence made good television because they meshed with science-fiction images of chemicals that turn Jekyll into Hyde.

What does it mean that we are willing to believe that intent to commit suicide or homicide can be induced by a pill, perhaps (as in the McLean case studies) even in the absence of a change in mood? Thoughts about suicide—much less the killing of others—are intimate and complex. They encompass moral and religious tenets, beliefs about the value of life and about self-worth, and sentiments concerning friends and family. Yet the idea that medication can cause people to ruminate about suicide and homicide is commonly accepted.

The television talk show title, "Medication That Makes You Kill," says something not only about medication but about "You." Within you is evil: not the evil of the conflicted unconscious but the evil of an animal—an injured, ostracized, low-status, impulsive cur who turns against his own kind and then himself. You have a personality that is readily subject to biological influence. Medication can reshape you in quite particular ways.

If these fantasies are credible, it is because medication has shaped our beliefs about how the self is constituted. In the final analysis, the uproar about Prozac and violence represents further testimony to our focus on biologically determined feelings and behaviors. The scare about violence contains a backhanded tribute to Prozac, an acknowledgment, albeit in nightmare form, that Prozac can transform the self.

Afterword

To the 1997 Edition

Listening to Prozac was due to be published in June of 1993. In the last week of May, I attended a psychiatric congress in San Francisco. Knowing that books had shipped early to the coasts, at lunch I left the Moscone Center to visit a nearby store. The staff had unpacked some copies that morning, but they were sold out; would I come back toward evening and autograph the next batch? When I returned, the reshipments had come and gone. I never did manage to catch the books; as soon as they arrived, they were snatched up. I phoned my editor and left a message on her voice mail. I said, I know you are tired of hearing this sort of thing from authors, but something unusual is happening out here.

That "something unusual" was a serious book by an unknown writer becoming a best-seller and, more than a best-seller, the talk of the nation. Coverage spanned the media, including *People, The Washington Post, Oprah, Good Morning America,* and National Public Radio. At *The New Yorker,* the book inspired one cartoon after another— cartoons about listening to over-the-counter medications (Tums, Tylenol) and about how Prozac might have affected the personality of Karl Marx or Edgar Allan Poe. Woody Allen and Bette Midler cracked Prozac-and-temperament jokes. "Better than well" and "cosmetic psychopharmacology" became catch phrases, along with "rejection-sensitivity," "pharmacological Calvinism," and "listening to" anything. *The New York Times'* banner headline for its year-end summary of the arts was "Listening to 1993."

No book endures this sort of career without alteration. Like the medication it discusses, *Listening to Prozac* was transformed into a cultural icon, though of what was less clear. In some quarters, it stood for hope that medication and its effects could be integrated into a new humane view of the self; in others, it stood for the fecklessness of physicians or for the ominous power of technology. Even for those who read it, the book came to serve diverse functions. For certain readers, it was a guide to the minor depressions, perhaps offering a fresh perspective on their own condition or that of a friend. Some readers used it as a how-to book or a whether-to book, a source of advice about taking a medication. There were readers who approached the book as popular science, news about the state of knowledge about mind and brain or disease and wellness. For others *Listening to Prozac* was a celebrity biography—what is this substance people are talking about? The book was not one thing but many.

This heterogeneity of use, both symbolic and practical, poses a problem in the writing of an afterword. Yes, it might be desirable, in the face of such a profound response, to update or at least relocate the book—but which book?

I do know which book I set out to write. I had been moved by patients' stories, their courage in adversity, their dramatic gains and subtle losses on medication. In particular I was struck by what they told me when they responded to Prozac—how it caused them to reassess their lives, how this new product of our culture became a lens through which they viewed the self. I wanted to capture their experience and, if possible, something broader, the effect of living in a society where such change is possible. This much I have written in the introduction to this book.

What I did not discuss there was how I hoped to carry out that task. Writers write in genres, and in imagining my own book I had a model in mind. There is a type of non-fiction in which the author simply describes a product of our culture, its origin and its uses. But though the technology may be humble and the details ordinary, the author views it from so many perspectives that the object develops a certain resonance—it seems to say something about the self that such a society supports and demands. John McPhee's writing about frozen orange juice has some of this quality, as do Tracy Kidder's account of the production of a new computer and Verlyn Klinkenborg's description of the way hay is made in the late twentieth century. "Resonant" nonfiction has some of the aspirations of fiction. Often it does what Milan Kundera says novels do: create "terrain where moral judgment is suspended." The products depicted are not so much good or bad as reflections of the society that creates them. The products and the societies are at once admirable and worrisome, serious and foolish. Though this genre is overstuffed with facts, those facts are mere dots in a pointillist portrayal of a greater truth, about who we are—except that this greater truth tends to be, in the manner of fiction, simultaneously stated and undermined.

I hoped to write that sort of book, using Prozac as the resonant subject. Soon I realized I was focused on a single aspect of what Prozac does—how on occasion it seems to affect personality in fairly healthy people—so it might equally be said that the product I was writing about was self, how we make or remake self at the end of the twentieth century. And I knew there were important ways in which my book would have to differ from the nonfiction I admire. As a doctor—a practitioner, and not just an observer—I had a different role than does the inquiring essayist, who is freer to stand at a distance from his subject. *Listening to Prozac* would depend in part on my clinical observations; it would necessarily have a personal and an openly speculative quality. Still, that "resonant" genre was my "deep model." My aim was not to settle a moral debate but to make such a debate seem unavoidable, unsettling, and difficult to resolve. I wanted simultaneously to state and undermine a contemporary perspective on the self.

Though I knew that I would need to introduce readers to the subcultures that comprise modern psychiatry—psychopharmacology, personality theory, animal ethology, cellular physiology, and the rest were the perspectives I would bring to bear—my intention was not to write "medical nonfiction." *Listening to Prozac* was never about scientific disciplines, nor about doctorly stories, nor even about a medication, but only and always about the culture and the self, though written with the hope that expertise, stories, and the constant exposure of facets of a medication would shed evocative and suggestive light on those central subjects. To my mind, resonance remains the standard by which the book succeeds or fails. Still, it is true that if you describe your hopes with such words as resonant, speculative, stated and undermined, evocative, and suggestive, you forfeit the right to complain when readers (and even nonreaders) use the book in unintended ways. Or rather, you can complain of certain misuses, ones that evince bad faith, but you must always end by admitting that, as regards morality, practical utility, and the like, what your book lacks is precisely intent to enforce a particular conclusion.

Looking back after four years, and judging in terms of my own goals, I would say the book has held up reasonably well. It continues to stimulate a discussion about perspectives on the self—as I write, I have received word of a new philosophy course at Notre Dame built around the imaginary dialogue the book proposes with Walker Percy. And the book has been the basis, at scientific conferences here and in Europe (where it was also a best-seller), for a reevaluation of the relation of psychotherapy to pharmacotherapy. Readers continue to correspond, often to say that a category proposed in the book—say, "rejection-sensitivity"—strikes a chord; often as not, these readers understand that any such category is tentative and culture-bound, as reliable and unreliable in our day as hysteria was in Freud's.

The book forecasts our entry into an era of biological reductionism, in which the self and others will increasingly be experienced and understood in external terms. If a child is shy or impulsive, parents will less often look for unconscious or spiritual causes and more often settle for the belief that the child "just is" shy or impulsive, presumably on the basis of brain biology. *Listening to Prozac* predicted a bull market for psychophysiology, in which we, as inhabitants of that era, will attend ever more to animal and genetic models and ascribe ever more of personality to neuroanatomically sustained temperament.

A new reader might find that *Listening to Prozac* does not so much imagine a future as describe the present. Each edition of the daily paper brings news of biological inevitability. We read that the sum of happiness a person will enjoy in life is set at birth or in childhood—without regard to the person's eventual successes or failures. Or we read that the violence of rogue (human) males stems from their chimpanzee heritage or the state of their sex hormones. Urban violence is understood to relate to ghetto youths' "low serotonin" states. Neuroticism is attributed (in part) to a "Woody Allen gene" that determines how the brain handles serotonin. And the Pope embraces Darwin! In journalism and sitcoms and comic strips alike, physiological explanations of personality and behavior have replaced psychological and spiritual ones. So that in reevaluating my book at this short but event-filled distance, I might say simply that the sort of discussion—the sort of active uncertainty—the book proposes is today yet more necessary than it was four years ago.

The book's principal speculation is that medication on occasion alters aspects of personality. This view is now widely accepted among clinicians. As regards both seriously depressed patients and those with dysthymia, the effects of medication on personality and social functioning are now staples of the research literature. Clinically, doctors no longer consider remission of acute symptoms to be a marker of adequate treatment; they expect to see personality change as well. I am often called upon to consult regarding depressed patients who have had an "incomplete response to medication." Typically, a colleague will phone and say, the medication ended the episode of depression but the patient continues to suffer from low self-esteem, social anxiety, and a limited ability to experience pleasure. And I will remind myself that a decade ago that more limited result—relief from tearfulness, insomnia, and grief—was understood as a complete response. There was no expectation that medication would mitigate melancholic personality traits.

Whether SSRIs affect "normals" is a question I avoided answering in the book. There is still no large-scale, definitive research on that topic, although leading scientists have proposed the critical studies that would settle the matter. The small studies that have come to my attention all point in one direction: these medications do have the power to affect "normals"—people without any psychiatric diagnosis.

The study that is most on point has just come across my desk and is not yet published. Scientists at the Langley Porter Institute of the University of California (Brian Knutson [now at the National Institutes of Health], Owen Wolkowitz, and others) looked at the social functioning of normal people—that is, people judged to be free of mood or personality disorders—before and after a month on an SSRI. The subjects were asked to perform a negotiating task in which they and a stranger had to approach a stressful problem. On medication, the normal subjects were less negative and more collaborative, and they tended from this posture to succeed in their negotiations; this result, the researchers suggested, resembles an effect SSRIs have in male vervet monkeys, increasing "prosocial" behaviors that can raise status in the troop hierarchy. On antidepressants, these normal subjects displayed altered personality traits, and the degree of alteration correlated with the blood levels of the medication. If I were writing *Listening to Prozac* today, I would say that there is suggestive evidence that medication like Prozac can affect normal people, even that it can alter their social behavior—and it may be that these effects are the rule, not the exception.

In the absence of direct evidence, *Listening to Prozac* proposed a chain of reasoning for assuming that our culture was or soon would be facing the prospect of cosmetic psychopharmacology. First, most psychoactive substances, from stimulants to anxiolytics, alter attitudes and capabilities of normal people. Second, medications such as SSRIs affect normal lower primates, who respond with changes in social behavior. Third, though developed to treat illness, psychotherapeutic medications target the same neurotransmitters, receptors, and brain regions that are implicated in the biology of personality. And fourth, mood disorders occur on a spectrum with normality such that, however illnesses are defined, there will always be someone just beyond the boundary who has a similar biological makeup to those within.

Every link in that chain has been strengthened by subsequent research and theorizing. It is just vanishingly unlikely that medications that affect the personality and behavior of depressed—and dysthymic, and obsessional, and anxious, and eating-disordered, and impulsively aggressive—patients will not affect certain people who carry no diagnosis at all. Parenthetically, I would add that the identical debate—about whether when we medicate for cases of less severe dysfunction we are treating illness or changing normality in response to social demands—is now being played out with regard to Ritalin and attention deficits. Very likely it will be played out with regard to many future biological interventions, including genetic engineering.

For the moment, anxiety over cosmetic psychopharmacology has been muted by an acceleration of the "diagnostic bracket creep" predicted in *Listening to Prozac.* That is, rather than say that medications affect patients without defined mental illness, the profession's tendency has been to consider ever more patients to be "dysthymic" or to suffer a minor variant of an anxiety syndrome. This change, which I cannot document but believe to be real enough, is not a matter of cynicism but of altered perception—a different paradigm for illness. Someone who is habitually diffident, listless, anhedonic, pessimistic, unassertive, perfectionistic, and emotionally vulnerable (in short, someone with the melancholic temperament) is likely to be diagnosed dysthymic and treated on that basis, even in the absence of discrete episodes of depression.

Recently, researchers have been studying people with isolated symptoms of depression. It turns out that having even a few depressive symptoms for a few weeks puts people at risk for a variety of social failures. This research is pushing psychiatry toward the treatment of ever more minor levels of mood disruption; there is, in other words, an empirical rationale for expanding the range of psychiatric diagnosis. It may be appropriate to medicate patients whose level of depression is "subsyndromal"—certainly a melancholic person may be a fit candidate for that other mental health technology, psychotherapy—but I would say that an honest labeling of this use of antidepressants would deem it an attempt, through pharmacology, to replace a normal if unrewarded personality style with another normal style that is more comfortable or better socially rewarded.

As a culture, we will increasingly face this dilemma: whether to broaden the definition of illness or to concede that biological treatments are being used to influence normal mental states. As scientists characterize the human genome, as they improve their ability through ever-better scanners to image the structure and physiological activity of the brain, as they discover more subtle chemical markers of brain processes, they will characterize variants in brain functioning that have effects on mood and behavior and that might prove suitable targets for one or another intervention. The question in each case will be whether the variant is to be considered health or illness—and whether altering the variant is a legitimate doctorly function. (For individuals, the parallel question will be how they understand their own behavioral style and personal idiosyncrasies.) Though it focuses only on one medication, *Listening to Prozac* served to place this debate on the national agenda.

• • •

The book's speculative themes—transformation, cosmetic psycho-pharmacology, biological reductionism—remain current and, if anything, are more important elements of the culture than they were when I was writing. But what of the underlying science? As *Listening to Prozac* became popular, I realized I had a difficult choice. I could attempt to follow developments in the many fields the book draws upon: psychopharmacology, animal ethology, child development, medical ethics, and the rest. Or I could return to old habits—reading random articles that caught my interest and pursuing topics related to the problems of patients I was treating. I chose the latter course. I had other writing projects in mind, and to try scrupulously to track so many disciplines would make me a prisoner of Prozac. I told myself I might revise the book in fifteen years or so, my guess as to the interval needed to develop a class of medications different enough to pose new questions about the self.

In preparing *Listening to Prozac* I had interviewed researchers about work that was still "in the pipeline," and I asked them about their theoretical models—their sense of how disparate data add up. Since much of what has appeared in the recent scientific literature is the fruit of those pending studies and that extrapolation, *Listening to Prozac* remains fairly current. An attempt to digest new research might result in a slightly rebalanced book—more decisive in some areas, more ambiguous in others. But I doubt that the occasional change in a pointillist dot would alter the overall picture. The biogenic amine hypothesis, rejection-sensitivity, pharmacological dissection, kindling, harm avoidance, social inhibition, dominance hierarchy, stress hormones, *formes frustes* of major mental illness, "cerebral joy-juice," consummatory and appetitive pleasure, hysteroid dysphoria, hyperthymia, reactivity, learned helplessness, mood brighteners, hedonic capacity, functional autonomy, evolutionary adaptation, affect tolerance, post-synaptic hypersensitivity, conservation of mood, "free choice under pressure"—these are still the concepts through which psychiatrists consider the minor variants of depression and their consequences.

As I spend more time writing, my psychiatric practice has contracted, but I continue on occasion to see the sort of "transformational" responses I described in *Listening to Prozac.* Often these occur in psychotherapy patients who return for further treatment, this time with the addition of a trial of medication. One of the most influential essays in modern psychotherapy is called "The Two Analyses of Mr. Z"; in it, a master analyst, Heinz Kohut, describes a patient who has responded well to a rigorous Freudian psychoanalysis but who experiences more profound change—a repair of deficits in the self—in an empathic treatment of Kohut's devising. A paper that would bear writing today is "The Two Therapies of Ms. Z"—one before and one after the availability of the new antidepressants.

Typically, Ms. Z will have suffered a loss in childhood—let us say, the death of her mother. In adolescence, Ms. Z will have been especially obedient with her stepmother, out of fear of abandonment and because the stepmother was stern or preoccupied. In adult life, Ms. Z will complain of social inhibition and a lack of self-confidence. Her first psychotherapy relates those traits to the results of childhood trauma: fear that she will be abandoned because she is not lovable. Ms. Z begins to assert herself in her marriage and at work; she declares herself satisfied with her progress.

After a few years, Ms. Z returns for a consultation. Her assertiveness has brought her husband around—he is now the man she hoped he would turn out to be—and she has achieved career advancement; but still she takes little pleasure in life. Her state is assessed as anhedonia or dysthymia, and she begins a trial of Prozac or another antidepressant. She responds well and reports that in retrospect she had not known what it is to feel self-esteem. What she understood in the past as confidence was only a hesitant move toward what she experiences on medication. In retrospect she has been bitter and angry for years. Only now can she truly enjoy her family. She is ever more prone to see herself as having been damaged in the past. She wants further psychotherapy, to understand that damage: to "put it all together."

In her second psychotherapy, Ms. Z is unexpectedly willing to own responsibility for her contribution to her social troubles in adult life: she acknowledges that she made the marriage difficult. She does so with a spirit of forgiveness toward the self, based on a keener sense of her early deprivation. What is most extraordinary is Ms. Z's ability to express ambivalence about her beloved mother. Ms. Z recalls incidents in which the mother was quite as rejecting as the stepmother. It is not so much that Ms. Z has captured new memories as that old ones have a fuller emotional coloration, and she is strong enough to face them. Her social inhibitions are diminished, and at the same time they make more emotional sense to her than they did before.

This sequence raises questions on a number of levels. How much of each therapy is necessary? Perhaps it is best for Ms. Z to have struggled in her first treatment with her demoralization, her social anxiety, her sense of vulnerability. (Perhaps it is that therapy that allows the medicine to work so well.) But can Ms. Z's therapy be said to be complete without the more freewheeling assessment of the past that becomes possible once she feels emotionally stable on medication? And who is the true Ms. Z? My contribution, as a clinician, to a revised *Listening to Prozac* would be an expression of wonder at the resilience of psychotherapy as a technology, as well as further insistence on the need to integrate psychotherapy with the new pharmacotherapy.

Here is where an afterword to the book I intended to write would end. But such an afterword ignores the career of the book—its iconic life, its place in the culture. The sort of afterword I have so far proposed does not address important ways in which *Listening to Prozac* has been used.

Regarding some of those uses, it is hard to know how to respond. Should a given person take Prozac? How do the effects and side effects of Prozac compare to those of other antidepressants? I know from conversations in my travels that these sorts of questions are urgent to certain readers. To answer them would require not revising this book but writing a new one and, to my mind, betraying the old one that tried, with some insistence, to resist the medical advisory role. I am thinking, for example, of the paragraph in the introduction that says, "even if Prozac were shown to cause one or another serious physical illness, that reality would have little to say about this other question: how is it that taking a capsule for depression can so alter a person's sense of self?" Besides, with the advent of new medications and increased experience in combining them, the art of psychopharmacology has become quite subtle; it is increasingly true that the only adequate answer to a practical personal question is a consultation with an experienced psychiatrist.

That being said, perhaps the following brief update is in order. Concerning efficacy: throughout *Listening to Prozac*, I cited circumstantial reasons for believing SSRIs might be especially useful for dysthymia, atypical depression, and depressive personality; that speculation has been confirmed by subsequent research. Concerning safety: millions more people have taken Prozac than had when I wrote the book. And the news, in terms of side effects, is good. For a medicine this potent, Prozac is well tolerated. The same can be said, though on the basis of smaller samples and time periods, of all the new antidepressants (Zoloft, Paxil, Wellbutrin, Luvox, Effexor, Serzone, and Remeron to date), although each appears to have its own, slightly different, "personality."

Regarding Prozac, more is known now about side effects. *Listening to Prozac* was early in mentioning Prozac's effects on sexual function. Today, it is clearly established that the medication can diminish libido and delay orgasm. The theoretical issue those side effects raise for psychoanalysis, which places such stress on libido as the basis for pleasure and health, is more starkly framed: How is it that a medication that tempers sex drive can enhance the sense of well-being?

More generally, writing today I would want to underscore the warning in *Listening to Prozac* about late-appearing side effects and effects following upon long-term use. Prozac is young as medications go. Especially in light of a new standard for the treatment of recurrent depression—some patients are kept on medication "indefinitely"—more research is needed on chronic usage. And much more work is needed on the effects of this medication on the developing brains of children and adolescents.

And writing today, I would repeat the plea I made in the book on behalf of psychotherapy, which I characterized as "the single most helpful technology for the treatment of minor depression and anxiety." *Listening to Prozac* anticipated that cost-cutters would cynically misuse the availability of new medications to deprive patients of needed psychotherapy, a treatment that increasingly appears to have its own physiological effects. My fantasy is that, in an enlightened psychiatry of the future, pharmacotherapy will be a subdiscipline of psychotherapy, one of many means of enhancing flexibility of perspective.

One other aspect of the book's career is hard to ignore—namely, the "controversy" surrounding *Listening to Prozac.* I use quotation marks because I have never believed the book to be controversial. The book's originality lay in the attempt to juxtapose perspectives, and to combine evidence from disparate subdisciplines in a way that researchers, bound by stricter rules of evidence, are often prevented from doing in public. But I had faith that my portrait of the field expressed what both researchers and clinicians believed in their hearts or would believe if they took the time to look about. For the most part, responses to *Listening to Prozac* confirmed this faith. The book was well received by my fellow clinicians and by experts in the disciplines—psychopharmacology, medical ethics, and the rest—whose perspectives I had attempted to characterize. And the vast majority of reviews was enthusiastic.

But the response to *Listening to Prozac* included two types of discussion that had at least the form of controversy. The first objections came from a group I think of as radical skeptics or intellectual anarchists. Initially these were Scientologists and ex-Scientologists who oppose the premises of modern psychiatry. They argued that Prozac is not a successful treatment for major depression, but simultaneously they maintained that major depression is not an illness and that much of neurobiology is wholesale fraud. Addressing this objection is like confronting the claim that a given satellite will not go into orbit, a discussion whose nature changes when you discover that you are having it with someone who believes the earth is flat.

That being said, elements of the skeptical critique have merit. As I indicate in *Listening to Prozac,* psychiatric diagnosis is flawed, culture-bound, and sometimes arbitrary. Like the skeptics, I want to challenge any simple definition of depression. Also, a fuller account of the skeptical position includes profound respect for the power of medications, in the sense that while the skeptics doubt that Prozac can treat depression, they have no trouble believing that it alters personality, albeit for the worse. And the radical skeptics (partly) agree with me when they argue that contemporary biological views of the mind give an incomplete account of human capabilities.

In my public discussions, I tried to avoid the radical skeptics. They frightened me, and not because of the force of their ideas. But when, as happened rarely, I was forced into debate, I found myself in an uncomfortable posture. I did not want to fall prey to the temptation to define my position in strict opposition to theirs.

I avoided the radical skeptics for another reason as well. They seemed to hope that the popularity of *Listening to Prozac* would provide a way for them to get on television. For my part, I did not want to provide a forum for fringe groups to promote dubious views that might cause depressed patients to avoid psychiatrists or medication. In any event, I thought I was the wrong person to enter into a debate. I had not written a book about how to manage serious depression— had declared, in my book's introduction, that I had no intention of addressing Prozac's results in treating major mental illness. As my public role grew, I did find myself sometimes discussing treatments for a variety of mood disorders. Still, that public health function had little to do with what I had written. The radical skeptics raised a general attack on modern science, but they did not join the particular issues—about medication and the contemporary sense of self—raised by *Listening to Prozac.*

More insidious was "controversy" coming from the opposite direction. Here, the contenders were often professionals or academicians. They believed that Prozac ameliorates major depression, but they claimed that that is all it does—and if it does do more, the book and its author were too enthusiastic over that prospect. I call the proponents of this view strict constructionists. In contrast to the radical skeptics, strict constructionists had no interest in debate, perhaps because some of them knew little about psychiatry except that they liked it well circumscribed and walled off from the public. Nor did they deign to ground their position in specifics. They merely branded the book anathema.

It took me some time to figure out the strict constructionists. It seemed to me they had overlooked the worried tone of much of the book—missed the book's intention simultaneously to state and question the perspectives of psychiatry. They acted as if the book promotes the very thing it attacks—that is, certainty about the social worth of new medications. Sometimes their essays contained what looked like a summary of my positions, except that the author would attribute my concerns about medication to himself. One diatribe claimed that *Listening to Prozac* is replete with scientific errors—but gave not a single example of such an error. Instead, the author pontificated about the "criteria by which the work of any physician should be judged." That phrase resolved my puzzlement. The strict constructionists were not critiquing the book's ideas. They were acting as defenders of the guild. Their objection was to what they saw as a corruption of the doctorly persona. Doctors ought not to speculate in public: saying aloud what researchers and clinicians believe in private risks damage to the reputation of the profession. Or to put the matter in my terms, medication is not a fit subject for the sort of resonant nonfiction *Listening to Prozac* emulates.

One response to such an objection is pragmatic: Just what has been the effect of *Listening to Prozac?* Hard to say—in a mass culture, does the written word still have the power to move? My impression is that if the book has had any effect (beyond its intended one, to illuminate self and culture through examining the artifact Prozac), it has been to place on the public agenda the question of the proper use of psychotherapeutic medication and incidentally to destigmatize the taking of medication to treat mental illness. Whether due to the book's influence or not, open discussion of mental illness as illness has flourished in the last few years as never before in human history. As for the honor of the guild, in their reviews the most relevant professional journals, *Depression* and *The American Journal of Psychiatry,* recommended the book as a way to introduce psychiatry to the general public.

Regarding the strict constructionists' public health concerns, there has never been evidence that the new antidepressants are overused. Prescribing of Prozac has continued to increase, although similar and newer medicines have accelerated faster in the race for "market share." Depression is so underdiagnosed, and when diagnosed it is so undertreated, that researchers have suggested current prescribing could double or even quadruple just to meet basic public health needs. Rumors abound of flagrant "cosmetic psychopharmacology"; but I receive hundreds of requests for consultation regarding antidepressant use, and I have yet to encounter a case that appears frivolous. The more important dilemma concerns diagnostic bracket creep. The expansion of diagnostic categories has legitimated prescribing antidepressants for more minor indications. Here, I think, the book raised the relevant issue: How shall we understand and delimit the use of psychopharmacology to treat socially handicapping minor conditions that exist on a spectrum with clear-cut mental illness?

Colleagues in clinical practice tell me that *Listening to Prozac* has brought into treatment people who previously had no name for what troubled them and who consequently did not know that there was anywhere to turn for help. News of the book's practical utility is particularly gratifying because the career of the book has made me appreciate how little influence a writer has over the use and misuse of his ideas. Although I believe that the book contributed to the public health, I never meant for it to be prescriptive. It would seem impossibly inhibiting to require writers as they compose their work to anticipate all aspects of the subsequent discussion; for the most part, writers' ethical responsibility is limited to what they have, in fact, written.

Faced with the criticism that *Listening to Prozac* does not meet a doctorly criterion, I prefer to answer at a more conceptual level. Just what is doctorly? Perhaps the strict constructionists are right to feel threatened or offended. *Listening to Prozac* does break rules: rules to speculate in private, to keep doubts to oneself, to think in discrete disciplinary categories. These are useful rules, and often we want our doctors to honor them.

"Listening" can be taken as a metaphor for rule-breaking. Listening to medication implies a crossing of boundaries, a mixing of categories—approaching pharmacology with the tools of the psychotherapist. And the therapist's posture is speculative and doubting. The book arises from that posture and from the writerly one, which often demands that internal mental processes be made public.

Here is where I differ most profoundly with the strict constructionists. I want to say that psychotherapy and speculative writing are doctorly. This book is a public example of how a doctor thinks. Not every doctor. We have need of strict constructionists and defenders of the guild; their categorical thought is responsible for some of what is best in medicine. But much of the doctor's role is not reached through certainty. It is "empirical" in the odd usage of that word that means impressionistic—based on trial-and-error, anecdotal experience, and pattern recognition. Faced with the unique patient, the doctor brings to bear every talent, every memory, every inspiration he can call upon, without suffering limitation by discipline, convention, or the strict requirements of scientific proof. Or rather, the doctor oscillates between perspectives, the eclectic and the conventional. I believe that the notion of "criteria" for the guild needs, like other grand categories, to be both stated and undermined. There is a "medical" perspective, and at the same time medicine must embrace foreign perspectives. The writerly must be the doctorly.

However necessary, this digression into "controversy" may give a false impression of my response to the public fate of my book. I am deeply grateful, I stand in nervous awe before my own good fortune. I had hoped my book might elicit a response from a handful of readers; instead, it "struck a chord," which is to say set off a special sort of resonance, with an entire culture, indeed many cultures.

The self, how it fares in a world where personality is understood as "biological" and subject to biological influence, is a central issue for our time, and people know it, to use the language of the book, viscerally. Who are we, if we can be so altered by medication? And why should the medicated self on occasion feel more "true" than the unmedicated? What is melancholy anyway, and how separable is it from our sense of self? What does it signify that so many who have shaped our manner of thought—philosophers, novelists, poets, the unacknowledged legislators of the world—have been depressives? Does our pain and anxiety speak to us and summon us to quest, or is what we feel so much static, a Darwinian residue, without special meaning? What is normal? What does our culture demand of us, and ought we to comply? With time, these questions have only become more urgent—not urgent in the way that treatment of depression is urgent, but urgent in the profound sense of demanding constant attention if we are to know ourselves and our place in nature and society.

The acceleration of neuropsychological research and the increasing use of a widening array of medication for the mind give an air of inevitability to *Listening to Prozac*. The "controversy" over the book finds its dialectical opposite in the sense, which I sometimes had in the midst of the national discussion, that in writing it I was less an autonomous thinker than an instrument of the zeitgeist. I am skeptical over impersonal forces—what I felt on the book tour was probably just jet lag—but I do suspect that if *Listening to Prozac* had not been written four years ago, it would need to be written today.

Notes

INTRODUCTION

ix   the antidepressant drug Prozac: The generic name for Prozac is fluoxetine. Regarding proprietary and generic names for drugs, I have used whichever I thought would cause least trouble for the reader. When discussing a series of related drugs (imipramine, desipramine, clomipramine), I use the generic names. But where the proprietary (trade) name is a household word, I take advantage of that familiarity—Valium, for example, rather than diazepam. All drugs are cross-referenced under both generic and the most common proprietary name in the index.

In referring to prescribed, licit substances, I have used the words "medication," "medicine," and "drug" interchangeably.

ix   I had occasion to treat an architect: This is a simplified account of a case I have described in detail elsewhere ("Metamorphosis," *Psychiatric Times*, May 1989, p. 3ff). Sam's illness was complex, as was his course of treatment; among other things, when he first fully responded to Prozac, Sam was also on an antianxiety medication, Xanax; later in the course of treatment, the Xanax became unnecessary. In general, I have not simplified other case vignettes in this book to this degree, but I have altered identifying details in order to protect privacy. One case (Philip, chapter 9) is a composite.

Freud noted the paradox "that it is far easier to divulge the patient's most intimate secrets than the most innocent and trivial facts about him; for, whereas the former would not throw any light on his identity, the latter, by which he is generally recognized, would make it obvious to everyone" ("Notes upon a

Case of Obsessional Neurosis (1909)," James Strachey, ed., *The Standard Edition of the Complete Psychological Works of Sigmund Freud*, vol X [London: Hogarth Press, 1955], p. 156). Since truth is in the details, this tension between the requirements of accuracy and privacy is an impossible one; to this difficulty are added the inevitable flaws in all communication. A colleague has phrased well what I believe is the proper disclaimer regarding case examples: "Any departure from 'real' events is in part intended, in part unintended: details are deliberately disguised to protect the privacy of patients; and the distortions of human perception and memory are unavoidable" (Byram T. Karasu, *Wisdom in the Practice of Psychotherapy* [New York: Basic Books, 1992], p. xix).

x he enjoyed sex as much as ever: I mention this detail because a common side effect of Prozac is change in sexual function, usually difficulty achieving orgasm. (See note to p. 265, on p. 366.) Sam did not experience this side effect.

Subsequent to my treatment of Sam, preliminary objective evidence has emerged that Prozac can, indeed, diminish sexual obsessions and compulsions (Dan J. Stein, Eric Hollander, et al., "Serotonergic Medications for Sexual Obsessions, Sexual Addictions, and Paraphilias," *Journal of Clinical Psychiatry*, vol. 53 [1992], pp. 267–71). I believe Sam was right—the interest in pornography was something like an obsession or a compulsion—but even if the truth is different, what remains interesting is Sam's willingness to turn to the medication for definition of the self.

xii like Kierkegaard and Heidegger: This issue is approached in the chapter "Philosophical Roots" of Robert Coles's book *Walker Percy: An American Search* (Boston: Atlantic-Little, Brown, 1978), especially pp. 22, 32. I return to the philosophical implications of a biological view of affect in chapter 9.

xii assuming a patient's anxiety was meaningless: The concept of meaningless anxiety is not restricted to assumptions about patients on medication; it is central to the biological theory of panic anxiety. I take this matter up in some detail in chapter 4.

xiii the genes for . . . asking directions: Since I wrote that sentence, a report of a serious study on this issue appeared in *The New York Times:* Sandra Blakeslee, "Why Don't Men Ask Directions? They Don't Feel Lost: Each Sex Has Its Own Way of Navigating, Study Finds," May 26, 1992, p. C1f.

xiii "half the difference in individuals' IQs": *Newsweek*, October 29, 1990, p. 69,

xiv such disorders as manic-depressive illness: This disorder is now properly called "bipolar affective disorder," but it remains "manic depression" in popular speech. (For instance, the relevant patient advocacy group is the National Depressive and Manic-Depressive Association.) For the sake of readability, I have chosen for the most part to call various conditions by their popular names. As in the case of drug names, the popular and scientific names are cross-referenced in the index.

Also, I have not scrupled to employ "manic-depressive," "schizophrenic," and, for that matter, "obsessive" or "dysthymic" as substantives. Occasionally I receive letters saying this usage is pejorative (on the grounds that no one *is*, globally, schizophrenic, but that people can *have* an illness, schizophrenia) and is restricted to mental illnesses. Given the examples of "asthmatic" and "diabetic," and the long history of reference to consumptives, I find this assertion unconvincing. I hope it is clear that no disparagement is intended when I try to avoid awkward locutions by using such terms as "manic-depressive."

xiv the studies proved impossible to replicate: Richard C. Lewontin expresses a yet stronger opinion:

> The rage for genes reminds us of Tulipomania and the South Sea Bubble in McKay's *Great Popular Delusions of* [sic] *the Madness of Crowds.* Claims for the definitive location of a gene for schizophrenia and manic depressive syndrome using DNA markers have been followed repeatedly by retraction of the claims and contrary claims as a few more members of a family tree have been observed, or a different set of families examined. In one notorious case, a claimed gene for manic depression, for which there was strong statistical evidence, was nowhere to be found when two members of the same family group developed symptoms. The original claim and its retraction both were published in the international journal *Nature,* causing David Baltimore to cry out at a scientific meeting, "Setting myself up as an average reader of *Nature,* what am I to believe?" Nothing.

("The Dream of the Human Genome," *New York Review of Books,* May 28, 1992, pp. 31–40; quotation on p. 37.)

xiv Carl Degler: See Carl N. Degler, *In Search of Human Nature: The Decline and Revival of Darwinism in American Social Thought* (New York: Oxford University Press, 1991).

xvi "cosmetic psychopharmacology": The essay is "The New You," *Psychiatric Times,* March 1990, pp. 45–46.

xvi cover story in *Newsweek:* March 26, 1990. One of my favorite Prozac media pieces appeared in the French magazine *Santé* (April 1990, p. 56). Under a reproduction of the *Newsweek* cover run these story headers: "Pilule Anti-Cafard: La Folie Américaine. L'Amérique est tombée amoureuse d'une pilule. Ses fans l'ont surnommé BBB (Bye Bye Blues: adieu cafard). Tout un programme. Mais est-ce pour autant la panacée?"

xvi definitive contemporary article for physicians: William Z. Potter, Matthew V. Rudorfer, and Husseini Manji, "The Pharmacologic Treatment of Depression," *New England Journal of Medicine,* vol. 325 (1991), pp. 633–42.

xvi green-and-off-white capsule: Officially it is a "pulvule." I asked the public-relations officer for Prozac's manufacturer what a pulvule is. She said the word is a registered trademark that refers to a capsule one of whose ends is slightly tapered, a characteristic Prozac has in common with a few other drugs, such as Darvon, also manufactured by Eli Lilly. It is so like Prozac-the-media-phenomenon to have this special, and meaningless, word associated with it.

xvii an ominous report had appeared: Martin H. Teicher, Carol Glod, and Jonathan O. Cole, "Emergence of Intense Suicidal Preoccupation During Fluoxetine Treatment," *American Journal of Psychiatry,* vol. 147 (1990), pp. 207–10. The issue of suicide, other violence, and Prozac is discussed in the appendix.

xvii Geraldo . . . Donahue: The most inflammatory television program may have been the February 27, 1991, "Donahue": "Prozac—Medication That Makes You Kill." On that show, Leanne Westover, widow of Del Shannon, claimed that Prozac-induced agitation led to his suicide.

xvii *Newsweek* again: "Violence Goes Mainstream," April 1, 1991.

xviii cover exposé of the Scientologists: *Time,* May 6, 1991.

xviii "60 Minutes": October 27, 1991.

xviii clinician after clinician had written: For example, Theodore Nadelson, "The Use of Adjunctive Fluoxetine in Analytic Psychotherapy with High Functioning Outpatients," unpublished, 1991, 24 pp. Nadelson, a psychoanalyst and nationally renowned consultation-liaison psychiatrist based at Tufts University, found that the best Prozac responders were often patients who were also good candidates for psychoanalysis, including those who had formed a strong relationship to the therapist and who had achieved a degree of social and career success. The types of positive results Nadelson noted included "increased satisfaction [and] disappearance of sensitivity to social criticism" as well as elevation of mood and a decrease in pessimism.

CHAPTER 1: MAKEOVER

1   a woman I worked with only around issues of medication: The issue of what is often called "medication backup" is a complicated one for psychiatry. There are psychiatrists who believe that it is unprofessional to do less than the whole job—that psychiatrists should not medicate patients whom social workers and psychologists see in psychotherapy. I prefer to do both aspects of treatment, but I have come to trust a handful of psychologists and social workers in my community—and they me—with the result that we work comfortably with patients whose care we share. These nonphysician psychotherapists are all women, which helps explain something the reader will notice about this book—namely, that most of the patients are women.

Women have always been overrepresented in the taking of antidepressants, for at least two, and probably three, reasons. First, most depression occurs in women. The best current understanding of this gender difference is that it is partly "biological" (broadly speaking, genetic, and in some way related to the cyclicity of women's biological functions, hormonal differences, and perhaps a stronger innate propensity to bond and therefore to suffer losses more deeply) but more predominantly psychological, related to the stresses and losses in women's lives. We will consider a complex interactive model of the causes of mood disorder, in chapter 5 and elsewhere. Second, women seek help more often than men do, so doctors see depressed women out of proportion to their presence in the population. A third likelihood is that, all things being equal, doctors may prescribe antidepressants somewhat more often for women than they do for men.

Along with two women colleagues in public health, I once investigated these issues by analyzing a sample of ninety thousand visits to doctors (not just psychiatrists), representative of all visits to doctors' private offices in the United States in 1980–81. In that study, 60 percent of all office visits to a doctor, for any reason, were by women. Sixty-four percent of visits for a psychiatric diagnosis were by women. And 70 percent of visits in which therapeutic listening was employed were for women. Even so, we found that, controlling for diagnosis and many other factors, a female patient visiting her physician for mental-health care had a 28-percent chance of receiving a psychotherapeutic drug, compared with a 24-percent chance for a virtually identical male patient. My impression is that women are more likely to be listened to and more likely to be medicated—they are just more likely to be treated than are men, and this is on top of any increased vulnerability to depression. (Rachel A. Schurman, Peter D. Kramer, and Janet B. Mitchell, "The Hidden Mental Health Network: Treatment of Mental Illness by Nonpsychiatric Physicians," *Archives of General Psychiatry*, vol. 42 [1985], pp. 89–94; Rachel A. Schurman, Peter D. Kramer, and Janet B. Mitchell, "The Hidden Mental Health Network: Provision of Mental Health Services by Non-Psychiatrist Physicians," research report, supported by contract 232-81-0039 from Division of Health Professional Analysis, DHHS, 1983.)

However, the *minor* mood disorders we will discuss in this book may be different from major depression. There are some researchers who believe these conditions—particularly "dysthymia," a category we will turn to in chapter 6—are biologically most like manic-depressive illness, which occurs with *equal* frequency in men and women.

My sense is that the number of medicated women in my practice is influenced by "medication-backup" referrals from women therapists whose caseloads are predominantly women and who are sensitive to issues of biological treatment for minor depression. In terms of the patients I see for both psychotherapy and pharmacotherapy, a group that is more equally men and women, the gender distribution of patients on medication is fairly even.

8 "People on the sidewalk ask me for directions!": I have since heard this identical report from other people on Prozac. In all cases, the medicine must have stimulated the patient to display subtle cues of accessibility. None of these people was manic or exhibitionistic. The alteration was subtle but thorough.

16 mental condition called "hyperthymia": Even the term "hyperthymia" is sometimes used to refer to a rather extreme condition (see chapter 6). I am borrowing the word to indicate a characteristic exuberance and quickness without implying overexpansiveness.

19 But who had she been . . . if not herself: We do occasionally make such claims. Here is a snippet of dialogue from Anne Tyler's novel *The Accidental Tourist* (New York: Alfred A. Knopf, 1985), p. 249. The first speaker is the brother of a man who has been transformed by his interactions with a woman; the second speaker, Macon, is the man transformed:

"You're not yourself these days. . . . Everybody says so."
"I'm more myself than I've been my whole life long," Macon told him.
"What kind of remark is that? It doesn't even make sense!"

CHAPTER 2: COMPULSION

22 a magazine article I had written about psychopharmacology: "Is Everybody Happy?," *Good Health Magazine,* supplement to Boston *Globe,* October 7, 1990, p. 15ff.

25 "for most of the day . . .": American Psychiatric Association, *Diagnostic and Statistical Manual of Mental Disorders,* 3rd ed., rev. (Washington, D.C.: American Psychiatric Association, 1987), p. 230 (DSM-III-R). (I turn to dysthymia in detail in chapter 6.) The definitions of "obsession" and "compulsion," as elements of OCD, are on p. 247; that of "obsessive compulsive personality disorder" (formerly "compulsive personality disorder") on p. 356. In the description of the personality disorder, I have chosen the language of DSM III (1980, pp. 326–28) because it is more expressive. The patient would equally fail to meet the criteria for DSM-III-R, which include certain other interesting considerations, such as "inability to discard worn-out or worthless objects" and "lack of generosity in giving time, money, or gifts when no personal gain is likely to result." There have been changes in the definition of compulsion, obsession, OCD, and the related personality disorder between DSM-III (1980) and DSM-III-R (1987), and changes are anticipated for DSM-IV (in progress). Some of the instability in diagnosis is due to a new focus on these disorders in light of their responsivity to medication.

28 I raised the dose: The majority of patients who respond do so on twenty milligrams per day. Prozac has a long half-life—it is degraded and excreted only slowly by the body. As a result, the patient taking twenty milligrams is, in effect, on a low dose for a number of days; it is often not for two weeks that the therapeutic level has been reached in the blood and brain, the result of the residual contributions of early doses added together. (With most other antidepressants, it is necessary to give a low dose for a few days, and then, when the body is acclimated, to add more. Someone taking imipramine may begin with twenty-five or fifty milligrams and end up needing two or three hundred milligrams daily.)

The manufacturer of Prozac made the brilliant marketing decision at first to manufacture only one form of Prozac, the twenty-milligram capsule. Then all doctors could be taught to dose their patients with one pill a day—so simple, as the pharmacists say, that even an internist can do it. This marketing decision was one factor in the enormous popularity of Prozac.

In fact, different patients do respond to different doses. For those prone to anxiety, twenty milligrams may be a high starting dose. Psychiatrists soon learned to have patients break open the capsule, dissolve it in water or juice, stir well, and drink half the solution to get a ten-milligram dose. Patients with panic anxiety are often started on a two-and-a-half-milligram dose, one ounce of the solution made from dissolving contents of the capsule in eight ounces of water.

Julia did well on forty milligrams—two pills in the morning—whereas Tess had been on the more usual dose of twenty milligrams. Eighty milligrams is the highest dose recommended by the manufacturer, but some patients with OCD do not respond until the dose reaches 160 milligrams.

32   Large numbers . . . are not "diagnosable": See Leon Eisenberg, "Treating Depression and Anxiety in Primary Care: Closing the Gap Between Knowledge and Practice," *New England Journal of Medicine,* vol. 326 (1992), pp. 1080–84; and James E. Barrett, Jane A. Barrett, et al., "The Prevalence of Psychiatric Disorders in a Primary Care Practice," *Archives of General Psychiatry,* vol. 45 (1988), pp. 1100–1106.

33   to encompass . . . personal idiosyncrasy: Not only the neat are obsessional. Clinicians recognize a category one might call the "sloppy obsessional." Behaviorally, the sloppy obsessional seems the opposite of Julia. He never cleans, and he scorns those who clean up for him; but his behavior is equally based on paralysis of choice, a strong superego (this is where some of the contempt for time wasted in cleaning arises), and a generally inflexible approach to life. Neat obsessives who fall into despair may also become slovenly in a decided, almost aggressive way.

33   I had described Tess: The full sentence is: "She was a hard-working executive so attentive to detail in her professional life that she found little time to socialize, and that she devoted to a hopeless attachment to a married man" ("Is Everybody Happy?," p. 15).

40   "Masochism is as unfashionable . . .": John Updike, "Falling Asleep Up North," *New Yorker,* May 6, 1991, pp. 36–39; quotation on p. 39.

41   an influential critique of capitalist society: See Daniel Burston, *The Legacy of Erich Fromm* (Cambridge, Mass.: Harvard University Press, 1991), pp. 33–34 and elsewhere.

41   like compulsiveness or . . . like depression: Before this century, this question would have been meaningless. Throughout most of history, obsessive-compulsive disorder was understood as a form or part of melancholia. For example, the early-seventeenth-century physician and clergyman Richard Napier described this typical picture in one of his melancholic patients:

Extreme melancholy, possessing her for a long time, with fear; and
sorely tempted not to touch anything for fear that then she shall be
tempted to wash her clothes, even upon her back. Is tortured until that
she be forced to wash her clothes, be them never so good and new.
Will not suffer her husband, child, nor any of the household to have
any new clothes until they wash them for fear the dust of them will
fall upon her. Dareth not to go to the church for treading on the ground,
fearing any dust should fall upon them.

(Michael MacDonald, *Mystical Bedlam: Madness, Anxiety, and Healing in
Seventeenth-Century England* [Cambridge: Cambridge University Press, 1981],
quoted in Stanley W. Jackson, *Melancholia and Depression: From Hippocratic Times
to Modern Times* [New Haven: Yale University Press, 1986], p. 106.)

From ancient times, a degree of compulsiveness was considered typical of
minor depression. Melancholics were understood to be driven. They had little
energy, but that little they could often channel effectively. (This point is
emphasized by Hagop Akiskal, whose work we will consider in chapter 6.) It
is only in recent decades that the minor disorders have been subdivided into
many distinct categories.

42 Freud's contemporary Emil Kraepelin: For a clear and masterful discussion
of Kraepelin's contribution, and of manic depression and schizophrenia, see
"Objective-Descriptive Psychiatry: Emil Kraepelin," in Leston Havens, *Approaches to the Mind: Movement of the Psychiatric Schools from Sects to Science* (Cambridge, Mass.: Harvard University Press, 1973), pp. 13–34.

42 ". . . essentially the same in quality . . .": Karl Menninger, *The Vital
Balance* (New York: Viking, 1963), p. 2.

42 "The predominant American psychiatric theory . . .": Donald F. Klein,
"Anxiety Reconceptualized," in Donald F. Klein and Judith G. Rabkin, eds.,
Anxiety: New Research and Changing Concepts (New York: Raven Press, 1981),
pp. 235–61; quotation on p. 235. This essay, one of the most important in
modern biological psychiatry, appears also in Donald F. Klein, ed., *Anxiety*
(Basel: Karger, 1987).

43 The landmark "U.S.-U.K. study": J. E. Cooper, R. E. Kendell, et al.,
*Psychiatric Diagnosis in New York and London: A Comparative Study of Mental
Hospital Admissions* (London: Oxford University Press, 1972), p. 103.

44 "an unknown psychiatrist . . .": Quotation and accompanying history are
from Cade's wonderful brief memoir, "The Story of Lithium," in Frank J. Ayd
and Barry Blackwell, eds., *Discoveries in Biological Psychiatry* (Philadelphia:

J. B. Lippincott, 1970). The serendipity is discussed in Barry Blackwell's essay "The Process of Discovery," in ibid., pp. 11–29.

44 "pharmacological dissection": The phrase is in Klein, "Anxiety Reconceptualized," p. 235.

45 attempts to elucidate links between them: See the discussion of the functional theory of psychopathology, p. 182. One example of the backlash against splitting is a recent article by Michael Alan Taylor, "Are Schizophrenia and Affective Disorder Related? A Selective Literature Review," *American Journal of Psychiatry*, vol. 149 (1992), pp. 22–32. Its abstract begins: "Although most modern investigators accept the Kraepelinian view that schizophrenia and affective disorder are biologically distinct, others have suggested the psychoses are on a continuum of liability. This article is a selective review of evidence for the continuum model." (p. 22.) Affective disorder, of course, includes manic depression, so the monograph is a reconsideration of Kraepelin's seminal diagnostic distinction. A second, quite different example is an important study demonstrating common genetic factors in depression and an anxiety disorder in women: Kenneth S. Kendler, Michael C. Neale, et al., "Major Depression and Generalized Anxiety Disorder: Same Genes, (Partly) Different Environments?," *Archives of General Psychiatry*, vol. 49 (1992), pp. 716–22.

CHAPTER 3: ANTIDEPRESSANTS

47 Associated Press photograph of 1953: Mark Caldwell, *The Last Crusade: The War on Consumption, 1862–1954* (New York: Atheneum, 1988), opposite p. 245.

47 "psychic energizer": Nathan S. Kline, "Monoamine Oxidase Inhibitors: An Unfinished Picaresque Tale," in Frank J. Ayd and Barry Blackwell, eds., *Discoveries in Biological Psychiatry* (Philadelphia: J. B. Lippincott, 1970), pp. 194–204.

48 "The plethora of id energy . . .": Ibid., p. 197.

48 "Probably no drug in history . . .": Ibid., p. 202.

48 a more potent antidepressant coming to market: The newer antidepressant, isocarboxazid, carries a "less-than-effective" indication from the Food and Drug Administration.

49 the most effective drug treatment . . . opium: Ronald Kuhn, "The Imipramine Story," in Ayd and Blackwell, eds., *Discoveries*, pp. 205–17. It turns out that medications that treat almost any mental condition can have a positive effect in depressed people. Today we criticize general practitioners for using anxiolytic (antianxiety) agents, like Valium, or neuroleptic (antipsychotic) agents, like Thorazine, or simple stimulants, like amphetamine, for depressed patients. There are good reasons to avoid these medications: the anxiolytics and stimulants can be habituating, and the neuroleptics can cause late-appearing and irreversible neurological damage. But studies show that all these classes of medication make depressed people feel better. One reason depressed patients improve on the "wrong" drugs is that depression results in, or comprises, a variety of symptoms—sadness, sleeplessness, feelings of guilt, loss of appetite, diminished concentration, listlessness—each of which can be terrible in itself. A medicine that, for example, allows a depressed patient to sleep better will be welcome, even if the underlying condition remains unaltered. But the individual brain is unique and complex; many brain pathways can become deranged in depression, and it seems now that some of these "wrong" drugs alleviate depression directly, through their effects on neurotransmitters other than norepinephrine and serotonin, in selected patients.

49   "to find a drug . . .": Ibid., p. 207.

50   "We have achieved a specific treatment . . .": Kuhn, "Imipramine Story," pp. 216–17.

50   "We knew that amphetamine . . .": Donald F. Klein, "Anxiety Reconceptualized," in Donald F. Klein and Judith G. Rabkin, eds., *Anxiety: New Research and Changing Concepts* (New York: Raven Press, 1981), pp. 235–61; quotation on p. 235.

52   the biogenic-amine theory of depression: A helpful review of both the strengths and flaws of this theory appears in Solomon H. Snyder, *The New Biology of Mood* (New York: Pfizer, 1988).

52   inactivated by "janitorial" enzymes: This metaphor was coined by Ross Baldessarini, a psychopharmacologist at Harvard Medical School and McLean Hospital.
    A fuller account of iproniazid's effect is: Neurotransmitter cells release biogenic amines into the synapse in discrete packets. When the janitorial enzyme (monoamine oxidase; see p. 55) fails to digest excess biogenic amine, two consequences result. First, the transmitting cell stuffs more neurotransmitter into each packet; and, second, in subsequent firings, not only does the transmitting cell release the packaged amine, it also allows the undisposed-of loose amine to pass into the synapse. The cell whose enzyme has been inhibited thus

provides more of the body's own excitatory neurotransmitters to the synapse and, therefore, to the receiving nerve cell.

52   This finding was taken as strong support: Of course, there was much other evidence for the biogenic-amine hypothesis, such as the fact that assays of the chemical content of the spinal fluid, blood, and urine of depressed people sometimes showed deficiencies in the breakdown products of biogenic amines. But some of these studies were contradictory, and all of them were equivocal. For instance, the biogenic amines are used *outside* the brain, and in much greater absolute amount than they are used within the brain; perhaps the low levels of breakdown products of biogenic amines in the urine of depressed patients is due to their lethargy and general lack of activity, not to a deficit of amines in the central nervous system. The strongest, most consistent evidence for the amine hypothesis remained the efficacy in treating depression of chemicals that increased the presence or effectiveness of biogenic amines.

53   a deficiency, depression: More precisely, depression relates to a deficiency in aminergic *transmission*. Scientists talk loosely about the "level" of biogenic amine as being high or low, or about a drug "acting on" or "raising" or "lowering" a given amine. It is hard to avoid falling into these locutions (and I will do so occasionally), but the issue is less the absolute amount of amine than the level of activity in the neural pathways in which amines are used as transmitters.

53   But it takes about four weeks: It generally takes two weeks to achieve an adequate blood (and brain) level of the antidepressant. Regarding the second two weeks, theories are now emerging, involving cellular regulation of amine production, that attempt to explain this time lag. One of the challenges in psychopharmacology remains the development of an antidepressant that does not take weeks to work.

53   only in about 20 percent: See Frederick K. Goodwin and William E. Bunney, Jr., "Depressions Following Reserpine: A Reevaluation," *Seminars in Psychiatry*, vol. 3 (1971), pp. 435–48.

54   drug development takes place by homology . . . analogy: I take these concepts from Ross Baldessarini, "Psychopharmacology for Psychosis and Affective Disorders: Receptors and Ligands," lecture, U.S. Psychiatric Congress, New York, November 1991.

54   70 percent . . . will improve on imipramine: However, they may not be free of depression. Many people classified in traditional studies as responders to drugs like imipramine are "better but not well." See Jerrold F. Rosenbaum,

"Depression and Polypharmacy," *Massachusetts General Hospital Clinical Psycho-pharmacology Unit Progress Notes,* vol. 3, no. 1 (1992).

56   MAOIs make blood pressure skyrocket: See Barry Blackwell, "The Process of Discovery," in Ayd and Blackwell, eds., *Discoveries,* pp. 11–29. Blackwell's reports appeared in 1964. The substance found in cheese is the amino acid tyramine. Other chemicals can also cause patients on MAOIs to develop hypertension. (In retrospect, perhaps physicians should have paid more heed to early reports of treated tubercular patients who suffered throbbing headaches and high blood pressure.)

56   American doctors remained wary of them: American psychiatrists, whose primary identity was often linked to psychotherapy, were traditionally highly concerned about physical side effects, relative to colleagues in countries where the identity of psychiatrists was clearly as physicians first and psychotherapists only secondarily. Even imipramine was very conservatively prescribed in the U.S. I do not want to leave the impression that MAOIs are impossibly dangerous drugs. They have a place today in the treatment of a variety of conditions and can be used safely by those who monitor their diet and avoid interacting medications. More selective MAOIs, including ones that do not cause the "cheese reaction," will likely be available here shortly.

57   *serotonin:* In the 1940s, a substance was identified in the blood serum that increased the constriction (tone) of blood vessels—hence, "serotonin." Serotonin was then found to be identical to an earlier-discovered substance known to be active in the gastrointestinal tract. Recognition of serotonin's role in the brain came only later.

57   came to be called "tricyclics": Some of the later-developed drugs had four carbon rings, so the class of drugs is more properly, but less commonly, called "heterocyclics."

60   the development of Prozac required serendipity: As Barry Blackwell pointed out when assessing Cade's work with lithium, "serendipity" originally referred not to blind luck but to deductions made by prepared minds. The fairy tale of the three princes of Serendip (an older name than Ceylon for Sri Lanka) told, for instance how one of them deduced "that a mule, blind in the right eye, had traveled the same road frequently because the grass was eaten only on the left side of the path." The word was apparently coined by Horace Walpole in 1754. (T. G. Remer, *Serendipity and the Three Princes* [Norman, Okla.: University of Oklahoma Press, 1965], cited in Blackwell, "Process of Discovery," pp. 14–15.)

60   The story begins in the 1960s: This history is based on a conversation with Ray W. Fuller, Brian B. Molloy, and David T. Wong at Eli Lilly's international headquarters in Indianapolis on December 9, 1991, and on a narrative provided me by Wong: David T. Wong, "History of Fluoxetine, a Selective Inhibitor of Serotonin Uptake and Antidepressant Drug (Prozac): My Recollection of the Formative Year," unpublished, 1991, 8 pp.

60   Fuller had worked with a method: Fuller's model was the chloroamphetamine-treated rat. Ironically, the model bore little fruit; it led to the development of an irreversible nerve toxin, useful in some basic research, but not to pharmaceuticals.

60   minimize the acetylcholine-related side effects: No one knew whether such a substance would affect depression. All antidepressants discovered to that time were anticholinergic, and it was thought that this property might be essential to antidepressants.

61   A particular book had caught Wong's attention: H. Weil-Malherbe and S. I. Szara, *The Biochemistry of Functional and Experimental Psychosis* (Springfield, Ill.: Charles C. Thomas, 1971).

61   a role for serotonin: The evidence, developed in the 1960s, was equivocal, but it seemed to show that there were lower levels of serotonin and its breakdown products in the brains of suicides than in those of people dying from heart disease. There was also evidence of low serotonin turnover in depressed patients. Evidence was also emerging from Europe of brain tracts that used serotonin, as opposed to norepinephrine, as the primary neurotransmitter. And, of course, it was known that both imipramine and the MAO inhibitors, in addition to affecting norepinephrine, had various effects on the breakdown or efficient use of serotonin.

63   In June 1974: David T. Wong, Jong S. Horng, et al., "A Selective Inhibitor of Serotonin Uptake: Lilly 110140, 3-(p-Trifluoromethylphenoxy-)-N-Methyl-3-Phenylpropylamine," *Life Sciences*, vol. 15 (1974), pp. 471–79. In the understated way that is typical of scientific reporting, they wrote: "We believe the discovery of specific inhibitors of 5HT reuptake like 110140 will help in elucidating the function of 5HT in brain and the importance of reuptake as an inactivating mechanism in 5HT neurotransmission. In addition, such an agent may find clinical use as a therapeutic agent." ("5HT" is the usual abbreviation for serotonin, whose chemical name is "5-hydroxytryptamine.") LY 110140 (fluoxetine hydrochloride, or Prozac) was probably the first selective serotonin-reuptake inhibitor, although others were soon developed, using independent lines of research, in Sweden, Holland, and elsewhere.

64 Prozac is a designed drug: That is, it was selected on the basis of a sought neurochemical effect. Today, drugs are "designed" structurally—molecules are selected based on their three-dimensional geometry, to fit particular chemical receptors.

66 reduced likelihood of effects on the heart: At about the time Prozac was released here, I had occasion to talk with the chairman of the psychiatry department of the University of Amsterdam. He told me that as a group psychiatrists in the Netherlands had decided to make a selective serotonin-reuptake inhibitor (like Prozac—perhaps not coincidentally, the one chosen in Holland is made by a Dutch manufacturer) the drug of first use in depression; their decision was based almost solely on the drug's lack of cardiac effects, and he said that, after the policy was instituted, they had in fact observed a decrease in successful suicides with antidepressants.

The case of a woman who took approximately one hundred Prozac capsules (two thousand milligrams) without adverse effects beyond nausea and drowsiness is reported in Jeffrey L. Moore and Robert Rodriguez, "Toxicity of Fluoxetine in Overdose," *American Journal of Psychiatry,* vol. 147 (1990), p. 1089 (letter).

66 patients . . . for whom Prozac is most helpful: For suggestive evidence that Prozac is especially effective in treating those with atypical and minor depression, see pp. 86–89 and 125–27.

CHAPTER 4: SENSITIVITY

72 To Klein, a number of hospitalized patients: See Donald F. Klein, "Psychiatric Diagnosis and a Typology of Clinical Drug Effects," *Psychopharmacologia* (Berlin), vol. 13 (1968), pp. 359–86; and Donald F. Klein, "Who Should Not Be Treated with Neuroleptics, but Often Are," in Frank Ayd, ed., *Rational Psychopharmacotherapy and the Right to Treatment* (Baltimore, Md.: Ayd Medical Communications, 1974). The monographs by Klein referred to in the notes on page 330 are also relevant.

73 the renowned analyst Elizabeth Zetzel: "On the So-Called Good Hysteric," in Elizabeth R. Zetzel, *The Capacity for Emotional Growth* (New York: International Universities Press, 1970), pp. 229–45. Zetzel ended her essay with this cautionary ditty:

There are many little girls
Whose complaints are little pearls

Of the classical hysterical neurotic.
And when this is true
Analysis can and should ensue,
But when this is false
'Twill be chaotic.

74 "These patients are usually females . . .": Donald F. Klein, "Approaches to Measuring the Efficacy of Drug Treatment of Personality Disorders: An Analysis and Program," in *Principles and Problems in Establishing the Efficacy of Psychotropic Agents* (Washington, D.C.: U.S. Department of HEW, Public Health Service No. 2138, 1971), pp. 187–204; quotation on pp. 194–95. For a similar description, see also Donald F. Klein, "Psychopharmacological Treatment and Delineation of Borderline Disorders," in Peter Hartocollis, ed., *Borderline Personality Disorders: The Concept, the Syndrome, the Patient* (New York: International Universities Press, 1977), pp. 365–83, especially pp. 372–73; Donald F. Klein, Rachel Gittelman, et al., *Diagnosis and Drug Treatment of Psychiatric Disorders: Adults and Children*, 2nd ed. (Baltimore, Md.: Williams & Wilkins, 1980), pp. 243–45. See also Michael R. Liebowitz and Donald F. Klein, "Hysteroid Dysphoria," *Psychiatric Clinics of North America*, vol. 2 (1979), pp. 555–75; Michael R. Liebowitz and Donald F. Klein, "Interrelationship of Hysteroid Dysphoria and Borderline Personality Disorder," *Psychiatric Clinics of North America*, vol. 4 (1981), pp. 67–87.

75 "a cause engenders an adaptive response . . .": Donald F. Klein, "Cybernetics, Activation, and Drug Effects," in R. H. Van den Hoofdakker, ed., "Biological Measures: Their Theoretical and Diagnostic Value in Psychiatry," *Acta Psychiatrica Scandinavica*, vol. 77, suppl. 341 (1988), pp. 126–37.

76 ". . . no need for these hypotheses": Klein made this assertion in the context of a discussion of panic anxiety, but he seems to hold the same position regarding rejection-sensitivity (Donald F. Klein, "Anxiety Reconceptualized," in Donald F. Klein and Judith G. Rabkin, eds., *Anxiety: New Research and Changing Concepts* [New York: Raven Press, 1981], pp. 235–61; quotation on p. 260).

77 "A crucial consequence . . .": Donald F. Klein, "Psychopharmacological Treatment and Delineation of Borderline Disorders," in Hartocollis, ed., *Borderline Personality Disorders*, p. 375. See also Klein, Gittelman, et al., *Diagnosis and Drug Treatment*, p. 440.

78 In 1895: "On the Grounds for Detaching a Particular Syndrome from Neurasthenia Under the Description 'Anxiety Neurosis,' " in James Strachey, ed., *The Standard Edition of the Complete Psychological Works of Sigmund Freud*,

vol. III (London: Hogarth Press, 1962), pp. 85–115. See also Sigmund Freud, "A Reply to Criticisms of My Paper on Anxiety Neurosis," in ibid., pp. 119–39.

78 "does not originate . . .": Ibid., p. 97.

79 One of my favorite footnotes: Sigmund Freud, "Miss Lucy R., Age 30," in Josef Breuer and Sigmund Freud, *Studies on Hysteria*, in Strachey, ed., *Standard Edition of Freud*, vol II (1955), pp. 106–24; footnote on 112–14. The footnote is a wonderful example of the early Freud—condensed, compelling, and amusing.

79 "neurosis" even encompassed conditions: According to the manual that defined official American psychiatric diagnoses from the late sixties until 1980, "neurosis" included conditions in which anxiety was "controlled unconsciously and automatically by conversion, displacement, and various other psychological mechanisms"—that is, in which it was out of the sufferer's awareness (American Psychiatric Association, *Diagnostic and Statistical Manual of Mental Disorders*, 2nd ed. [Washington, D.C.: American Psychiatric Association, 1968], p. 39). The definition of anxiety neurosis does use the word "panic," but in practice the diagnosis was applied promiscuously.

80 his followers, came to see meaningful anxiety: I am here simplifying what is in fact a diverse literature. As early as 1941, the respected psychoanalyst Phyllis Greenacre argued for a return to acknowledgment of a substantial biological and genetic component to anxiety. She distinguished unanalyzable (basic, blind, or amorphous) anxiety (also called the "essential" neurosis) from experiential and secondary anxieties; she advocated a modified psychoanalysis for severely anxious patients, one that would take into account the irreducible nature of aspects of their ailment. In these regards, she anticipated contemporary models of etiology and treatment. (See "The Predisposition to Anxiety," in Phyllis Greenacre, *Trauma, Growth, and Personality* [New York: W. W. Norton, 1952], pp. 27–82.) I want to thank Donald Klein for pointing me in the direction of Greenacre's work.

80 "The predominant American psychiatric theory . . .": Klein, "Anxiety Reconceptualized," p. 235.

81 "By the third week . . .": Klein, "Anxiety Reconceptualized," p. 238.

82 Klein did hypothesize about the origin: Donald F. Klein and Hilary M. Klein, "The Definition and Psychopharmacology of Spontaneous Panic and Phobia," in P. J. Tyrer, ed., *Psychopharmacology of Anxiety* (London: Oxford University Press, 1989), pp. 135–62; Donald F. Klein and Hilary M. Klein,

"The Nosology, Genetics, and Theory of Spontaneous Panic and Phobia," in ibid., pp. 163–95; Rachel Gittelman and Donald F. Klein, "Relationship Between Separation Anxiety and Panic and Agoraphobic Disorder," *Psychopathology*, vol. 17, suppl. 1 (1984), pp. 56–65; Donald F. Klein and Michael R. Liebowitz, "Psychotherapeutic Attitudes in the Drug Treatment of Anxiety and Phobic Reactions," in Maurice H. Greenhill and Alexander Gralnick, eds., *Psychopharmacology and Psychotherapy* (New York: Free Press, 1982), pp. 145–63; Donald F. Klein, "False Suffocation Alarms and Spontaneous Panics: Subsuming the CO_2 Hypersensitivity Theory," unpublished, draft of August 7, 1991, 85 pp.

84   lecture by an eminent psychoanalyst: John Nemiah, "The Psychoanalytic View of Anxiety," in Klein and Rabkin, *Anxiety*, pp. 291–330. The Nemiah talk was gracious but unyielding and could have been written at any time in the prior fifty years. His core statement is: "Anxiety is the reaction of the individual's ego . . . to the threatened emergence into conscious awareness of unpleasant, forbidden, unwanted, frightening impulses, feelings, and thoughts" (p. 294).

86   Donald Klein's model of panic anxiety now prevails: A curious side effect of the carving out of panic anxiety from generalized anxiety was the reopening of a lacuna on the diagnostic map; now that the anxiety disorders had specific meanings and "anxiety neurosis" had disappeared, there was no category to deal with "nervous exhaustion." Into this gap stepped . . . neurasthenia, which is now making a comeback! An entire issue of *Psychiatric Annals* (vol. 22, no. 4 [April 1992]), guest-edited by Joe Yamamoto, is dedicated to "Neurasthenia Revisited."

87   converging evidence of diverse sorts: Here I am relying heavily on research reported at the Neurobiology of Affective Disorders conference at Yale University School of Medicine, New Haven, Conn., October 25–26, 1991. The dietary L-tryptophan deprivation studies are the work of a team headed by Pedro Delgado and Dennis Charney at Yale (see Pedro L. Delgado, Dennis S. Charney, et al., "Serotonin Function and the Mechanism of Antidepressant Action: Reversal of Antidepressant-Induced Remission by Rapid Depletion of Plasma Tryptophan," *Archives of General Psychiatry*, vol. 47 [1990], pp. 411–18). The cellular-level research results are from Claude de Montigny of McGill University; the anatomical research is by Alan Frazer of the University of Pennsylvania.

The preliminary report on Prozac's effectiveness in atypical depression was given by Atul C. Pande, of the University of Michigan, at the Annual Meeting of the American Psychiatric Association, May 2–7, 1992, in Washington, D.C.

The issues are, of course, more complex than I have so far indicated. Considering only the question of where in the brain these medications act, even within a drug class there is variability. That is, different MAOIs are most active in different parts of the brain. This result should not surprise us, since sometimes a patient will respond to one MAOI but not another.

Researchers have identified subtypes of the monoamine-oxidase enzyme, just as they have identified numerous distinct subtypes of the serotonin receptor. There are already experimental medications that are selective for one or another subtype of MAO, as well as medications that selectively affect uptake at cells with specific serotonin-receptor subtypes. These laboratory findings are rapidly being translated into marketed drugs, so the story I am presenting here will soon have complex subplots.

91   "the interpersonal tactics . . .": Klein, Gittelman, et al., *Diagnosis and Drug Treatment*, p. 245.

91   Klein did twice rename: See Donald F. Klein, "Endogenomorphic Depression: A Conceptual and Terminological Revision," *Archives of General Psychiatry*, vol. 31 (1974), pp. 447–54; Klein, "Psychopharmacological Treatment," pp. 372–75. Klein's descriptions of hysteroid dysphoria, chronic overreactive dysphoria, and rejection-sensitive dysphoria are for all purposes identical. I have corresponded with Klein on the question whether people who are not histrionic can, in his diagnostic system, be rejection-sensitive. They can, but Klein limits rejection-sensitivity to a fairly small group—those diagnosed with hysteroid dysphoria and those in its immediate penumbra. Rejection-sensitivity, for Klein, always entails both vulnerability to loss and a strong drive for positive attention; even nonhysteroid rejection-sensitivity is characterized by touchiness rather than clinging in relationships. My definition is broader: I have come to see rejection-sensitivity as applying to people who respond to loss with symptoms of atypical depression, whether or not applause hunger is a prominent feature. Klein would characterize some of these people as having separation anxiety, even though their symptoms entail depression rather than panic. I reserve separation anxiety for the infantile behavior that serves as a possible model for panic in adults.

96   "aloneness affect": Ronald M. Winchel, "Self-Mutilation and Aloneness," *Academy Forum* (of the American Academy of Psychoanalysis), vol. 35 (1991), pp. 10–12.

97   a particular element of personality: That element of personality, under differing names, has long been a focus of psychotherapy. Psychoanalysis pays great attention to the patient's reaction to brief interruptions in the relationship, not least the analyst's famous August vacation. Brief separations test the patient's ability to tolerate loss. And the end of therapy—the termination phase—is the subject of an extensive literature. Some brief therapies, especially ones used for healthy college students, rely heavily on the stress of termination. Patient and therapist agree to meet for twelve sessions, and half of the therapy concerns the patient's inability to tolerate that agreement—that is, to experience the end of a relationship without the usual distortions that result from his or her customary style of avoiding the pain of separation. See James Mann, *Time-Limited Psychotherapy* (Cambridge, Mass.: Harvard University Press, 1973).

CHAPTER 5: STRESS

108 "rapid cycling": Much of this material is from Robert M. Post and James C. Ballenger, eds., *Neurobiology of Mood Disorders* (Baltimore, Md.: Williams & Wilkins, 1984), especially Post's own contributions to that book. I have also relied on a lecture, Robert M. Post, "Episode and Stress Sensitization in the Longitudinal Course of Affective Disorders: Role of Proto-Oncogenes and Other Transcription Factors," Neurobiology of Affective Disorders conference, Yale University School of Medicine, New Haven, Conn., October 25–26, 1991.

See also Robert M. Post, Keith G. Kramlinger, et al., "Treatment of Rapid Cycling Bipolar Illness," *Psychopharmacology Bulletin,* vol. 26 (1990), pp. 37–47; R. M. Post, "Sensitization and Kindling Perspectives for the Course of Affective Illness: Toward a New Treatment with the Anticonvulsant Carbamazepine," *Pharmacopsychiatry,* vol. 23 (1990), pp. 3–17; Robert M. Post, David R. Rubinow, and James C. Ballenger, "Conditioning and Sensitization in the Longitudinal Course of Affective Illness," *British Journal of Psychiatry,* vol. 149 (1986), pp. 191–201; Robert M. Post, "Transduction of Psychosocial Stress into the Neurobiology of Recurrent Affective Disorder," *American Journal of Psychiatry,* in press; Robert M. Post, "Prophylaxis of Bipolar Affective Disorders," *International Review of Psychiatry,* vol. 2 (1990), pp. 277–320; Robert M. Post, Gabriele S. Leverich, et al., "Carbamazepine Prophylaxis in Refractory Affective Disorders: A Focus on Long-Term Follow-Up," *Journal of Clinical Psychopharmacology,* vol. 10 (1990), pp. 318–27.

The trend toward increasing frequency and severity of episodes with recurrence is almost certainly not limited to manic-depressive illness but occurs in "unipolar" (i.e., without mania) depression as well. See, for example, Mario Maj, Franco Veltro, et al., "Pattern of Recurrence of Illness After Recovery from an Episode of Major Depression: A Prospective Study," *American Journal of Psychiatry,* vol. 149 (1992), pp. 795–800.

110 "negative feedback loop": More precisely, a negative feedback system is one in which output of a product inhibits further production of that product—for example, a rising level of thyroid hormone inhibits the production and release of thyroid hormone. This is the most common homeostatic mechanism in biology. See, for example, Peter C. Whybrow, Hagop S. Akiskal, and William T. McKinney, Jr., *Mood Disorder: Toward a New Psychobiology* (New York: Plenum Publishing, 1984), pp. 98–101.

110 Seizures are "kindled" in an experimental animal: The reader may be made uncomfortable or even outraged by some of the animal experiments I describe. My own less judgmental attitude arises from having spent many hours with seriously depressed patients in the search for whose cure I would willingly sacrifice any number of rats and mice, or separate monkey infants from their mothers. Though crucial to our understanding of human mental disorder, animal research can be cruel.

One of the oddities of research is that, though antidepressants are used mostly in depressed human females, they are tested mostly in healthy male rats: the estrus cycle in rats is four to five days, creating constant hormonal variability in females, which makes data analysis difficult and adds greatly to the complexity of experimental design and the number of animals needed. However, testing of female rats would be of interest, because they appear to differ from male rats in terms of stress responses and brain anatomy. (I thank Dr. Huda Akil of the University of Michigan for answering my inquiry on these points.) In earlier decades, "reserpinized" rats—ones whose biogenic amines had been depleted to produce "depression"—were widely used for drug testing; in recent years, this model has been dropped as unwieldy.

112 Some cells . . . change shape: Other animal models, using various sorts of stress to change brain-hormone levels, also show anatomical changes, including cell atrophy and death. There are, in fact, numerous models of stress that cause changes in cell shape, synapse numbers, and local synapse density. See in particular the work of Bruce S. McEwen, of Rockefeller University.

114 Thereafter, antiepileptic drugs, such as Tegretol: Depakote is another anticonvulsant, more recently studied, that may be especially effective in refractory, late-stage manic-depressive illness. It is interesting that antidepressants and anticonvulsants act in a stabilizing way at two levels: at the organismic level, they affect mood balance in response to stress; at the cellular level, they affect the cell's protein production in response to stress. It is not known whether this second effect is a result of the first.

116 Cortisol levels . . . high in many acutely depressed adults: But not in acutely depressed adolescents, a finding that reverberates with our theme of kindling: the human organism becomes less flexible—less able to recuperate— with aging and repeated injury.

116 according to imaging studies: See, for example, Charles B. Nemeroff, K. Ranga, R. Krishnan, et al., "Adrenal Gland Enlargement in Major Depression: A Computed Tomographic Study," *Archives of General Psychiatry*, vol. 49 (1992), pp. 384–87.

116 Rats can be stressed: I have taken much of this material from a lecture by Bruce S. McEwen, "Glucocorticoid Actions in the Hippocampus: Implications for Affective Disorders," Neurobiology of Affective Disorders conference, Yale University School of Medicine, New Haven, Conn., October 25– 26, 1991. See also Whybrow, Akiskal, and McKinney, *Mood Disorder*.

118 160 girls: This study, headed by Frank Putnam, was reported on in *Clinical Psychiatry News*, vol. 19, no. 12 (December 1991), p. 3ff.

118 research on mood in rhesus monkeys: I am here largely reviewing the work of Stephen J. Suomi. See especially Stephen J. Suomi, "Primate Separation Models of Affective Disorder," in John Madden IV, ed., *Neurobiology of Learning, Emotion, and Affect* (New York: Raven Press, 1991), pp. 195–214; Stephen J. Suomi, "Early Stress and Adult Emotional Reactivity in Rhesus Monkeys," in *The Childhood Environment and Adult Disease*, Ciba Foundation Symposium 156 (Chichester: Wiley, 1991), pp. 171–88. See also Stephen J. Suomi, "Uptight and Laid-Back Monkeys: Individual Differences in the Response to Social Challenges," in S. Branch, W. Hall, and E. Dooling, eds., *Plasticity of Development* (Cambridge, Mass.: M.I.T. Press, 1991), pp. 27–55; J. Dee Higley, Stephen J. Suomi, and Markuu Linnoila, "Developmental Influences on the Serotonergic System and Timidity in the Nonhuman Primate," in Emil F. Coccaro and Dennis L. Murphy, eds., *Serotonin in Major Psychiatric Disorders* (Washington, D.C.: American Psychiatric Press, 1990), pp. 29–46; Stephen J. Suomi, Harry F. Harlow, and Carol J. Domek, "Effect of Repetitive Infant-Infant Separation of Young Monkeys," *Journal of Abnormal Psychology*, vol. 76 (1970), pp. 161– 72; Stephen J. Suomi, Stephen F. Seaman, et al., "Effects of Imipramine Treatment of Separation-Induced Social Disorders in Rhesus Monkeys," *Archives of General Psychiatry*, vol. 35 (1978), pp. 321–25; J. D. Higley, S. J. Suomi, and M. Linnoila, "CSF Monoamine Metabolite Concentrations Vary According to Age, Rearing, and Sex, and Are Influenced by the Stressor of Social Separation in Rhesus Monkeys," *Psychopharmacology*, vol. 103 (1991), pp. 551–56.

119 rapidly become attached to their peers: At eleven weeks, a monkey infant will interact as often with other monkey infants as with his or her mother, and by the age of six months, young monkeys have four or five times as many contacts with age-mates as with their mothers. Except in unusual circumstances, fathering is much less important to young rhesus monkeys than are ties to mother and peers.

119 best-known study: Harry F. Harlow and Robert R. Zimmerman, "Affectional Responses in the Infant Monkey," *Science,* vol. 130 (1959), pp. 421–32.

121 "Moreover, the same basic pattern . . .": Suomi, "Early Stress and Adult Emotional Reactivity," p. 177. See also Higley, Suomi, and Linnoila, "Developmental Influences."

124 "the memory of the body": I think here of a passage from the Jane Smiley novella "Ordinary Love." To a brother who has witnessed suffering, a young man asks: "Would you prefer not to have seen it?" The affected brother replies: "I would prefer not to be shaped by experiences. I would like just to have them, not to incorporate them." (*Ordinary Love and Good Will* [New York: Ballantine, 1989], p. 80.) Our troubling experiences are not just known to us; they become us.

I think also of dialogue in Smiley's short story "Long Distance" (*The Age of Grief* [New York: Ballantine, 1987], pp. 61–79), in which a man who is hurting over a love affair says, "It seems so dramatic to say that I will never get over this." His sister-in-law replies, "Does it? To me it seems like saying that what people do is important." To say that loss is biologically encoded, perhaps irreversibly, is to say that what people do and experience is important.

125 This new method: The role of antidepressants in prevention of recurrence, while now widely accepted, remains controversial. Important contrary research, pioneered by Frederick K. Goodwin at the National Institute of Mental Health, shows that, in patients prone to recurrent depression, tricyclics—and perhaps all antidepressants—can *hasten* the onset of subsequent episodes and increase cyclicity. The field has not reconciled the two contradictory bodies of evidence.

126 universities in Denmark: Danish University Antidepressant Group, "Citalopram: Clinical Effect Profile in Comparison with Clomipramine: A Controlled Multicenter Study," *Psychopharmacology,* vol. 90 (1986), pp. 131–38; Danish University Antidepressant Group, "Paroxetine: A Selective Serotonin Reuptake Inhibitor Showing Better Tolerance, but Weaker Antidepressant Effect than Clomipramine in a Controlled Multicenter Study," *Journal of Affective Disorders,* vol. 18 (1990), pp. 289–99.

126 A group at Indiana University: Stephen R. Dunlop, Bruce E. Dornseif, et al., "Pattern Analysis Shows Beneficial Effect of Fluoxetine Treatment in Mild Depression," *Psychopharmacology Bulletin*, vol. 26 (1990), pp. 173–80.

126 Psychiatrists at the University of Utah: Fred W. Reimherr, David R. Wood, et al., "Characteristics of Responders to Fluoxetine," *Psychopharmacology Bulletin*, vol. 20 (1984), pp. 70–72. The Prozac responders also tended to meet Donald Klein's criteria for atypical depression.

126 Taken together, these studies: J. Craig Nelson, of Yale University, juxtaposed these four articles and brought them to my attention.

127 psychotherapy will affect neural structure: Biological technologies are only just beginning to be applied to the study of psychotherapy. An intriguing preliminary report, albeit still far from the level of cellular repair, is Lewis R. Baxter, Jr., Jeffrey M. Schwartz, et al., "Caudate Glucose Metabolic Rate Changes with Both Drug and Behavior Therapy for Obsessive-Compulsive Disorder," *Archives of General Psychiatry*, vol. 49 (1992), pp. 681–89. In this experiment, ten weeks of behavioral instruction, supplemented by cognitive therapy, was shown to resemble Prozac in its ability to change metabolism in a part of the brain thought to be affected by OCD.

127 exposed to "therapists": Suomi, "Early Stress and Adult Emotional Reactivity."

128 the great hypnotist Milton Erickson: See Jay Haley, *Uncommon Therapy: The Psychiatric Techniques of Milton Erickson* (New York: W. W. Norton, 1973).

128 those that emphasize empathy: I have in mind self psychology. The central image of healing in self psychology is "transmuting internalization": the patient takes in a function previously provided by the therapist, and this taking in, rather than insight, results in a changed structure of mind. A typical jibe at self psychology goes, "The couch is not a bassinet" (George Vaillant, "Managing Defense Mechanisms in Personality Disorders," lecture, U.S. Psychiatric Congress, New York, November 1991). That is, although self psychology does rely on interpretations and insight as techniques, its critics see it as fundamentally an attempt at reparenting and nothing more.

130 prone to repeated alcohol consumption: J. D. Higley, M. F. Hasert, et al., "Nonhuman Primate Model of Alcohol Abuse: Effects of Early Experience, Personality, and Stress on Alcohol Consumption," *Proceedings of the National Academy of Sciences, U.S.A.* (Psychology), vol. 88 (1991), pp. 7261–65. The "not specialized" quip is from Vaillant, "Managing Defense Mechanisms."

131 In the mid-1960s: See William E. Bunney and John M. Davis, "Nor-epinephrine in Depressive Reactions: A Review," *Archives of General Psychiatry*, vol. 13 (1965), pp. 483–94; Joseph J. Schildkraut, "The Catecholamine Hypothesis of Affective Disorders: A Review of Supporting Evidence," *American Journal of Psychiatry*, vol. 122 (1965), pp. 509–22. These were enormously influential publications.

131 By the mid-1970s: James W. Maas, "Biogenic Amines and Depression: Biochemical and Pharmacological Separation of Two Types of Depression," *Archives of General Psychiatry*, vol. 32 (1975), pp. 1357–61.

131 in the 1980s: Dennis S. Charney, David B. Menkes, and George R. Heninger, "Receptor Sensitivity and the Mechanisms of Action of Antidepressant Treatment: Implications for the Etiology and Therapy of Depression," *Archives of General Psychiatry*, vol. 38 (1981), pp. 1160–80; Dennis S. Charney, Pedro L. Delgado, et al., "The Receptor Sensitivity Hypothesis of Antidepressant Action: A Review of Antidepressant Effects on Serotonin Function," in Serena-Lynn Brown and Herman M. van Praag, eds., *The Role of Serotonin in Psychiatric Disorders* (New York: Brunner/Mazel, 1991), pp. 27–56.

132 meshes well with the animal studies: I have presented the postsynaptic-receptor-sensitivity model in highly simplified form. But see Robert M. Cohen and Iain C. Campbell, "Receptor Adaptation in Animal Models of Mood Disorders: A State Change Approach to Psychiatric Illness," in Post and Ballenger, eds., *Neurobiology of Mood Disorders*, pp. 572–86.

133 Prozac does not downregulate norepinephrine receptors: In almost all experimental models in which tricyclics downregulate norepinephrine receptors, Prozac fails to do so, although, as always, there is an exception, and in one line of research Prozac *has* been shown to downregulate a receptor in one part of the brain. It does seem that, when the drugs are given in combination, Prozac quickens desipramine's downregulation of norepinephrine receptors; this may be due to an interesting pharmacologic synergy at the cellular level, or it may be an artefact related to Prozac's interference with the metabolism of desipramine.

134 "Maybe serotonin is the police . . .": There is a serious scientific model that in some regards corresponds to serotonin-as-police: the "permissive biogenic amine hypothesis" proposed by A. J. Prange. According to this theory, serotonin deficiency permits depression but is an insufficient cause; the emergence of overt depression depends on changes in norepinephrine or other transmitters. (That is, low serotonin + normal norepinephrine = normal affective state; low serotonin + low norepinephrine = depression; and low serotonin + high

norepinephrine = mania. But, again, this model is too simple to explain a variety of phenomena.) See Arthur J. Prange, Jr., Ian C. Wilson, et al., "L-Tryptophan in Mania: Contribution to a Permissive Hypothesis of Affective Disorders," *Archives of General Psychiatry*, vol. 30 (1974), pp. 56–62. What I have in mind when I refer to serotonin-as-police goes beyond the permissive hypothesis and implies that serotonin has a role in the maintenance of confidence, assertiveness, and overall social and emotional resilience.

136 "late-onset depression": An excellent summary, albeit by authors who doubt the validity of the late-onset/early-onset distinction, is Henry Brodaty, Karin Peters, et al., "Age and Depression," *Journal of Affective Disorders*, vol. 23 (1991), pp. 137–49.

142 So unwilling was a distant friend of Levi's: Esther B. Fein, "Book Notes: A British Doctor Casts Doubt on Primo Levi's Suicide . . . ," *New York Times*, December 11, 1991, p. C26. The background material is from an essay in *The New York Times Book Review* by Alexander Stille. For a relevant perspective on judgmental views of suicide, see Alexander Gralnick, "Is Suicide a Cause of Death?," *American Journal of Social Psychiatry*, vol. 5 (1985), pp. 24–28.

CHAPTER 6: RISK

147 mania is an infrequent bad outcome: Although there are scant data on the subject, many psychiatrists believe Prozac causes this side effect more frequently than do tricyclic antidepressants.

147 half a capsule per day (ten milligrams): Regarding dosage, see the note to p. 28, on pp. 321–22.

148 the words used to describe: Here I am relying mostly on the usage of Hagop Akiskal. See his chapter, "Validating Affective Personality Types," in Lee N. Robins and James E. Barrett, *The Validity of Psychiatric Diagnosis* (New York: Raven Press, 1989), pp. 217–27. I have added in concepts from Alexander Thomas and Stella Chess, *Temperament and Development* (New York: Brunner/Mazel, 1977), and others. This particular usage of "temperament" (nature), "character" (nurture), and "personality" (both) was employed by David Riesman in *The Lonely Crowd* (New Haven, Conn.: Yale University Press, 1950), and before that in psychiatry by Erich Fromm. See Daniel Burston, *The Legacy of Erich Fromm* (Cambridge, Mass.: Harvard University Press, 1991).

149 temperament . . . the tar pit of psychological research: A notable exception is the acceptance, especially in the field of child development, of the

work of Alexander Thomas and Stella Chess. In addition to *Temperament and Development*, cited above, see Stella Chess and Alexander Thomas, *Temperament in Clinical Practice* (New York: Guilford Press, 1986). The authors have summarized their research in a book for a general audience, Stella Chess and Alexander Thomas, *Know Your Child: An Authoritative Guide for Today's Parents* (New York: Basic Books, 1987). Their key concept is the importance of "goodness of fit" between the child and the family in which he or she is raised.

150 Kagan began with three hundred: Jerome Kagan, J. Steven Reznick, and Nancy Snidman, "Biological Basis of Childhood Shyness," *Science*, vol. 240 (1988), pp. 167–71; Cynthia Garcia Coll, Jerome Kagan, and J. Steven Reznick, "Behavioral Inhibition in Young Children," *Child Development*, vol. 55 (1984), pp. 1005–19; Jerome Kagan, J. Steven Reznick, et al., "Behavioral Inhibition to the Unfamiliar," *Child Development*, vol. 55 (1984), pp. 2212–25.

151 "A frequent scene . . .": Kagan, Reznick, and Snidman, "Biological Basis," p. 168.

151 *lack* of inhibition was not a special category: In some of the studies, extreme lack of inhibition did look like a discontinuous, distinct category.

151 15 percent of children are born inhibited: Ruth M. Galvin, "The Nature of Shyness," *Harvard Magazine*, vol. 94 (1992), pp. 40–45; see especially p. 41. Just what this statement means is not perfectly clear. Kagan has observed that 10 to 15 percent of two- and three-year-olds are inhibited. Whether these come from a larger pool with predispositions to be inhibited, or from a smaller pool which is then supplemented by children who are traumatized, is unclear; a much smaller percentage of adults is openly shy.

151 In his study: Garcia Coll, Kagan, and Reznick, "Behavioral Inhibition," and Kagan, Reznick, et al., "Behavioral Inhibition."

151 "for every ten children . . .": Galvin, "The Nature of Shyness," p. 45. (Here Galvin is paraphrasing Kagan.)

152 even when asleep: Jerome Kagan, Grand Rounds, Bradley Hospital, Providence, R.I., December 1987.

153 "most of the children . . ." and subsequent quotations: Kagan, Reznick, and Snidman, "Biological Basis," p. 171.

153 before having studied: Kagan had shown some behavioral continuity in relation to inhibited play in infants as young as fourteen months—he could pick out a group half of whom still looked inhibited on retesting at age four years. Kagan, Reznick, and Snidman, "Biological Bases," p. 169.

154 In the 1960s, Kagan was a leader: Kagan was a figure to whom television anchors and other media reporters turned for comments in the IQ controversy. That debate was sparked by an article by the psychologist Arthur Jensen in a 1969 issue of the *Harvard Educational Review*, vol. 39, pp. 1–123. In reply, Kagan contended that the concept of intelligence is culturally defined and that IQ tests are culturally biased. He emphasized mother-child interaction as a key environmental contributor to intelligence. Kagan concluded that, although genetic constitution might set "a range of mental ability," the genetic contribution to IQ was unknown, and that this uncertainty applied even more strongly to the vague concept "intelligence." See Jerome S. Kagan, "Inadequate Evidence and Illogical Conclusions," *Harvard Educational Review*, vol. 39 (1969), pp. 274–77, a reply to the Jensen essay; Jerome Kagan, "IQ: Fair Science for Dark Deeds," *Radcliffe Quarterly*, vol. 56 (1972), pp. 3–5. For an overview of popular coverage and impact of the debate, see Mark Snyderman and Stanley Rothman, *The IQ Controversy, the Media and Public Policy* (New Brunswick, N.J.: Transaction Books, 1988).

155 Among white children: See Jerome Kagan and Nancy Snidman, "Infant Predictors of Inhibited and Uninhibited Profiles," *Psychological Science*, vol. 2 (1991), pp. 40–44. Most of the subjects in the early studies were middle-to-upper-class white children.

155 an excess of allergies: Jerome Kagan, Nancy Snidman, et al., "Temperament and Allergic Symptoms," *Psychosomatic Medicine*, vol. 53 (1991), pp. 332–40. There is suggestive evidence that, especially in women, migraine headaches and gastrointestinal symptoms are additional features associated with inhibition.

155 A group at Brown: L. La Gasse, C. Gruber, and L. P. Lipsett, "The Infantile Expression of Avidity in Relation to Later Assessments," in J. Steven Reznick, ed., *Perspectives on Behavioral Inhibition* (Chicago: University of Chicago Press, 1989), pp. 159–76.

155 Kagan's group tested four-month-olds: Kagan and Snidman, "Infant Predictors."

156 among mildly depressed adults: This result was reported by Radwan F. Haykal at the May 1992 Annual Meeting of the American Psychiatric Association in Washington, D.C., in conjunction with his presentation, "Is Early Onset Dysthymia More Treatable Today?" Haykal is a student and co-worker of Hagop Akiskal, whose research we will discuss later in this chapter.

156 Suomi . . . 20 percent: This and much of what follows is from Stephen J. Suomi, "Uptight and Laid-Back Monkeys: Individual Differences in the Response to Social Challenges," in S. Branch, W. Hall, and E. Dooling, eds., *Plasticity of Development* (Cambridge, Mass.: M.I.T. Press, 1991), pp. 27–55.

156 "differences in response to novelty . . .": Ibid., p. 38.

157 differences . . . only in response to novelty: The important role of novelty as a stimulus is crucial in humans, too. Kagan keeps pinned above his desk a note from a mother of one of the inhibited children he observed: "If something is new and different, his inclination is to be quiet and watch. . . . It's unfamiliarity that's the cause of his behavior. Not just new people, but *newness.*" (Quoted in Galvin, "Nature of Shyness," p. 41.) "Inhibition" in Kagan's usage is less social inhibition than inhibition to the unfamiliar, although in practice the two forms of inhibition seem linked.

157 earlier monkey studies: Summarized in Suomi, "Uptight and Laid-Back Monkeys," pp. 40–41.

157 in anticipation of irritating noise: In this model, infants are conditioned by being exposed to a steady tone followed by irritating white noise; in time, they show a conditioned response, a decrease in heart rate in response to the steady tone. Ibid. However, among unconditioned young monkeys, as in humans, those "who show extreme stress reactions typically have very high and stable heartrates relative to their less reactive counterparts faced with identical stressors, and these heartrate patterns are predictive of later extreme behavioral reactions with different kinds of stressors." Currents Interview, "In Our Wild: Studies from a Rhesus Colony" (interview with Stephen J. Suomi), *Currents in Affective Illness*, vol. 11 (1992), pp. 5–14, quotation p. 6.

157 among *half*-siblings: These studies have stood up to more recent replication. In addition, observations have found the fathers of reactive half-siblings themselves to be reactive on a variety of measures. (Stephen J. Suomi, "Primate Separation Models of Affective Disorders," in John Madden, ed., *Neurobiology of Learning, Emotion and Affect* [New York: Raven Press, 1991], pp. 195–214.)

157 second offspring . . . given to adoptive mothers: Merely being adopted out does not appear to increase reactivity in rhesus monkeys.

158 "Clearly, for these infants . . .": Suomi, "Uptight and Laid-Back Monkeys," p. 49. The style of the adoptive mothers did affect other traits and behaviors (particularly closeness to the mother when she was present) but not reactivity; as they grew, uptight infants appeared normal when with their mothers but more disturbed when separated.

More recent observations by Suomi suggest that nervous, shy infants foster-reared by unusually nurturant mothers grow up precocious and socially adept. In particular, when subjected to social stress these monkeys tend to recruit others to help—and this trait enhances their social status in the troop. (Currents Interview, "In Our Wild," p. 8.) It is interesting to speculate that the "reactive" trait may confer evolutionary fitness because it sometimes leads not to inhibition but to a particular coping skill: social collaboration. Perhaps social facilitation is the healthy version of reactivity and "people pleasing" is not so much a weakness as the characteristic strength of otherwise inhibited individuals.

158 become withdrawn or depressed: Suomi, "Uptight and Laid-Back Monkeys," p. 42.

158 parallel abnormalities in neurotransmitters: The uptight monkeys have higher-than-normal levels and turnover of stress hormones in their bloodstreams. In their spinal fluid, after separation they have lower levels of norepinephrine and higher levels of norepinephrine-breakdown products—preseumably a sign that they are exhausting the system—than do normally reactive monkeys. These abnormalities can be prevented with antidepressants, and the attenuation is most pronounced in the most uptight monkeys.

158 prone to both: Currents Interview, "In Our Wild," p. 6. Suomi believes the same individuals are at risk for both anxiety and depression, and the behavioral pattern elicited depends on which stressors the monkey encounters in life. Interestingly, both "reactivity" and the accompanying anxious and depressive patterns of behavior occur equally between the genders before puberty. But reactivity in males becomes blunted during adolescence, when for females it becomes more extreme. Ibid., pp. 7–8.

158 drink more when under stress: Ibid., p. 13.

159 to show allergic reactions: Ibid., p. 7.

159 they can be born uptight: In lower animals, there have been attempts to breed for temperament. For example, in mice the amount of activity displayed in a brightly lit open field is thought to be a marker for emotional reactivity. Mice were selectively bred to be high or low on this test trait. After thirty generations, the mice displayed a thirtyfold difference in terms of activity in this environment, with no overlap between the scores of the high and low line. (J. C. De Fries, J. C. Gervais, and E. A. Thomas, in *Behavioral Genetics*, vol. 8 [1978], p. 3, cited in Robert Plomin, "The Role of Inheritance in Behavior," *Science*, vol. 248 [1990], pp. 183–88.)

159 "consistently sociable . . .": Kagan and Snidman, "Infant Predictors."

159   "those reserved . . .": Carl Jung, *Psychological Types,* trans. R. F. C. Hull (Princeton, N.J.: Princeton University Press, 1971), p. 330. The subsequent quotes are from pp. 331–32.

160   in 1934: The complete quote is: "The Aryan unconscious has a higher potential than the Jewish; this is the advantage and the disadvantage of a youthfulness not yet fully escaped from barbarism. In my opinion it has been a great mistake of all previous medical psychology to apply Jewish categories which are not binding even to Jews, indiscriminately to Christians, Germans, or Slavs. In doing so, medical psychology has declared the most precious secret of the Germanic peoples—the creatively prophetic depths of soul—to be a childishly banal morass. . . ."

Whether Jung merely reflected the scientific racism of his times, or whether he contributed to it, is a difficult matter. My reading of *Psychological Types* is that it is dangerously, one might say irresponsibly, romantic. As for the editorship of the *Zentralblatt,* my sense is that Jung had a cultural contempt for the Nazis but was guilty of opportunism at Freud's and his colleagues' expense in a way that, because of what followed, reflects very badly on Jung. See my column, "Matters of Taste," *Psychiatric Times,* September 1988, p. 3ff; Vincent Brome, *Jung* (New York: Atheneum, 1978). However, many respected scholars consider Jung blameless and misunderstood; it appears he was helpful personally to certain Jewish physicians during the war. Those interested in the broader subject might consult Robert Jay Lifton's *The Nazi Doctors* (New York: Basic Books, 1986); and Geoffrey Cocks's eye-opening *Psychotherapy in the Third Reich* (Oxford: Oxford University Press, 1985).

160   her studies in the 1930s: Margaret Mead, *Sex and Temperament in Three Primitive Societies* (New York: William Morrow, 1963, orig. 1935), cited in Carl N. Degler, *In Search of Human Nature: The Decline and Revival of Darwinism in American Thought* (New York: Oxford University Press, 1991), p. 134.

161   "The main impetus . . .": Degler, *In Search,* p. viii. Degler points to many cultural and scientific factors that have led to the resurgence of interest in biology. One interesting minor detail (ibid., pp. 225, 232) is his tracing of the revival of interest among political scientists in biology to an article on ethology and psychopharmacology. Even though the author, Albert Somit, was not certain that antidepressants directly treated depression (he held open the possibility they might be facilitating psychotherapy), he believed that the effects of psychotherapeutic drugs in humans confirmed the relevance of animal ethology to human behavior. ("Toward a More Biologically-Oriented Political Science: Ethology and Pharmacology," *Midwest Journal of Political Science,* vol. 12 [1968], pp. 550–67.)

161   Kagan has speculated: Galvin, "Nature of Shyness," p. 44.

161   "The return of the idea of temperament . . .": Kagan and Snidman, "Infant Predictors," p. 332.

161   "all statements about the genetic basis . . .": R. C. Lewontin, Steven Rose, and Leon J. Kamin, *Not in Our Genes: Biology, Ideology, and Human Nature* (New York: Pantheon, 1984), p. 251. Lewontin's premise is slightly disingenuous; certainly major gene defects, like those producing phenylketonuria, Down's syndrome, and a number of other disorders associated with risk of mental retardation, have strong effects on human social behavior in ordinary, expectable environments. Still, it has been surprisingly difficult to link even major mental illness to specific genetic defects.

161   "what every parent knows": But we should remember that a previous generation of parents, certainly the educated middle class, knew differently. Degler, *In Search,* reminds us how recent is our new certainty about the power of temperament.

162   the theory of the humors: See Stanley Jackson, *Melancholia and Depression: From Hippocratic to Modern Times* (New Haven, Conn.: Yale University Press, 1986).

163   Aristotle asked: Jackson, *Melancholia and Depression,* p. 31. Regarding mood disorder and creativity, it is interesting to note, in light of our discussion in chapter 4, the observations of one of the great figures in public psychiatry, Philippe Pinel, at the close of the eighteenth century: "The excessive sensitivity that characterizes very talented people may become a cause for the loss of their reason. . . . Groups as diverse as investigators, artists, orators, poets, geometers, engineers, painters and sculptors pay an almost annual price to the hospice for the insane. . . . How many talents lost to society and what great efforts are needed to salvage them!" (Doris B. Weiner, "Philippe Pinel's 'Memoir on Madness' of December 11, 1794: A Fundamental Text of Modern Psychiatry," *American Journal of Psychiatry,* vol. 149 [1992], pp. 725–32; quotation on p. 728.)

163   the work of Hagop Akiskal: Hagop S. Akiskal, "Validating Affective Personality Types," in Lee N. Robins and James E. Barrett, eds., *The Validity of Psychiatric Diagnosis* (New York: Raven Press, 1989), pp. 217–27. See also Boghos I. Yerevanian and Hagop S. Akiskal, " 'Neurotic,' Characterological, and Dysthymic Depressions," *Psychiatric Clinics of North America,* vol. 2 (1979), pp. 595–617; Hagop S. Akiskal, Ted L. Rosenthal, et al., "Characterological Depressions: Clinical and Sleep EEG Findings Separating 'Subaffective Dys-

thymias' from 'Character Spectrum Disorders,' " *Archives of General Psychiatry*, vol. 37 (1980), pp. 777–83.

163 *forme fruste:* See note below, p. 352.

164 "These individuals . . .": Akiskal, "Validating Affective Personality Types," pp. 222–23.

164 Among the most enduring traits: Ibid., p. 221.

165 Elsewhere on the spectrum: "Euthymic" means "normal mood"; "hyperthymia" refers to a chronic elevation of mood that is less than hypomania, which is less than mania, the extreme perturbation of mood and level of energy in which a person may be so euphoric, irritable, impulsive, and fast-thinking as to be delusional. Theorists have argued about what a spectrum of these normal variants and disorders should look like. On first thought, it may seem that the proper ordering is depressed-dysthymic-euthymic-hyperthymic-hypomanic-manic. But there are those who believe that bipolar affective disorder is in effect a severe form of depression, so that depression lies between normality and mania. Others believe the sequence includes a number of distinct diseases, and that spectrum-ordering misrepresents reality: perhaps hyperthymic personality and recurrent depression are just different entities with distinct relations to mind and brain, in the way that asthma and tuberculosis are both lung diseases but do not sit on a spectrum.

165 hyperthymics are habitually "irritable": Akiskal, "Validating Affective Personality Types," p. 219.

166 both temperaments relate to manic-depressive illness: Akiskal refers to a "soft bipolar spectrum." See Hagop S. Akiskal, John Downs, et al., "Affective Disorders in Referred Children and Younger Siblings of Manic Depressives: Mode of Onset and Prospective Course," *Archives of General Psychiatry*, vol. 42 (1985), pp. 996–1003; Hagop S. Akiskal and Gopinath M. Mallya, "Criteria for the 'Soft' Bipolar Spectrum: Treatment Implications," *Psychopharmacology Bulletin*, vol. 23 (1987), pp. 68–73; Hagop S. Akiskal, "The Milder Spectrum of Bipolar Disorders: Diagnostic, Characterologic, and Pharmacologic Aspects," *Psychiatric Annals*, vol. 17 (1987), pp. 33–37.

166 subaffective dysthymia sits in the penumbra of the penumbra: Though some of the patients we have met are probably dysthymic or subaffectively dysthymic, my impression is that the patients Akiskal describes in his monographs tend chronically and recurrently to suffer more distinct periods of depressed mood than do the Prozac responders whose lives we have glimpsed in these pages. Perhaps this difference is due to the sorts of people who attend

the Mood Clinic in Memphis. Not just in Akiskal's reports but in general, although the words "dysthymia" and "depressive personality" appear in the research literature, little work has been done with people whose mood disorder or personality variant is chronic and mild. Most studies of dysthymia involve subjects who, at the time of the study, are suffering "double depression," major depression superimposed on chronic depressive symptoms. This tendency in the literature is easy to understand: people seek out doctors when they are in the midst of a depression, and it is in this state that patients are most willing to participate in drug trials.

Regarding the degree of illness of Akiskal's patients, a trade paper recently reported on a study of the use of Prozac in dysthymia conducted at Charter Lakeside Hospital in Memphis by Akiskal with Radwan Haykal ("Fluoxetine Found Effective for Dysthymia," *Clinical Psychiatry News,* vol. 20, no. 2 [February 1992], p. 4f. Of thirty-nine dysthymic outpatients under study, nineteen had been hospitalized previously for mental illness, and ten had made prior suicide attempts. This is greater past pathology than occurs in the typical history of patients with major depression—and much greater pathology than is reported by the patients we have discussed in this book. Of interest in Haykal and Akiskal's study is that a much higher percentage of dysthymic women than men responded to Prozac (fourteen of sixteen women responded to Prozac, versus six of fourteen men), whereas the ratio was more nearly equal for tricyclics.

167   Psychiatrists who are skeptical: William Z. Potter, Matthew V. Rudorfer, and Husseni Manji, "The Pharmacologic Treatment of Depression," *New England Journal of Medicine,* vol. 325 (1991), pp. 633–42. Potter and his colleagues express doubt about any special role for Prozac in treating dysthymia.

167   which is primary: Perhaps a unified concept of temperament would contain a more equal weighting of social and affective components, taking into account the ordinary social observation that few people are euphoric and inhibited, just as few are gloomy and gregarious. Arguing against a relationship between inhibition and dysthymia is the greater prevalence of anxiety, as opposed to depressive, disorders in relatives of inhibited infants. In favor of a relationship are: the overlap of traits related to both disorders in uptight monkeys, the apparent increased prevalence of inhibition in the history of dysthymics, the similarity in neurotransmitters and parts of the brain implicated, the prominence of social maladroitness in dysthymics between depressive episodes—and a fascinating theory, discussed next in the chapter, linking inhibition with subsequent dysthymia.

168   he gave a preview: Michael T. McGuire, "Can Evolutionary Theory Help Us Understand the Proximate Mechanism and Symptom Changes Characteristic

of Persons with Dysthymic Disorder?," American Psychiatric Association Annual Meeting in New York City, May 14, 1990. I thank Dr. McGuire for sharing his notes with me. It is interesting to see that in the pilot phase of this study the women were diagnosed as having "neurotic depression." The designations for minor and chronic depression are impossibly fluid.

168 the researchers could not differentiate: The lack of memory difference confirms that the experimental subjects were not deeply depressed, since memory and concentration are so often impaired in major depression. The dysthymic women had one interesting trait I do not mention in the text: they tended to attribute their frustration to chance or circumstance, and to engage in various forms of self-deception. This failure to organize experience in a usable way results in repetition of dysfunctional behavior. Internal locus of control—the belief that a person causes his own good or ill fortune—demands a constant re-examination of failed strategies; these women's external attribution of control caused them to persist in their maladaptive approaches. See also Michael T. McGuire and Alfonso Troisi, "Unrealistic Wishes and Physiological Change: An Overview," *Psychotherapy and Psychosomatics,* vol. 47 (1987), pp. 82–94.

175 Studies from a variety of perspectives: I should make it clear that this synthesis of the work of Kagan, Suomi, Akiskal, McGuire, and, in the background, Klein, Post, and others is my own, and that it brings together material the researchers themselves might consider incompatible. For example, Akiskal seems to see subaffective dysthymia as a discrete disorder in which social inhibition is a secondary feature; and Kagan implies that inhibited children will likely grow up to be anxious rather than depressed. Conventionally, social inhibition is thought to relate to the anxiety disorders, whereas dysthymia relates to the depressive disorders. But the prevalence of social inhibition as the (temporally) primary trait in McGuire's dysthymics points to the overlap of categories.

My own view is that the whole "affective spectrum" is tightly linked. The commonality of these prevalent minor conditions is supported not only by the common responsiveness of a range of anxiety and depressive disorders, from panic and OCD to dysthymia and depression, to the same drugs, but also by a growing body of basic research. See, for example, Kenneth S. Kendler, Michael C. Neale, et al., "Major Depression and Generalized Anxiety Disorder: Same Genes, (Partly) Different Environments?," *Archives of General Psychiatry,* vol. 49 (1992), pp. 716–22. This work meshes well with Suomi's speculation that a genetic predisposition to reactivity can give rise, depending on the nature of stressors encountered, to either anxiety or depression.

179   Klein's group looked at about two hundred: Jonathan W. Stewart, Frederic M. Quitkin, et al., "Social Functioning in Chronic Depression: Effect of 6 Weeks of Antidepressant Treatment," *Psychiatry Research,* vol. 25 (1988), pp. 213–22. A good summary of the research on the relationship of dysthymia to personality disorder can be found in James H. Kocsis and Allen J. Frances, "A Critical Discussion of *DSM-III* Dysthymic Disorder," *American Journal of Psychiatry,* vol. 144 (1987), pp. 1534–42.

180   Akiskal no longer divides patients: This change in his point of view was apparent in a number of Akiskal's presentations at the 1992 Annual Meeting of the American Psychiatric Association, and Akiskal confirmed it in response to a question I asked him at that meeting. See also Haykal, "Early Onset Dysthymia."

183   "the functional theory of psychopathology": Herman M. van Praag, Serena-Lynn Brown, et al., "Beyond Serotonin: A Multiaminergic Perspective on Abnormal Behavior," in Herman M. van Praag and Serena-Lynn Brown, eds., *The Role of Serotonin in Psychiatric Disorders* (New York: Brunner/Mazel, 1991), pp. 302–32.

183   Likewise, panic anxiety: These examples are mine.

184   "The greater the biochemical specificity . . .": Van Praag, Brown, et al., "Beyond Serotonin," p. 325.

185   C. Robert Cloninger: "A Unified Biosocial Theory of Personality and Its Role in the Development of Anxiety States," *Psychiatric Developments,* vol. 3 (1986), pp. 167–226; "A Systematic Method for Clinical Description and Classification of Personality Variants: A Proposal," *Archives of General Psychiatry,* vol. 44 (1987), pp. 573–88.

185   "reward dependence" and related quotations: Cloninger, "Systematic Method," p. 578.

186   "harm avoidance": Ibid., p. 577.

187   "novelty seeking"; "Consistently . . .": Ibid., p. 576. This axis was the subject of the title essay of the popular book by the anthropologist-physician Melvin Konner, *Why the Reckless Survive: And Other Secrets of Human Nature* (New York: Viking, 1990), in which Konner argues that both risk-takers and risk-avoiders contribute to the survival of the species.

187   These three axes: Cloninger, "Unified Biosocial Theory," p. 185; Cloninger, "Systematic Method," p. 579.
     As if three axes were not enough, other researchers have proposed a fourth,

based on how people take in stimuli such as pain. Some people seem neurologically, when tested by means of brain-wave tests (electroencephalograms), to have exaggerated reactions to loud noises or flashes of light. They are called "augmenters"; the opposite end of the axis of "perceptual reactance" is "reducing." Theorists have especially discussed combinations of novelty seeking and perceptual reactance. High novelty seeking and augmenting seems a bad combination—the person is drawn to stimuli he or she cannot tolerate, and the result is an excess of mental illness. High stimulus-seeking and reducing leads to successful risk-taking, and so on. Cloninger argues that perceptual reactance is not a separate axis, and that he can cover the same territory more parsimoniously with his one-neurotransmitter/one-trait model.

Not only social ease, mood, and level of energy, but other qualities we have not mentioned, such as propensity toward anger and violence, have been shown in one or another experimental model to be influenced by transmitters and receptors.

187 "passive avoidance . . . gullible": Cloninger, "Systematic Method," p. 579.

191 the "Ideas" story in *Newsweek:* Sharon Begley, "Brother Sun, Sister Moon," *Newsweek,* October 29, 1990, p. 69, a discussion of Judy Dunn and Robert Plomin, *Separate Lives: Why Siblings Are So Different* (New York: Basic Books, 1990).

191 A geneticist would deem . . . meaningless: The reporting of the percent contribution of genes to behavioral traits is critiqued effectively by Richard Lewontin in his book *Human Diversity* (New York: Scientific American, 1982). Hidden in most twin studies, upon which percentage statements of this sort are often based, is the truth that most "adopted-out" twins are raised by aunts and uncles, not by people from vastly different cultural backgrounds.

191 *The Glass Menagerie:* Trinity Repertory Company, Providence, R.I., fall 1991.

193 a recent genetic study of white twin girls: Kenneth S. Kendler, Michael C. Neale, et al., "Childhood Parental Loss and Adult Psychopathology in Women: A Twin Study Perspective," *Archives of General Psychiatry,* vol. 49 (1992), pp. 109–16. This study is complex and has a number of interesting results. For instance, panic anxiety was found to be associated with both parental death and separation, but only if the separation was from the mother. This sort of result speaks against a nonspecific diagnosis such as neurosis, and indicates that panic anxiety and major depression may be distinct entities arising in response to differing social stressors. In aggregate, this twin study found a

variety of mental illnesses in the sample to correlate much more with genetic than environmental factors, though both sorts of effects were discernible.

196   personality extends far beyond: The effects of medication on inhibited people may also change our conception of "social skills" and social development. It is my observation that patients who say they have not grown since early childhood, and who in fact appear immature or socially stunted, often do quite well when properly medicated—and without the need for any social-skills training. Having observed people in the school or workplace, and watched television shows and read books that model social behavior, and dreamed of social competency, seems to be enough for them. Once they are less inhibited, they interact with surprising success. The limiting factor in their past failures was social anxiety or a missetting of the sensor for interpersonal distance, and not any failure to have matured.

196   Is Sally's fiancé truly marrying: There is an ethical aspect to this question: Are the psychiatrist and the patient colluding to deceive the prospective mate? Is the "real" Sally the woman off medication, as she was and may perhaps again be? Of course, similar issues are hidden in psychotherapy: a patient who is supported by therapy may appear socially more stable than he or she was in the past, or than he or she may be in the future.

My sense is that a good deal of marrying takes place around changes in affective state. One classic instance is marriage "on the rebound." Generally, a person may be more susceptible to marrying when depressed (and therefore needy) or when euphoric. The altered state may be helpful, in that it pushes a person past his or her inhibitions, or it may be a prelude to unhappiness. An empirically based assumption of marriage counseling is that both partners are probably in about the same state of maturity (more exactly, that they have the same level of "differentiation of self," or ability to resist regressive social and family forces). My sense is that many marital troubles arise when a depressed woman marries a man who is at her level of social competence at the time of her weakness; when she recovers from depression, she finds herself mismatched, but, afraid she may sink back into depression in response to a separation, unable to extricate herself.

CHAPTER 7: *FORMES FRUSTES:* LOW SELF-ESTEEM

197   A reviewer of a recent book: Elaine Showalter, "Ladies Sing the Blues," *New Republic,* vol. 206, no. 10 (March 9, 1992), pp. 44–45. The section cited

refers to Colette Dowling, *You Mean I Don't Have to Feel This Way?* (New York: Scribner's, 1992).

197   now most often called *formes frustes:* Regarding Freud's view of partial presentations of anxiety neurosis, see chapter 4. The classic example of a *forme fruste* is "migraine without migraine": migraine headaches are often accompanied or preceded by diverse symptoms, such as the illusion of flashing lights, queasiness in the stomach, numbness over one side of the face, and weakness or paralysis of one arm; people can suffer, on the same physiological basis as migraine, only the accompanying features without ever having a headache. For example, a patient may consult a gastroenterologist for recurrent queasiness when the problem is really "migraine without migraine." In discussing *formes frustes* of minor depression, I am saying that there is also "dysthymia without dysthymia."

In medical school, I was told that a *forme fruste* was a "frustrated form" of an illness, and *Stedman's Medical Dictionary* supports this assertion, tracing *fruste* to the Latin *frustra,* "without effect" or "in vain." But a "frust," in the eighteenth-century English of *Tristram Shandy,* was a fragment; the *Oxford English Dictionary* relates the word to the Latin *frustum,* "a piece." In French, *fruste* refers specifically to something worn away by friction. A *forme fruste* is thus not a frustrated but a partial illness.

198   an earlier era stressed building character: My daughter for some years attended a girls' school based on Quaker principles one of whose mottoes was "lowliness," a thoroughly unmodern virtue and one that presupposes an unmodern mix of self-worth, self-doubt, and humility. The school stressed the inculcation of confidence, assertiveness, and leadership. I believe it is fair to say that the goal of instilling lowliness in girls was not especially talked up in the school's contacts with parents of prospective pupils.

I think in this context of an Ed Koren cartoon that shows a mother, with an unhappy preschooler beside her standing in front of a school, addressing another mother with a child in a stroller: "Can you believe this is happening to me? Her scores are very low in self-esteem." (*New Yorker,* April 6, 1992, p. 35.)

An interesting critique of self-esteem, and also of psychoanalysis as a clinical modality, is Christopher Lasch, "For Shame: Why Americans Should Be Wary of Self-Esteem," *New Republic,* August 10, 1992, pp. 29–34. Lasch's essay is in part a skeptical commentary on Gloria Steinem's *Revolution from Within: A Book of Self-Esteem* (Boston: Little, Brown, 1992), and the state of California's Task Force to Promote Self-Esteem, which Steinem praises (pp. 26–30). Regarding self-esteem as autobiographical, Steinem quotes psychiatrists to the effect that self-valuation in adults is "the inner child of the past" or "the child within" (pp. 34–39, 65–69, and throughout).

199   rather odd theories of Alfred Adler: Alfred Adler, *Study of Organ Inferiority and Its Psychical Compensation: A Contribution to Clinical Medicine* (1907), trans. Smith Ely Jelliffe (New York: Nervous and Mental Disease Publishing Co., 1917); Alfred Adler, *The Neurotic Constitution: Outlines of a Comparative Individualistic Psychology and Psychotherapy* (1912), trans. Bernard Glueck and John E. Lind (New York: Moffat, Yard and Co., 1917). In his early years, Adler was a major and beneficent figure in Viennese community medicine, taking an interest, for instance, in the ocular problems of tailors; in later years, he became a popularizer of psychology, focusing especially on people's innate social interest (not unlike the "aloneness affect" we have discussed) and their strivings for success.

199   a variant form of guilt: "But the major part of the sense of inferiority derives from the ego's relation to its super-ego. . . . Altogether, it is hard to separate the sense of inferiority from the sense of guilt." (Sigmund Freud, *New Introductory Lectures on Psycho-Analysis* [1933], in James Strachey, ed., *The Standard Edition of the Complete Psychological Works of Sigmund Freud*, vol. 22 [London: Hogarth Press, 1964], pp. 65–66. Although Freud emphasized the role of the superego, he also had a complex view of the development of self-worth, and a healthy respect for the role of maternal nurturance. And he had a modern understanding of the role of the cross-generational transmission of pathology, saying that, in the development of the superego, the child responded less to the parent than to the parent's superego—that is, the mother or father's recollection of the grandparents' (often severe) child-rearing practices.

200   The new guiding metaphor: In this and the following paragraph, I am relying on the theories of the modern school of psychoanalysis called "self psychology," whose emphasis on the self is evident in its very name.

202   Donald Klein has written: Paul H. Wender and Donald F. Klein, *Mind, Mood, and Medicine* (New York: Farrar, Straus & Giroux, 1981), especially pp. 39–66; the case of William M. is on pp. 46–48. Paul Wender is a psychiatrist best known for his work on attention-deficit hyperactivity disorder, a phenomenon we will encounter in chapter 9.

204   altered emotional proprioception—a neurological distortion: I find it hard to avoid words like "altered" or "distortion," but it may be more reasonable to think of self-esteem as a spectrum trait that differs among normal people. William M. may be not damaged but just different, with a sense of self that is logically defensible but socially maladaptive.

208 self-image changes overnight: Recent work on dysthymia indicates that not all responses are of this sort. An unpublished study from Cornell University finds that good antidepressant responders fall into two groups as regards personality. Some seem cured outright, like the patients we have met. Others also report dramatic change but find the change dislocating. In these patients, although the change in feeling about the self is strong, cognition (and organization of the defenses) lags; they generally need psychotherapy to deal with the success of medication. The study, by a group headed by James Kocsis, was cited in Arnold Cooper, "The Relevance of Psychotherapy to Clinical Practice Today," address, Rhode Island Psychiatric Society, Butler Hospital, Providence, R.I., March 2, 1992, 27 pp.

210 The classic experience of college students: This point is made by Wender and Klein, *Mind, Mood, and Medicine,* p. 202.

212 including Michael McGuire: Michael J. Raleigh and Michael T. McGuire, "Social and Environmental Influences on Blood Serotonin Concentrations in Monkeys," *Archives of General Psychiatry,* vol. 41 (1984), pp. 405–10. "Troop" is an inexact but convenient word for referring to groups of captive monkeys.

Dominance and submission are not difficult to identify in vervets. A dominant male will win over 90 percent of his aggressive contacts (threatening, slapping and pushing, or "displaying"—bouncing, circling the tail, and swinging the penis) with other males, whereas no submissive male will win more than half of his encounters. Submissive behaviors are: avoiding or retreating from threat; signaling submission by squealing, hopping backward, and pawing the ground; and standing rigidly vigilant.

213 To investigate this issue: Michael J. Raleigh, Michael T. McGuire, et al., "Serotonergic Mechanisms Promote Dominance Acquisition in Adult Male Vervet Monkeys," *Brain Research,* vol. 559 (1991), pp. 181–90. It is important to note that the monkeys on serotonin-depleting or -elevating medication did not appear drugged; they engaged in all the normal behaviors of vervet males.

214 serotonic mechanisms . . . : Ibid., p. 188.

214 studies of serotonin levels in man: A political scientist at the University of Iowa has performed two preliminary experiments using blood serotonin levels to assess the influence of biology on power-seeking behavior in humans. Based on a study of male undergraduates placed in a stressful competitive situation, he concludes that serotonin levels correlate with self-assessed social rank and leadership qualities, albeit complexly. Among aggressive, ambitious, manipulative, and self-centered young men (the majority of the sample), high blood serotonin correlated with high status; among deferential, nonaggressive, moralistic young men, high serotonin correlated with low status. Interestingly, serotonin levels, and social status, existed on a continuous spectrum in aggressive young men (as opposed to the discontinuous submissive-dominant dichotomy in vervets). Douglas Madsen, "Blood Serotonin and Social Rank Among Human Males," in Roger Masters and Michael McGuire, eds., *The Neurotransmitter Revolution* (unpublished).

Madsen had earlier found that very strong type A ("Machiavellian") behavior in young men—encompassing drive, aggressiveness, mistrust, and competitiveness—correlates with high blood serotonin levels. Madsen believes any relationship between hierarchy and serotonin levels in humans must necessarily be complex because humans achieve power through various means (money, inheritance, a group decision to compromise on a weak leader who won't rock the boat) that have little to do with biologically mediated leadership traits. Douglas Madsen, "A Biochemical Property Relating to Power Seeking in Humans," *American Political Science Review*, vol. 79 (1985), pp. 448–57.

215   maintained by the serotonin system: Serotonin is hardly likely to be the whole story. Researchers have also looked at stress hormones in relation to dominance hierarchy. To mention only two results: When male monkeys compete for dominance, their blood-norepinephrine and stress-hormone levels rise. Once the battle is decided, the stress-hormone levels in the newly dominant monkey fall; in the defeated monkey, they remain high. Likewise, aroused females have high stress-hormone levels that, however, "fall precipitously if they come under the protection of a dominant male" (Peter C. Whybrow, Hagop S. Akiskal, and William T. McKinney, Jr., *Mood Disorder: Toward a New Psychobiology* [New York: Plenum, 1984], p. 115). The norepinephrine and stress-hormone results are less impressive than the work on serotonin. Blood levels of norepinephrine and stress hormones vary widely in individuals over time—they are state variables. But serotonin levels are so stable that they appear to be trait variables, and to show that a trait variable changes according to social status is remarkable. Testosterone and other hormones almost certainly also play a role in dominance.

There was, by the way, an interesting article by Natalie Angier in *The New York Times* of November 12, 1991 (p. C1), referring to a study showing that a particular area of the brains of African cichlid fish increases in size when they achieve dominance. It is interesting to see dominance anatomically encoded, in any species.

215   often cited study of children in Connecticut: Stanley Coopersmith, *The Antecedents of Self-Esteem* (San Francisco: Freeman, 1967).

220 increase in his tolerance for strong, disturbing emotions: This increase, under the influence of pharmacotherapy, parallels a change certain theorists consider crucial in the psychotherapy of depression—namely, a replacement of the clinical syndrome of depression (which can include a deadening of affect, and is therefore called a "nonfeeling state") by the experiencing of sadness (a feeling state). See Irene Pierce Stiver and Jean Baker Miller, "From Depression to Sadness in Women's Psychotherapy," *Work in Progress* (The Stone Center, Wellesley College), vol. 36 (1988), pp. 1–12. Stiver and Miller consider a growing affective awareness of disappointment to be central to recovery from depression in women. The essay contains a useful review of social factors contributory to depression in women in our culture.

222 psychiatry's "loss of mind": Morton F. Reiser, "Are Psychiatric Educators 'Losing the Mind?,' " *American Journal of Psychiatry*, vol. 145 (1988), pp. 148–53.

CHAPTER 8: *FORMES FRUSTES:* INHIBITION OF PLEASURE, SLUGGISHNESS OF THOUGHT

223 *Annie Hall . . . Anhedonia:* Eric Lax, *Woody Allen: A Biography* (New York, Vintage, 1992), p. 284.

225 Graham Greene . . . felt such ennui: The following passage is from the autobiography of his early years, *A Sort of Life* (New York: Simon and Schuster, 1971), pp. 157–58:

> . . . the oppression of boredom soon began to descend. Once on my free day I walked over the hills to Chesterfield and found a dentist. I described to him the symptoms, which I knew well, of an abscess. He tapped a perfectly good tooth with his little mirror and I reacted in the correct way. "Better have it out," he advised.
> "Yes," I said, "but with ether."
> A few minutes' unconsciousness was like a holiday from the world. I had lost a good tooth, but the boredom was for the time being dispersed.

Greene is someone Jerome Kagan mentions as having come to social inhibition on an environmental basis, through having been hazed in school. But I wonder whether Greene did not suffer as well, or even primarily, from anhedonia, self-treated by means of extreme adventure and expressed in the remarkable laconic distance of his authorial voice. Kagan is quoted on Greene in Ruth M. Galvin, "The Nature of Shyness," *Harvard Magazine,* vol. 94 (1992), pp. 40–45.

228   A variety of neurochemical systems: Norepinephrine in particular has been proposed as key to "hedonic capacity," as, for example, in Herman van Praag's theory, referred to in chapter 6, of reward-coupling. Dopamine, through its relationship to schizophrenia, Parkinsonism, and the effects of amphetamine, has been proposed as a major factor in the regulation of pleasure. There is also interest in the endorphins, the internally produced substances whose effects heroin and morphine mimic. The encoding of pleasure in the brain probably extends far beyond the limbic system, where the biological correlates of depression are most often studied. See Nancy Andreason, "Affective Flattening: Evaluation and Diagnostic Significance," in David C. Clark and Jan Fawcett, eds., *Anhedonia and Affect Deficit States* (New York: PMA Publishing Corp., 1987), pp. 15–31.

228   Paul Meehl . . . published a critique: Paul E. Meehl, "Hedonic Capacity: Some Conjectures," *Bulletin of the Menninger Clinic,* vol. 39 (1975), pp. 295–307; reprinted in Clark and Fawcett, eds., *Anhedonia,* pp. 33–45. The various quotes from Meehl are all from this essay. Meehl quotes Sandor Rado in the phrase "scarcity economy of pleasure." See also Paul E. Meehl, " 'Hedonic Capacity' Ten Years Later: Some Clarifications," in ibid., pp. 47–50.

229   depression may result: Such depression is generally described, in a term favored by the behavioral psychologist B. F. Skinner, as "extinction depression." Michael McGuire's account of dysthymia as resulting from the effects of behavioral inflexibility—women who stand on long lines end up with few friends and cramped lodgings—is an extinction-depression model.

230   the work of . . . Jan Fawcett . . . and David Clark: See David Clark and Jan Fawcett, "Anhedonia, Hypohedonia and Pleasure Capacity in Major Depressive Disorders," in Clark and Fawcett, eds., *Anhedonia,* pp. 51–63.

230   fewer signs of neurotic conflict: The anhedonic subjects showed less indecision, pessimism, irritability, and hypochondriasis—the more neurotic depressive traits.

231   Klein had just published: Donald F. Klein, "Endogenomorphic Depression: A Conceptual and Terminological Revision," *Archives of General Psychiatry,* vol. 31 (1974), pp. 447–54. The ideas in that early monograph are expanded on and clarified in Donald F. Klein, "Depression and Anhedonia," in Clark and Fawcett, eds., *Anhedonia,* pp. 1–14. Much of what appears in the following paragraphs constitutes a condensation of that second monograph.

The reader will recognize the "central comparator" as conceptual kin to the "emotional thermostat" in Klein's theory of rejection-sensitivity, summarized in chapter 4.

232 consummatory anhedonia: Klein said consummatory anhedonia was mostly primary—perhaps the central problem in typical depression. More rarely, consummatory anhedonia might occur secondarily, as a result of severe and chronic appetitive anhedonia.

233 Klein's account . . . contrasted to Meehl's: If Meehl is right, anhedonia should be chronic and result primarily in "character pathology." If Klein is right, the most pervasive anhedonia (consummatory, which includes appetitive) should be a feature of the deepest major depressions. But this contrast is partly specious. When we talk about anhedonia, we tend to mean what Klein would call an appetitive disorder—boredom, lethargy, indifference to a variety of activities. And as regards appetitive dysfunction, Klein and Meehl are very largely in agreement.

Fawcett and Clark's research was in part an attempt to settle the apparent disagreement between Meehl and Klein. Fawcett and Clark's results shed doubt on Klein's account of comsummatory anhedonia. In their study, anhedonia is absent in the vast majority of depressed patients. The minority of patients who score high on Fawcett and Clark's measure of anhedonia appear to have a chronic trait that remains when depression subsides. Klein has argued that the researchers' scale measures appetitive anhedonia, because testing necessarily asks respondents to *imagine how they will feel*—and appetitive anhedonia is a disorder of *imagining* pleasure. Klein may well be right, but if consummatory anhedonia presupposes appetitive anhedonia, Fawcett and Clark's net ought to catch a more varied group of depressives—both pure appetitive anhedonics with atypical depression and those suffering from deep, acute, typical depression, of which appetitive anhedonia, as well as consummatory, is necessarily a feature.

233 And once Prozac works: Why Prozac? I have no good explanation. If anhedonia is a matter of problems with norepinephrine, dopamine, and the endorphins, Hillary should have responded to anything except Prozac. Hillary's initial short-lived success on Prozac sounds like a favorable reaction to the "amphetaminelike effect," except that it lasted weeks rather than days. That response, along with certain of Hillary's symptoms, including lethargy and a lack of follow-through that might be interpreted as a sign of attention-deficit disorder, would lead some biological psychiatrists to prescribe a stimulant, such as Ritalin or an amphetamine (which affects norepinephrine and dopamine). The noradrenergic drug desipramine would be a likely candidate on theoretical

grounds—except that Klein's clinical experience showed the tricyclics to be relatively ineffective for anhedonia.

My guess is that serotonin plays a role in anhedonia, perhaps through something like Klein's comparator or center for appetitive pleasure. To reverse the issue, any adequate theory of anhedonia will have to explain the efficacy of Prozac and the MAOIs in treating the condition, which is to say that any adequate model will have to say something about serotonin.

235   "self-medication hypothesis . . .": Edward Khantzian, "The Self-Medication Hypothesis of Addictive Disorders: Focus on Heroin and Cocaine Dependence," *American Journal of Psychiatry*, vol. 142 (1985), pp. 1259–64; Edward Khantzian, "Self-Regulation and Self-Medication Factors in Alcoholism and the Addictions: Similarities and Differences," in Marc Galanter, ed., *Recent Developments in Alcoholism*, vol. 8 (New York: Plenum Publishing, 1990).

237   graphic artist: I discussed this case in an essay, "Medication Consultation," in *Psychiatric Times*, June 1991, pp. 4–5.

239   Attention-deficit disorder: I have drawn on American Psychiatric Association, *Diagnostic and Statistical Manual of Mental Disorders*, 3rd ed. (Washington, D.C.: American Psychiatric Association, 1980). By 1987, attention-deficit disorder without hyperactivity was considered rare; the revised manual (DSM III-R) recognizes only attention-deficit hyperactivity disorder (ADHD) and adds a minor category (undifferentiated attention-deficit disorder) as a sop to those clinicians who still distinguish attention-deficit disorder from ADHD. The point is that the complete syndrome (ADHD) is more common, and the incomplete may be merely a *forme fruste*.

A more recent overview of the topic is Russell A. Barkley, "Attention Deficit Hyperactivity Disorder," *Psychiatric Annals*, vol. 21 (1991), pp. 725–33. A major longitudinal study of hyperactive children which finds they do not have an excess of depression in later life is: Salvatore Mannuzza, Rachel G. Klein, et al., "Hyperactive Boys Almost Grown Up: V. Replication of Psychiatric Status," *Archives of General Psychiatry*, vol. 48 (1992), pp. 77–83. My description of ADHD is far from exhaustive. I have included primarily traits related to (mostly contrasting with) characteristics of dysthymia that we have discussed.

ADHD is often confused with learning disabilities, such as the various reading or decoding disorders, the dyslexias. Children with ADHD often have learning disorders, perhaps on the basis of a broad minor impairment of neurological development. But it seems the learning disorders occur on a different biological basis, in different parts of the brain, from the attention deficits. As opposed to ADHD, learning disorders may be associated with depression, perhaps even because of a relationship between the biological substrates of learning and mood disorders. See, for example, Drake D. Duane, "Dyslexia: Neurobiological and Behavioral Correlates," *Psychiatric Annals*, vol. 21 (1991), pp. 703–8.

240 But it sometimes continues into adult life: See Paul H. Wender, *The Hyperactive Child, Adolescent, and Adult: Attention Deficit Disorder Through the Lifespan* (New York: Oxford University Press, 1987), especially chapter 6, "Attention Deficit Disorder in Adults," pp. 117–40.

241 demoralization paired with a subtle disorganization of thought: I have just said that hyperactive boys tend not to suffer depression in adulthood, so the reader may well wonder how it is possible to say that ADHD can be confused with dysthymia. The answer is twofold. First, what characterizes ADHD in adulthood is not depression as a diagnosable illness but, rather, mood swings. ADHD patients as adults are overexcited by success and bored or discontented when frustrated or understimulated. Even though the "down" moods may be on a quite different basis, the account an adult with ADHD gives of himself —easily bored, joyless, self-deprecating—may lead to confusion with the anhedonia or low self-worth of dysthymia. Those who favor ADHD as a diagnosis in depressed adults with poor concentration also argue that ADHD is so underdiagnosed that even research studies tend to miss quiet or withdrawn children who have the disorder. It is these patients, they say, who on reaching adulthood will present with stories like Sonia's or Hillary's—depression characterized by boredom, disorganization, and a sense of not "getting" some of what is obvious to others. See, for example John J. Ratey, "Paying Attention to Attention in Adults," *Chadder*, Fall–Winter 1991, pp. 13–14.

241 pharmacologic dissection: The area of most distinct difference is responsiveness to very low-dose antidepressants. Some ADHD patients feel much less blue and impulsive after a few days on ten to thirty milligrams of desipramine—whereas most depressed patients require 150 to 300 milligrams given for four weeks. But dysthymic patients of all stripes sometimes respond to low-dose antidepressants. ADHD and dysthymia are both poorly studied pharmacologically, and the area of possible overlap has barely been studied at all.

241 But stimulants are sometimes effective in depression: There are depressed patients who respond only to stimulants. The work of Jonathan Cole of Harvard University is of particular interest in this area. ADHD has been associated with disorders of dopamine; it is at least possible that ADHD patients benefit from stimulants' dopamine effects and depressed patients from their norepinephrine

effects. It is also possible that these disorders are more closely connected than the evidence I have adduced here would indicate. It is of particular interest that ADHD sometimes responds to SSRIs, which affect the "wrong" neurotransmitter system. One could imagine that ADHD and the concentration and memory deficits of depression are related, as mania may be to be depression, through an abnormality of a thermostat or comparator.

243 If the twins had been subtly injured: I do not mean to say that ADHD is always a result of traumatic or chemical damage to the brain. There is evidence that in some cases ADHD may be heritable. It is nonetheless generally understood as a dysfunction, more like illness than like a normal variant.

245 the management consultant Tom Peters: "The Quick and the Dead: Slow, Careful Decisions Aren't Always the Best," Providence *Business News*, March 2, 1992, p. 12. The essay refers to a study contrasting slow and fast decision-makers at microcomputer firms. The faster executives use more real-time information, consider more alternatives, thrive on conflict and uncertainty, and integrate strategy and tactics. Their decisions are more timely and, in part for that reason, better. The essay ends with a quote from one executive: "The '90s will be a . . . nanosecond culture. There'll be only two kinds of managers: the quick and the dead." See also Jay Bourgeois and Kathleen Eisenhardt, "Strategic Decision Processes in High-Velocity Environments: Four Cases in the Microcomputer Industry," *Management Science*, vol. 34 (1988), pp. 816–35.

246 This nightmare view: As a parent, I sometimes think I see these pressures in an area that is far from the pharmacologic arena, but near to the issue of mental achievement—in grade placement for elementary-school children, particularly in affluent school districts or private schools. First a few enlightened parents hold back their developmentally immature children from first grade; then normal, late-birthday children are held back; soon all the parents who want their children to be leaders decide the boys and girls should wait a year; and before you know it the whole first grade is filled with seven-year-olds, and a normal six-year-old is too immature to compete successfully. We are used to theories about the influence of technology on cultural norms but perhaps do not appreciate that in the modern, intelligence-driven economy such nonmechanical entities as school placement and medication are technologies.

246 Khantzian . . . wrote to ask: Personal correspondence, cited in Kramer, "Medication Consultation."

CHAPTER 9: THE MESSAGE IN THE CAPSULE

250 the last novel by . . . Walker Percy: *The Thanatos Syndrome* (New York: Farrar, Straus & Giroux, 1987). The quotes are from p. 6 (Dickinson) and 21.

251 I raised that question in . . . essays: The first two were "Metamorphosis," *Psychiatric Times,* May 1989, p. 3ff, and "The New You," *Psychiatric Times,* March 1990, pp. 45–46. I am, I say with a mixture of pride and amusement, the first doctor to have posed these questions in print—indeed, the first to write that Prozac's effect sometimes goes beyond treating depression to brightening mood or altering personality traits. This distinction is minor: I only reported what thousands of doctors had seen. My small claim to priority is testimony mostly to the profession's overreliance on experiment and its neglect of ordinary observation. The Prozac columns were part of a larger series I had written, stretching back to 1986, on the way medications, and antidepressants in particular, color psychiatrists' understanding of patients. (Some of the earlier thinking is summarized in the chapter "The Mind-Mind-Body-Problem Problem" in my book *Moments of Engagement: Intimate Psychotherapy in a Technological Age* [New York: W. W. Norton, 1989], pp. 43–65.)

Robert Aranow was working independently on similar ideas; just before my second essay appeared, he chaired a clinical case conference at McLean Hospital on "The Clinical and Ethical Issues Raised by the Possible Development of 'Mood Brighteners,' " based on two cases of patients on Prozac, indicating "that significant improvement in mood can be gained in individuals who do not meet criteria" for mood disorder. Richard Schwartz (see p. 253) spoke at that conference. In May 1991, I joined Aranow, Schwartz, and Mark Sullivan in a symposium on "Mood Brighteners: Clinical and Ethical Dilemmas" at the American Psychiatric Association's Annual Meeting in New Orleans. The level of activity Prozac immediately aroused within the field of medical ethics is remarkable. Within two or three years of Prozac's introduction, articles on its ethical implications began to appear in professional journals, testimony to the strong impression the drug made on doctors as soon as they saw patients respond to it.

251 "mood brighteners," a phrase he coined: The concept "mood brightener" has been wrongly attributed to me. See Randolph M. Nesse, "What Good Is Feeling Bad? The Evolutionary Benefits of Psychic Pain," *The Sciences,* November–December 1990, pp. 30–37.

251 "brighten the episodically down moods . . .": Robert Aranow quoted in Richard S. Schwartz, "Mood Brighteners, Affect Tolerance, and the Blues,"

Psychiatry, vol. 54 (1991), pp. 397–403; quotation on p. 397. The essay is a written version of the talk Schwartz presented at the May 1991 symposium.

252 "conservation of mood": Robert B. Aranow, Richard S. Schwartz, and Mark D. Sullivan, "Mood Brighteners," *American Journal of Psychiatry,* in press, draft of March 19, 1992, 16 pp.

252 "In effect, there has been . . .": Ibid, p. 1.

252 violate the principle of conservation of mood: It must seem ironic that such issues should arise around a medicine alleged to trigger impulses to commit suicide or homicide. But those allegations had just been made when Prozac caught the attention of the ethics community, and they have never dominated doctors' view of Prozac.

252 forty-four-year-old woman: Aranow, Schwartz, and Sullivan, "Mood Brighteners."

252 "reduce the common experiences . . .": Aranow quoted in Schwartz, "Mood Brighteners," p. 397.

253 "Recovery from a depressive illness . . .": Ibid., p. 398.

253 "an act of disconnection . . .": Ibid.

253 it is the "normal": Schwartz recounts the Russian story of two mice who fell into a bucket of milk. "Unable to swim, one mouse recognized the hopelessness of the situation, gave up, and drowned. The other became enraged, flailed at the milk, churned it to butter, and walked off." (Ibid., p. 399.)

254 "stand to feel . . .": Ibid., p. 400.

254 the contribution of . . . Zetzel: Elizabeth R. Zetzel, *The Capacity for Emotional Growth* (London: Hogarth Press, 1970), especially "Anxiety and the Capacity to Bear It," pp. 33–52, and "On the Incapacity to Bear Depression," pp. 82–114. This is the same Elizabeth Zetzel whom we met in chapter 4, in connection with the observation that, as psychoanalytic patients, hysterics can be either good or horrid.

254 "Here is a culture . . ." Schwartz, "Mood Brighteners," p. 401.

254 Nesse . . . has collaborated with Michael McGuire: Michael T. McGuire, Isaac Marks, et al., "Evolutionary Biology: A Basic Science for Psychiatry?," *Acta Psychiatrica Scandinavica,* in press, draft of February 22, 1992, 21 pp. I thank Dr. McGuire for sharing this manuscript with me.

254 criticized . . . from the viewpoint of evolutionary biology: Nesse, "What Good Is Feeling Bad?"

255 "The new perspective . . .": Ibid., p. 37.

256 Aranow . . . co-authored with Schwartz and Mark Sullivan: Aranow, Schwartz, and Sullivan, "Mood Brighteners."

256 Sullivan suggests "autonomy": Mark Sullivan, "Ethics and the Perfection of Psychopharmacology," unpublished, 10 pp.; Aranow, Schwartz, and Sullivan, "Mood Brighteners." Regarding "autonomy," Sullivan draws on the work of Eric Cassell and Gerald Dworkin.

259 ". . . a person grows . . ." Schwartz, "Mood Brighteners," p. 400.

259 pharmacological Calvinism: The phrase is Gerald Klerman's (Gerald L. Klerman, "Psychotropic Hedonism vs. Pharmacological Calvinism," *Hastings Center Report,* vol. 2, no. 4 [1972], pp. 1–3). This issue is discussed further on p. 274. In the 1980s, Klerman told me he wished he had instead used the phrase "pharmacologic puritanism," as more expressive of the judgmental and prohibitive quality of the objection to medication.

260 Prozac shifts people from dysthymia: I am here using "dysthymia" and "hyperthymia" to refer to spectrum traits. Akiskal sometimes uses the same words to refer to illnesses. Any such distinction is complicated by the possibility that normal temperament at either end of the spectrum can be an early stage of a kindled mood disorder. It is in any case explicit in the mood-brightener debate that such a drug moves people from one nonillness state to another.

260 "I used to be uncomfortable . . .": Nesse, "What Good Is Feeling Bad?," p. 30. I do not mean to deny that it can sometimes be useful to share with patients the impression that their social handicaps arise from normal variant traits. This viewpoint was, for example, quite helpful to Jerry, the surgeon whose treatment I discussed in chapter 6.

261 I will worry about Nesse's patient: I am not saying that Nesse believes all chronic sadness is inherited, only that in a clinical setting such a belief regarding a particular patient must come late in the evaluation process.

262 the rich can have it and the poor cannot: It might well be argued that access to a drug that enhances mood must be treated differently from access to a drug that enhances hair growth. Beyond issues of mood brightening, this argument (for greater equality of access to "enhancement" in the arena of mental functioning) would apply all the more strongly to a drug that improves mental agility or self-esteem. It strikes me as a peculiarity of our culture that this need for equal access seems more obvious when applied to medication than when applied to psychotherapy, even, or especially, when the therapy has similar goals.

262   enhancement (of normal people's mood, in which case it would not): Or perhaps medication for certain forms of normal depressed mood will come to be considered prevention of kindled mood disorder, and therefore not enhancement but prophylactic treatment.

262   Estrogen used: But see Ronni Sandroff, "Menopause: Is It a Medical Problem?," *Good Health*, suppl. to *New York Times*, April 26, 1992, p. 22ff. To treat menopause, must we define it as endocrinopathy, or are we free to enhance or transform normal functioning? Is medication an attack on normal women, at the behest of a youth-conscious society? The issues are parallel to those for mood brighteners. See also Robert Michels, "Doctors, Drugs, and the Medical Model," in Thomas H. Murray, Willard Gaylin, and Ruth Macklin, eds., *Feeling Good and Doing Better: Ethics and Nontherapeutic Drug Use* (Clifton, N.J.: Humana, 1984), pp. 175–85. This book came to my attention through Aranow, Schwartz, and Sullivan, "Mood Brighteners."

263   what . . . Brock has called: Dan W. Brock, "The Use of Drugs for Pleasure: Some Philosophical Issues," in Murray, Gaylin, and Macklin, eds., *Feeling Good*, pp. 83–106. Much of this section on hedonism is based on Brock's essay. Brock is of course not responsible for my application of his model to the case of Prozac.

264   drugs that draw people *toward:* This argument would be vastly complicated by a short-acting drug that allows people to take on sociability at will. The authors of a pharmacologic overview of drugs of abuse that act via serotonin report: "The unique behavioral properties of MDA, a popular recreational drug for about twenty years, and its more recently abused congeners MDMA (Ecstasy) and MDEA (Eve), do not involve profound sensory disruption, but instead produce powerful enhancement of emotions, empathy, and affiliative bonds with other persons" (Martin P. Paulus and Mark A. Geyer, "The Effects of MDMA and Other Methylenedioxy-Substituted Phenylalkylamines on the Structure of Rat Locomotor Activity," *Neuropsychopharmacology*, vol. 7 [1992], pp. 15–31; quotation on p. 16.

265   Prozac is different: As a side note to the discussion of hedonism: Prozac can cause difficulties in achieving orgasm, more noticeably in men but in women as well. Probably because it is underreported, this side effect is not listed in standard references as being frequent, but clinicians see it fairly often. I have never had a patient discontinue Prozac because of it. Colleagues I have asked,

including some who do much more prescribing than I do, have, with rare exception, said the same thing. Here is an odd circumstance: a drug prescribed for relatively well-put-together people, often for the complaint of anhedonia, but well tolerated by them even when it causes sexual dysfunction. Patients' willingness to tolerate anorgasmia says something about Prozac and its relationship to pleasure. Prozac does not feel good to take, and it can cause a discouraging, even embarrassing, form of impotence, and yet it is "hedonic" because it allows people to experience the vibrancy of pleasure in the ordinary course of life. The degree to which ejaculatory delay or anorgasmia is tolerated speaks both to the diversity of pleasures people value and to the relative invulnerability of biologically supported self-esteem to particular physical and social failures.

This observation finds support in the following remark by a psychiatrist who works with OCD patients: "Surprisingly, orgasmic difficulties that are common with clomipramine [Anafranil] and fluoxetine [Prozac] result in discontinuing treatment less commonly than one might suppose, presumably because patients strongly desire the beneficial effects of the drugs" (John S. March, "Pharmacotherapy Effective in Obsessive-Compulsive Disorder," *Psychiatric Times,* May 1992, pp. 44–46).

265   Ms. B.: Aranow, Schwartz, and Sullivan, "Mood Brighteners," p. 10.

266   He is Ronald Winchel: Aloneness affect was mentioned in chapter 4. The description of the woman with trichotillomania is in Ronald M. Winchel, "Self-Mutilation and Aloneness," *Academy Forum* (of the American Academy of Psychoanalysis), vol. 35 (1991), pp. 10–12; quotation on p. 11.

267   If Ms. B. had taken Prozac as a mood brightener: Actually, Winchel describes the woman as having been treated for both compulsive hair-pulling and dysthymia. This erases much of our unease about the outcome.

269   Consider the Greek widow: Schwartz takes the example of the Greek widow from Anthony Storr, *Solitude* (New York: Ballantine, 1989). Storr was referring to a lovely work of anthropology and photography, enhanced by the poetry of funeral laments: Loring M. Danforth, *The Death Rituals of Rural Greece,* photographs by Alexander Tsiaras (Princeton, N.J.: Princeton University Press, 1982). The degree of recovery of the bereaved Greek women is unclear, even after five years of formal mourning. Several years after a child's death, one surviving mother will not attend a daughter's wedding and becomes upset whenever a member of the household listens to music on the radio. She calls her pain the wound that never heals.

The five-year period of mourning is enforced, and is thus an imposition for some women. The prolonged rituals sometimes result in strife; for example, a daughter-in-law may not mourn adequately according to the standards of the widow. The restrictions placed on men are much less stringent and of shorter duration. In effect, prolonged mourning is an enforced duty of women, as well as an opportunity to experience profound affect and accept loss.

271   The Mexican poet and essayist: Octavio Paz, "Mexico and the United States," in Paz, *The Labyrinth of Solitude, The Other Mexico, Return to the Labyrinth of Solitude, Mexico and the United States, The Philanthropic Ogre*, trans. Lysander Kemp, Yara Milos, and Rachel Phillips Belash (New York: Grove, 1985), p. 366.

272   The poet James Merrill: As is evident in a fuller excerpt, Merrill uses Prozac as one of a series of indicators of the simultaneously amusing and deadening banality of modern communal life:

Still, not to paint a picture wholly black,
Some social highlights: Dead white males in malls.
Prayer breakfasts. Pay-phone sex. "Ring up as meat."
Oprah. The G.N.P. The contour sheet.
The painless death of History. The stick
Figures on Capitol Hill. Their rhetoric,
Gladly—no rapturously (on Prozac) suffered!
Gay studies. Right-to-Lifers. The laugh track.

("Self-Portrait in Tyvek™ Windbreaker," *New Yorker*, February 24, 1992, pp. 38–39.)

272   steroids in competitive sports: Much of what follows is influenced by Thomas H. Murray, "Drugs, Sports, and Ethics," in Murray, Gaylin, and Macklin, eds., *Feeling Good*, pp. 107–126; see also 197–200, a helpful discussion of Murray's essay by Ruth Macklin.

274   "a general distrust of drugs . . .": Klerman, "Psychotropic Hedonism," p. 3. I served under Klerman when Jimmy Carter was in the White House and Klerman was director of the Alcohol, Drug Abuse, and Mental Health Administration of the Department of Health and Human Services. It was then that I chaired a government work group investigating the issue of women's use of prescribed psychotherapeutic drugs. Among our findings were the conclusions expressed in the text here, about the moderate use of prescribed psychotropics by Americans. (Peter D. Kramer, Mitchell E. Balter, and Louise Richardson,

"Women and the Abuse of Prescribed Psychotropic Medication," signed and distributed by U.S. Surgeon General, April 1981.)

274   prescribing . . . is moderate: Ibid. This issue is most extensively researched with regard to antianxiety drugs. See Mitchell B. Balter, Jerome Levine, and Dean L. Manheimer, "Cross-National Study of the Extent of Anti-Anxiety/Sedative Drug Use," *New England Journal of Medicine*, vol. 290 (1974), pp. 769–74; M. B. Balter, D. L. Manheimer, G. D. Mellinger, et al., "A Cross-National Comparison of Anti-Anxiety/Sedative Drug Use," *Current Medical Research and Opinon*, vol. 8, supplement 4 (1984), pp. 5–30; and M. B. Balter and E. H. Uhlenhuth, "Benzodiazepine Use: 1990 Survey Data," symposium presentation, Fifth World Congress of Biological Psychiatry, Florence, Italy, June 1991. The trends are much the same for antidepressants: if anything, antidepressants appear to be underprescribed in the United States and elsewhere. See Ira D. Glick, Lorenzo Burti, Koji Suzuki, et al., "Effectiveness in Psychiatric Care: I. A Cross-National Study of the Process of Treatment and Outcomes of Major Depressive Disorder," *Journal of Nervous and Mental Disease*, vol. 179 (1991), pp. 55–63; Martin B. Keller, Philip W. Lavori, Gerald L. Klerman, et al., "Low Levels and Lack of Predictors of Somatotherapy and Psychotherapy Received by Depressed Patients," *Archives of General Psychiatry*, vol. 43 (1986), pp. 458–67; and Martin B. Keller, Gerald L. Klerman, Philip W. Lavori, et al., "Treatment Received by Depressed Patients," *JAMA*, vol. 248 (1982), pp. 1848–55.

274   erode our "Calvinism": Another issue is whether acceptance of licit drugs legitimizes the use of illicit drugs. Of course, the appropriate use of thymoleptics might diminish illicit drug use by treating the underlying states for which addicts self-medicate. (See the discussion of the self-medication hypothesis of drug abuse, in chapter 8.)

275   "the best thing . . .": Mary Deems Howland, *The Gift of the Other: Gabriel Marcel's Concept of Intersubjectivity in Walker Percy's Novels* (Pittsburgh: Duquesne University Press, 1990), p. 1. A slim volume that has been helpful to me in my thinking about Percy is Linda Whitney Hobson, *Understanding Walker Percy* (Columbia, S.C.: University of South Carolina, 1988). An extraordinarily deep and thorough appreciation of Percy, one that has influenced the discussion that follows, is Robert Coles's book, part biography, part literary criticism, and part original philosophical contribution, *Walker Percy: An American Search* (Boston: Atlantic–Little, Brown, 1978).

276   Edmund Wilson and Lionel Trilling: "Philoctetes: The Wound and the Bow," in Edmund Wilson, *The Wound and the Bow: Seven Studies in Literature*

(Cambridge, Mass.: Riverside Press [Houghton Mifflin], 1941), pp. 272–95; "Art and Neurosis," in Lionel Trilling, *The Liberal Imagination: Essays on Literature and Society* (New York: Viking, 1950), pp. 160–80. See also my column "Heartbreak House," *Psychiatric Times,* December 1987, p. 3ff.

277 "Thus if a drug . . .": Klerman, "Psychotropic Hedonism," p. 3. Klerman's concern was medical treatment of psychiatric illness. He made the point that mental-health professionals, most of whom were psychotherapists, opposed drugs on an arbitrary, often counterfactual, basis. The complete quote is: "Thus if a drug makes you feel good, it not only represents a secondary form of salvation but somehow it is morally wrong and the user is likely to suffer retribution with either dependence, liver damage, or chromosomal change, or some other form of medical-theological damnation. Implicit in this theory of therapeutic change is the philosophy of personal growth, basically a secular variant of the theological view of salvation through good works." We can see from this quote why Aranow formulated "mood brightener," in order to tease apart the issue of drug side effect from that of moral wrong; we have also seen, in our discussion of ethical objections to mood brighteners, how easy it is to slip into pharmacological Calvinism.

277 *"unable* to take account . . .": Walker Percy, "The Coming Crisis in Psychiatry" (1957), collected in his *Signposts in a Strange Land* (New York: Farrar, Straus & Giroux, 1991), pp. 251–62; quotations on pp. 252, 259. In the same volume, see also "The Fateful Rift: The San Andreas Fault in the Modern Mind" (1989), pp. 271–91.

279 "The Message in the Bottle": Collected in Walker Percy, *The Message in the Bottle* (New York: Farrar, Straus and Giroux, 1975), pp. 119–49.

279 "he regularly comes upon bottles . . .": Ibid., p. 120; the messages quoted are from pp. 120–23.

279 "In summary . . .": Ibid., p. 130.

280 "Come! I know your need . . .": Ibid., p. 134.

280 two commuters on a train: Ibid.

280 "To be a castaway . . .": Ibid., p. 144.

280 the resort to psychotherapy or to drugs: Ibid., p. 139.

280 "even if his symptoms": Ibid., p. 140.

285 principle of psychotherapy: Technically, neutrality applies to mental structures. The dynamic therapist should "sit equidistant" from the id, ego,

and superego. In practice, neutrality often entails avoiding assent to, and dissent from, the patient's criticism of people about whom the patient has ambivalent feelings. See my essay "Non-Neutrality," *Psychiatric Times,* September 1992, p. 4.

287 support for a concrete choice: Awareness of such categories as rejection-sensitivity tends to change the relationship between doctor and patient. In this case, I accepted my patient's stated wish to divorce and ignored any mixed feelings she might have had. At the most obvious level, this decision respects Susan's freedom of choice; but when compared with a treatment in which the doctor remains neutral and waits for the patient to initiate each action, this treatment moves the locus of control from the patient to the therapist.

The notion that a therapist is free to "take sides," in assessing a patient's choices in the world, raises profound ethical issues. For instance, we may worry that a therapist who supports a divorce is acting on his or her distorted beliefs about marriage or men or the rescue of vulnerable women. But psychotherapy, at its heart, is a matter of facing reality in good faith. A therapist who sees patients' handicaps partly in terms of relatively fixed aspects of personality—rejection-sensitivity, separation anxiety, inhibition to novelty—must use that perspective in his or her work, not just incidentally but integrally—because the therapist will hear patients' stories differently.

Of course, patients become aware of this change in the psychiatrist's focus. A patient of mine had the following dream: "I am going to a safe-deposit box. I am bringing jewels to deposit. When I open the box, all it contains is hundreds of capsules." I interpreted to her that she was bringing her precious emotions to this safe place, my office, but she feared all she would find was pills. She replied that she associated her growing dependence on me, and the safety of the office, with craziness, and that her engagement in therapy meant she would need many pills. It is natural that medication should become a metaphor in psychotherapies that are accompanied by pharmacotherapy. See also the chapter "The Mind-Mind-Body-Problem Problem," in my book *Moments of Engagement.*

287 psychoanalysts at the Payne Whitney Clinic: Fredric N. Busch, Arnold M. Cooper, et al., "Neurophysiological, Cognitive-Behavioral, and Psychoanalytic Approaches to Panic Disorder: Toward an Integration," *Psychoanalytic Inquiry,* vol. 11 (1991), pp. 316–30; Arnold M. Cooper, "The Relevance of Psychotherapy to Clinical Practice Today," address, Rhode Island Psychiatric Society, Butler Hospital, Providence, R.I., March 2, 1992, 27 pp. The quotations are from the text of Dr. Cooper's speech.

287 the analysts' understanding: I have not done justice to the complexities of the work of the Payne Whitney group. The analysts draw on the full ar-

mamentarium of psychoanalytic theory to integrate the biological findings. They speculate, for example, that the fearfully dependent and unsatisfied child becomes angry at the parent, and then, since the parent is also loved, guilt-ridden. "The child will therefore become fearful not only of loss, but of the arousal or expression of anger for fear of loss. Defenses are triggered, including denial and projection, the latter leading to a perception of the parent as even more rejecting." This perception makes the child feel even less supported, thus heightening the fearful dependency and separation anxiety, and reinforcing the cycle.

The Payne Whitney model makes predictions about the sorts of internal representation of others that adults with this disorder will have (controlling and rejecting) and the life events that will lead to periods of panic (threats to attachment). Such speculation, itself based on clinical observation, allows for further formal research, which can be confirming, disconfirming, or modifying of the original hypotheses—a wonderful event in psychoanalysis, and itself a sign of the predominance of the biological model.

288   impossibly complex and overly specific: Here, for example, is a diagnosis that merits two pages in the newest diagnostic manual, and which I hazard to predict will not stand the test of time: "Gender Identity Disorder of Adolescence or Adulthood, Nontranssexual Type (GIDAANT)." GIDAANT refers to people with anxiety about their masculine or feminine identity; they may cross-dress to lower their anxiety, but if they cross-dress to attain sexual excitation, they get a different diagnosis. (American Psychiatric Association, *Diagnostic and Statistical Manual of Mental Disorders,* 3rd ed., rev. [Washington, D.C.: American Psychiatric Association, 1987], pp. 76–77.)

288   no appropriate niche: James E. Barrett, Jane A. Barrett, et al., "The Prevalence of Psychiatric Disorders in a Primary Care Practice," *Archives of General Psychiatry,* vol. 45 (1988), pp. 1100–1106; Leon Eisenberg, "Treating Depression and Anxiety in Primary Care: Closing the Gap Between Knowledge and Practice," *New England Journal of Medicine,* vol. 326 (1992), pp. 1080–84.

289   a good case . . . for the return of "neurosis": Another possibility is the further expansion of "post-traumatic stress disorder" (PTSD), originally applied to people who had suffered recent trauma (like shell shock or railway spine), but now used also in reference to adults who suffered stresses at crucial developmental phases of childhood. The emergence of PTSD is, under a new name, and with more attention to biological damage, the rebirth of the traumatic theory of neurosis and personality disorder, a century after Freud first proposed it.

Apropos of neurosis, Arnold Cooper, the senior figure in the Payne Whitney group cited above, recently reminded colleagues: "British authors have suggested that the [American diagnostic] system inappropriately focuses on the symptom rather than the high degree of neuroticism out of which the symptom emerges" (Cooper, "Relevance of Psychotherapy," p. 16).

289   The coalescing of diagnoses: I have already mentioned, in connection with the concept of depressive temperament (chapter 6), a movement within descriptive psychiatry to do away with the concept of personality disorder and think only in terms of clinical syndromes, such as recurrent depression. The argument here is an extrapolation of Donald Klein's work with rejection-sensitivity, panic anxiety, and characterologic depression—the notion that much of what looks like disordered character is really a response to a chronic or recurrent mood disorder.

290   Allen's fantasy *Alice:* See my column "Wonderland," *Psychiatric Times,* April 1991, p. 4ff. The film's working title was *The Magical Herbs of Dr. Yang* (Eric Lax, *Woody Allen: A Biography* [New York: Vintage, 1992], p. 321).

292   Prozac works best: An unpublished study from Cornell University finds that good antidepressant responders fall into two groups as regards personality. Some seem cured outright, like many of the patients we have met. Others (like Philip) also report dramatic change, but find the change dislocating. In these patients, the change in feeling about the self is strong, but change in cognition (and organization of the defenses) lags; they generally need psychotherapy to deal with the success of medication. The study, by a group headed by James Kocsis, was described by Cooper in "Relevance of Psychotherapy."

296   spouse as a . . . neurotransmitter: ". . . the psychoanalyst actually *is* a neurotransmitter—a generator of signals, transduced by the receiver into neurochemical activity—initially just inhibiting 'aloneness affect,' but eventually helping to reset the homeostatic controls so that the system responds to a new level or frequency of input" (Winchel, "Self-Mutilation," p. 12). In this passage, Winchel is assuming the patient suffers from reversible damage and that psychoanalysis is equivalent to psychotherapeutic medication in its ability to alter transmitter levels.

297   the self-absorption of Goethe's Werther: Hans-Jurgen van Bose, a German composer, has written a new opera titled *The Sorrows of Young Werther,* but *The New York Times* reports: "The facts of Goethe's original have been reassembled to create something quite distant from it. The tenderness of grief, the sweet self-indulgence of despairing love have been bled away." (Bernard Holland, "New Setting of Goethe's Melancholy Love Story," *New York Times,* August

7, 1992, p. C3.) The review goes on to emphasize how the emotions in the modern opera do not parallel those of the eighteenth-century novel. The reviewer attributes this difference to opera's difficulty in addressing ambiguity, but I wonder whether the difference does not have also to do with a change over time in sensibility as regards affect.

297   Karl Marx and Freud: Daniel Burston, *The Legacy of Erich Fromm* (Cambridge, Mass.: Harvard University Press, 1991), pp. 30–52. The Freudo-Marxists misunderstood the modern trend. They were concerned that sexuality would be repressed. Walker Percy correctly understood it would instead be trivialized.

300   for Freud to have discovered the unconscious: This is, of course, shorthand. There was an unconscious before Freud. See Henri Ellenberger, *The Discovery of the Unconscious* (New York: Basic Books, 1970).

300   a whole climate of opinion: ". . . to us, he is no longer a person / now but a whole climate of opinion / under whom we conduct our different lives" (W. H. Auden, "In Memory of Sigmund Freud [d. Sept. 1939]," in W. H. Auden, *Collected Shorter Poems 1927–1957* [London: Faber & Faber, 1966], pp. 166–70.

APPENDIX: VIOLENCE

301   serotonin and aggression: There is a large literature on aggression and neurotransmitters in man and other animals. The discussion that follows is based largely on Michael J. Raleigh, Michael T. McGuire, et al., "Serotonergic Mechanisms Promote Dominance Acquisition in Adult Male Vervet Monkeys," *Brain Research*, vol. 559 (1991), pp. 181–90; and a series of articles in the *Archives of General Psychiatry*, vol. 49, no. 6 (June 1992). These include: J. Dee Higley, P. T. Mehlman, et al., "Cerebrospinal Fluid Monoamine and Adrenal Correlates of Aggression in Free-Ranging Rhesus Monkeys," pp. 436–41; Burr Eichelman, "Aggressive Behavior: From Laboratory to Clinic: Quo Vadit?," pp. 488–92; Markus J. P. Kruesi, Euthymia D. Hibbs, et al., "A 2-Year Prospective Follow-Up Study of Children and Adolescents with Disruptive Behavior Disorders: Prediction by Cerebrospinal Fluid 5-Hydroxyindolacetic Acid, Homovanillic Acid, and Autonomic Measures?," pp. 429–35; J. John Mann, Anne McBride, et al., "Relationship Between Central and Peripheral Serotonin Indexes in Depressed and Suicidal Psychiatric Inpatients," pp. 442–59. The studies involving serotonin-altering medication given to monkeys include work by Michael McGuire's group (on vervet monkeys);

the study of scarred wild rhesus monkeys is by Stephen Suomi's group. As in the case of depression, other neurotransmitters and hormones, not just serotonin, are implicated in aggression; the parts of the brain involved, although there is overlap, almost certainly differ between depression and aggression. Both are basic, widely and complexly encoded functions. The use of BuSpar for violent retarded patients is associated with John Ratey of Massachusetts General Hospital.

303 Prozac resulted in a marked decline: A study by Maurizio Fava, Jerrold Rosenbaum, and others at Harvard showed "a dramatic decline" in hostility and a decrease in "anger attacks" in eighty-four patients treated with Prozac. Interestingly, the presence of anger attacks predicted positive mood response to Prozac. ("Antidepressants Found to Prevent Depression-Related 'Anger Attacks,' " *Clinical Psychiatry News,* September 1992, p. 6.)

303 What distinguishes the suicides: Indeed, there is a "biological-catharsis" theory that "The act of attempting suicide may make a depressed individual feel better by increasing serotonin activity" (Kevin M. Malone, quoted in "Potential Clinical, Biological Predictors of Suicide Reattempts Identified," *Clinical Psychiatry News,* August 1992, p. 8). The supportive research (showing higher responsivity of serotonin systems in male suicide attempters whose attempts were recent than in those whose attempts occurred longer ago) was done at Western Psychiatric Institute, Pittsburgh, Pa., in conjunction with John J. Mann.

304 Teicher and two colleagues: Martin H. Teicher, Carol C. Glod, and Jonathan O. Cole, "Emergence of Intense Suicidal Preoccupation During Fluoxetine Treatment," *American Journal of Psychiatry,* vol. 147 (1990), pp. 207–10. See also Patricia Thomas, "Sad Attack: Prozac," *Harvard Health Letter,* vol. 16, no. 12 (1991), pp. 1–4.

305 the Teicher report aroused great interest: John J. Mann and Shitij Kapur, "The Emergence of Suicidal Ideation and Behavior During Antidepressant Therapy," *Archives of General Psychiatry,* vol. 48 (1991), pp. 1027–33; Cynthia E. Hoover, "Suicidal Ideation Not Associated with Fluoxetine" (letter), *American Journal of Psychiatry,* vol. 148 (1991), p. 543; Maurizio Fava and Jerrold F. Rosenbaum, "Suicidality and Fluoxetine: Is There a Relationship?," *Journal of Clinical Psychiatry,* vol. 52 (1991), pp. 108–11; Charles M. Beasley, Bruce E. Dornseif, et al., "Fluoxetine and Suicide: A Meta-Analysis of Controlled Trials of Treatment for Depression," *British Medical Journal,* vol. 303 (1991), pp. 685–92; William C. Wirshing, Theodore Van Putten, et al., "Fluoxetine,

Akathisia, and Suicidality: Is There a Causal Connection?" (letter), *Archives of General Psychiatry*, vol. 49 (1992), pp. 580–81.

306 "Examining large, placebo-controlled databases": Wirshing, Van Putten, et al., "Fluoxetine," p. 581.

307 akathisia: The theory is plausible, because the "pacing urge," most often seen as a side effect of antipsychotic medication, has been associated with homicidal and suicidal behavior in psychotic patients. See Teicher, Glod, and Cole, "Emergence of Suicidal Preoccupation," Mann and Kaplan, "Emergence of Suicidal Ideation," and Wirshing, Van Putten, et al., "Fluoxetine."

307 "Because patients seek treatment . . .": Mann and Kapur, "Emergence of Suicidal Ideation," p. 1031. In the elision, I have omitted a long discussion of further research required to clarify any association between Prozac and suicidality.

308 Wesbecker . . . on "Larry King Live": "Prozac: Painful Legacy?," September 26, 1990.

309 "Donahue": February 27, 1991.

309 "lifelong journey of disintegration": "And the horror that unfolded that Thursday morning was merely the final step of a lifelong journey of disintegration, an extreme reflection of the alienation, anger and sorrow with which Wesbecker had been wrestling all his life. The man who stepped off the elevator with the spitting AK-47 was Joe. Himself. Doing what he'd vowed to do." (John Filatreau, "A Life in Pieces" [also titled: "Little Boy Lost: The Emotional Life and Death of Joe Wesbecker"], *Louisville*, January 1990, pp. 26–41.) I have relied very largely on this essay, in conjunction with reporting in the Louisville *Courier-Journal* and other news reports, for the biographical sketch of Wesbecker. I have no knowledge of Wesbecker other than what appeared in the press and on television.

310 McStoots joined "Larry King Live": March 18, 1991. In my account of McStoots, I have relied also on the order dismissing the civil complaint by Judge J. David Francis, Warren [Kentucky] Circuit Court, November 6, 1991, and news stories in the Louisville *Courier-Journal*, Indianapolis *Star*, and the Bowling Green *Daily News*. I have no knowledge of McStoots other than what appeared in the court order, in the press, and on television. Prozac had been prescribed to McStoots not by Dr. Tapp but by another physician, Lawrence Green.

310   Many other cases have been publicized: On "60 Minutes," October 27, 1991, Lesley Stahl reported, "But what about the other 100 plus people they [the Scientologists] claim Prozac made suicidal? We decided to look into some of those cases and what we found were people who, like Wesbecker, had already shown signs of mental instability or suicidal behavior before they ever went on Prozac."

311   the Church of Scientology: See *Time* magazine's cover story of May 6, 1991 ("Scientology: The Cult of Greed," also titled "The Thriving Cult of Greed and Power," pp. 32–39), and the series of stories in the June, July, and September 1991 issues of the *Psychiatric Times* regarding the Scientologists' crusade against psychiatry.

311   people, . . . are often leery: This issue is difficult for doctors, too. Deciding when to discontinue medication is complicated by our ignorance regarding the biological process of healing. We have some sense of how stress, under the kindling model, causes anatomical damage in the brain even before a person experiences serious illness. But we do not know whether what takes place when people improve—through psychotherapy, medication, or change in circumstance—is cure or adaptation to injury. In the absence of good models of healing, we need to answer the pharmacologic issue through empirical observation: when can we stop the Prozac?

What evidence we have concerns the use of tricyclic antidepressants for episodes of major depression. Here a number of studies show that, if a person has not been entirely free of symptoms for a substantial period of time, at least five months and perhaps a year, then stopping medication will result in a swift relapse. These studies might be understood to say a patient can safely stop medication if he or she has been well for five to twelve months. But other, more controversial studies show that, if there is any tendency toward relapse, it may be wise to continue medication, probably at a full dose, for a good deal longer, perhaps indefinitely. Even patients who are are past the point where they will relapse immediately may benefit, in terms of the length of time before the next episode, from "continuation" or "maintenance" pharmacotherapy.

It is hard to know just how to apply these findings to the care of people with minor variants of depressive disorders or with the sorts of personality traits—compulsivity, inhibition, low self-esteem—we have discussed. My practice with "good responders" is to taper and stop Prozac after six or eight months. Some patients, those whose symptoms turn on and off as if in response to an electric switch, relapse almost immediately. Others notice a small deterioration in functioning off medication. A good number—over a third—ask to resume medication in the course of the next two or three years, and others may suffer recurrences of some of their problems without requesting medication. But there are people who continue to do very well off all medication, perhaps because of a stable resetting of neuronal functioning, perhaps because of the continuing effect of changes in career, friendships, and self-image, or perhaps for other biological and social reasons.

312   whether antidepressants . . . promote tumor growth: A team from the University of Manitoba injected susceptible rats with either cancer cells or a cancer-causing chemical. They then injected the same rats with salt water, Prozac, or a tricyclic antidepressant, amitriptyline. At certain stages in the brief study (in one model, at day 5 but not day 8), the antidepressant-injected rats had more tumors than the control rats. The study raised questions as to whether antidepressants might be dangerous to patients who already have cancer or who have high exposure to carcinogens. (Lorne J. Brandes, Randi J. Arron, et al., "Stimulation of Malignant Growth in Rodents by Antidepressant Drugs at Clinically Relevant Doses," *Cancer Research,* vol. 52 [1992], pp. 3796–3800.)

The study has a number of problems. For example, the control rats got suspiciously few tumors—fewer than rats on the same regimens in other studies. The number of rats tested was unusually small. And the data presented were scanty. For these and other reasons, it is unclear whether this study is of relevance to humans. The standard assays for carcinogenesis follow rats or mice liable to tumor formation for two years or until death, in the presence of high doses of medication. In those studies, Prozac did not cause cancer and may even have prevented it. A large series of studies in humans shows no connection between antidepressant use and cancer formation or progression, although antidepressants (and probably depression alone, without medication) can under some conditions affect immune function.

It is obviously important to know whether antidepressants promote tumor growth in cancer patients, who often are candidates for these drugs, or in those exposed to carcinogens, such as smokers. It is unclear whether the Brandes study is of clinical significance—it flies in the face of a large number of more thorough studies that failed to show an association between antidepressants and tumor progression—but it serves as a reminder that, despite extensive testing before drugs are introduced, concerns can arise about medications many years (in amitriptyline's case, almost forty years) after their introduction.

Acknowledgments

I could not have written this book without the generous help of patients, colleagues, friends, and family.

In particular, I want to thank the following researchers who discussed their work with me, answered queries, or shared material, often including unpublished monographs: Drs. Huda Akil (University of Michigan), Hagop Akiskal (National Institute of Mental Health), Robert Aranow (Harvard), Frank Ayd (West Virginia University), Ross Baldessarini (Harvard), Mitchell Balter (Tufts), Walter Brown (Brown), Jonathan Cole (Harvard), Arnold Cooper (Cornell), George Heninger (Yale), Jerome Kagan (Harvard), Edward Khanzian (Harvard), Donald Klein (Columbia), Douglas Madsen (University of Iowa), Michael T. McGuire (UCLA), Theodore Nadelson (Tufts), J. Craig Nelson (Yale), Robert Post (National Institute of Mental Health), Mark D. Sullivan (University of Washington, Seattle), Stephen J. Suomi (National Institute of Child Health and Human Development), and Ronald Winchel (Columbia). In addition, the following colleagues offered comments when this book was in manuscript: Drs. Jeffrey Blum, Walter Brown, and Alan Gruenberg.

My collaborators in treating certain of the patients whose stories I have told include: Anita Berger, M.S.W., Elena Gonzales, Ph.D.,

Diana Elliott Lidofsky, Ph.D., and Judith H. Puleston, M.S.W. They, as much as Prozac, are instruments of transformation.

Regarding a book written largely about one proprietary medication, questions will inevitably arise concerning the relationship between the author and the drug's manufacturer. I have had only one contact with Eli Lilly. I spent much of December 9, 1991, at Lilly's international headquarters in Indianapolis, Indiana. I paid for my own plane flight, hotel, and meals. In the morning, I spent two hours discussing the development of Prozac with Drs. Brian Molloy, Ray Fuller, and David Wong, the researchers who created the chemical twenty years earlier. In the afternoon, Ed West, Lilly's director of corporate communications, and his then assistant, Gerianne Hap, kindly permitted me to look through Lilly's library of newspaper clippings and television videotapes. Before that trip, Mr. West had sent me the "Clinical Investigation Brochure" for Prozac (the technical information relied on by drug researchers); subsequently he forwarded scientific reprints and photocopies of news clippings I had specifically requested. I have no relationship to Eli Lilly, and I have no financial stake in the company.

John Schwartz, editor of the *Psychiatric Times*, has printed my monthly column "Practicing" since 1985; though the essays are often speculative or controversial, John has never offered the least hint of editorial interference.

Nan Graham, my editor at Viking, supplied the warmth, enthusiasm, and clarity of judgment that every author hopes for. Courtney Hodell, Nan's assistant, read acutely and managed a host of important details. Going beyond the limited role of literary agent, Chuck Verrill provided valuable advice at each stage of the writing of this book.

Judith Henriques helped in the production of printed drafts from my computer files. Ruthann Gildea of the Isaac Ray Medical Library at Butler Hospital went out of her way to provide prompt assistance in locating technical materials.

My deepest thanks are to my patients. I have tried to protect their privacy, but I hope the spirit of our work together, and of their often heroic lives, is discernible in these pages.

Finally, I could never have written this book without the encouragement and support of my wife, Rachel Schwartz, and the indulgence of our three children, Sarah, Jacob, and Matthew. The drug will never be invented that sustains the spirit the way a family can.

Index

Abuse, 2, 16, 17, 120, 192, 261
  see also Masochism, social: Sexual
    abuse
Academy Forum, 351*n.*, 385*n.*
Accidental Tourist, The (Tyler), 320*n.*
Acetylcholine, 55, 57, 58, 60, 61, 65,
  66, 356
Acta Psychiatrica Scandinavica, 348*n.*,
  382*n.*
Adler, Alfred, 199, 221, 372*n.*
Adolescence, rejection-sensitivity in
  late, 100–101
Adoption, 157–58, 361*n.*, 362*n.*
"Adrenal Gland Enlargement in Major
  Depression: A Computed Tomo-
  graphic Study," 354*n.*
Adrenal glands, 115, 116
Adrenaline, 115
"Affectional Responses in the Infant
  Monkey," 355*n.*
"Affective Disorders in Referred Chil-
  dren and Younger Siblings of
  Manic Depressives: Mode of On-
  set and Prospective Course,"
  365*n.*
"Affective Flattening: Evaluation and
  Diagnostic Significance," 376*n.*
Affective loading, 14
Affect tolerance, 254, 256, 257, 258,
  269–70
  increase of, 259

"Age and Depression," 358*n.*
Aggression, 183, 271, 303, 373*n.*–
  374*n.*, 392*n.*–93*n.*
  affective, 302
  predatory, 302
  serotonin and, 301–4, 392*n.*–93*n.*
Agressive Behavior: From Laboratory to
  Clinic: Quo Vadit?," 392*n.*
Aging, 135–36
  late-onset depression, 136–43, 358*n.*
Agoraphobia, 78, 79, 82, 84
Akathisia, 307
Akil, Dr. Huda, 353*n.*
Akiskal, Hagop S., 163–66, 167, 178,
  179–80, 341*n.*, 353*n.*, 354*n.*,
  358*n.*, 364*n.*, 365*n.*–366*n.*,
  367*n.*, 368*n.*, 374*n.*, 383*n.*
Alcohol, 252, 265
Alcoholism, 1, 2, 13, 14, 158, 164, 178
  depression in near relatives and,
    14–15
  heredity and, xiv
  self-esteem and, 198
Alice, 290
Allen, Woody, 223, 290, 304
Allergies, 49, 155, 159
"Aloneness affect," 96, 278, 351*n.*,
  385*n.*, 391*n.*
Alprozam, *see* Xanax
American Journal of Psychiatry, 304,
  336*n.*, 342*n.*, 347*n.*, 352*n.*,

FOR THE BEST IN PAPERBACKS, LOOK FOR THE

In every corner of the world, on every subject under the sun, Penguin represents quality and variety—the very best in publishing today.

For complete information about books available from Penguin—including Puffins, Penguin Classics, and Arkana—and how to order them, write to us at the appropriate address below. Please note that for copyright reasons the selection of books varies from country to country.

In the United Kingdom: Please write to *Dept. JC, Penguin Books Ltd, FREEPOST, West Drayton, Middlesex UB7 0BR.*

If you have any difficulty in obtaining a title, please send your order with the correct money, plus ten percent for postage and packaging, to *P.O. Box No. 11, West Drayton, Middlesex UB7 0BR*

In the United States: Please write to *Consumer Sales, Penguin USA, P.O. Box 999, Dept. 17109, Bergenfield, New Jersey 07621-0120.* VISA and MasterCard holders call 1-800-253-6476 to order all Penguin titles

In Canada: Please write to *Penguin Books Canada Ltd, 10 Alcorn Avenue, Suite 300, Toronto, Ontario M4V 3B2*

In Australia: Please write to *Penguin Books Australia Ltd, P.O. Box 257, Ringwood, Victoria 3134*

In New Zealand: Please write to *Penguin Books (NZ) Ltd, Private Bag 102902, North Shore Mail Centre, Auckland 10*

In India: Please write to *Penguin Books India Pvt Ltd, 706 Eros Apartments, 56 Nehru Place, New Delhi 110 019*

In the Netherlands: Please write to *Penguin Books Netherlands bv, Postbus 3507, NL-1001 AH Amsterdam*

In Germany: Please write to *Penguin Books Deutschland GmbH, Metzlerstrasse 26, 60594 Frankfurt am Main*

In Spain: Please write to *Penguin Books S. A., Bravo Murillo 19, 1° B, 28015 Madrid*

In Italy: Please write to *Penguin Italia s.r.l., Via Felice Casati 20, I-20124 Milano*

In France: Please write to *Penguin France S. A., 17 rue Lejeune, F–31000 Toulouse*

In Japan: Please write to *Penguin Books Japan, Ishikiribashi Building, 2–5–4, Suido, Bunkyo-ku, Tokyo 112*

In Greece: Please write to *Penguin Hellas Ltd, Dimocritou 3, GR–106 71 Athens*

In South Africa: Please write to *Longman Penguin Southern Africa (Pty) Ltd, Private Bag X08, Bertsham 2013*